D0535801

THE HEALTHCARE QUALITY BOOK

SECOND EDITION

THE HEALTHCARE QUALITY BOOK

SECOND EDITION

VISION, STRATEGY, AND TOOLS

Elizabeth R. Ransom, Maulik S. Joshi, David B. Nash, and Scott B. Ransom, Editors

Health Administration Press, Chicago
AUPHA Press, Washington, DC

AUPHA

Your board, staff, or clients may also benefit from this book's insight. For more information on quantity discounts, contact the Health Administration Press Marketing Manager at (312) 424-9470.

Reprinting May 2013

Library of Congress Cataloging-in-Publication Data

The healthcare quality book : vision, strategy, and tools / [edited by] Elizabeth R. Ransom ... [et al.].—2nd ed.
   p. ; cm.
  Includes bibliographical references and index.
  ISBN 978-1-56793-301-7 (alk. paper)
   1. Medical care—United States—Quality control. 2. Health services administration—United States—Quality control. 3. Total quality management—United States. I. Ransom, Elizabeth R.
  [DNLM: 1. Quality of Health Care—organization & administration—United States. 2. Health Services Administration—United States. 3. Total Quality Management—organization & administration—United States. W 84 AA1 H443 2008]

RA399.A3H433 2008
362.11068—dc22

2008017268

The paper used in this publication meets the minimum requirements of American National Standard for Information Sciences-Permanence of Paper for Printed Library Materials, ANSI Z39.48-1984. ⊚™

Project manager: Jennifer Seibert; Acquisitions editor: Audrey Kaufman; Book designer: Scott R. Miller.

Health Administration Press
A division of the Foundation
  of the American College of
  Healthcare Executives
One North Franklin Street
Suite 1700
Chicago, IL 60606
(312) 424-2800

Association of University Programs
  in Health Administration
2000 14th Street North
Suite 780
Arlington, VA 22201
(703) 894-0940

CONTENTS IN BRIEF

DETAILED CONTENTS

III   Environment

FOREWORD

Nancy M. Schlichting

There has never been a more important and exciting time in the journey to achieve excellence in healthcare quality. After more than eight years since the Institute of Medicine released its groundbreaking report, *To Err Is Human: Building a Safer Health System,* on the poor state of healthcare quality in the United States, there is significant momentum for fundamental change to improve quality. The momentum is being felt in a number of important venues:

- In the government world, as legislators and administrators are working to increase the incentives for quality in governmental programs
- In the business world, as companies are redesigning health benefit plans to encourage more involvement of the employees in their choice of healthcare providers based on performance
- In the insurance world, as health plans are evaluating providers based on quality indicators
- In the provider world, as hospitals and physicians are investing in new information technology to provide more consistent and safer quality of care for their patients
- In the consumer world, as individuals are seeking out information about quality before choosing a physician, a hospital, or a health plan

The importance of this momentum cannot be overstated. It will create enormous opportunities for learning that can be spread across the country, more alignment of incentives among all stakeholders, more informed consumers, and greater availability of accurate and useful information for decision making.

The second edition of *The Healthcare Quality Book* is a resource for all learners and participants in this critical process of change. It is a guide for quality improvement that incorporates both theoretical models and practical approaches for implementation. The editors have brought together some of the best minds in healthcare to offer insights on leadership strategy, tools, organizational design, information technology, legal and regulatory issues, and, most important, the patient experience. *The Healthcare Quality Book* will serve all who have a passion for changing the quality paradigm and creating an ideal patient and family experience. Now is the time for action! The editors of *The Healthcare Quality Book* are providing the necessary resources. I am confident the readers will be part of the healthcare quality solution.

Nancy M. Schlichting
President and CEO
Henry Ford Health System
Detroit, Michigan

PREFACE

Change is constant, and no statement is more appropriate for the health-care industry. Since the first edition of this textbook, healthcare costs have increased beyond the rate of inflation, the number of uninsured individuals has grown dramatically, employers and consumers are facing a greater share of healthcare expenses, and navigation of the complex and complicated healthcare system has become a burden on the public. Our healthcare crisis permeates every aspect of the industry—the delivery of medical care, the financing of our system, and the quality of healthcare we receive.

In our fragmented, unsustainable, and uncertain healthcare system, one element remains steadfast—healthcare quality is paramount. Healthcare that is safe, effective, efficient, equitable, patient centered, and timely is fundamental to all potential healthcare reform plans—big or small, national or regional.

This textbook provides a framework, a context, strategies, and practical tactics for all stakeholders to understand, learn, teach, and lead healthcare improvement. We have assembled an internationally prominent group of contributors for the best available current thinking and practices in each of their disciplines.

This edition has evolved from the first. New case studies have been added, up-to-date content has been included, new study questions have been posed, and a new chapter has been added. The framework of the book remains constant. Chapters 1 through 4 discuss foundational healthcare quality principles. Chapters 5 through 16 discuss critical quality issues at the organizational and microsystem levels. Chapters 17 through 19 detail the influence the environment has on the organizations, teams, and individuals delivering healthcare services and products.

In Chapter 1, Maulik Joshi and Donald Berwick center on the patient and articulate key findings from national, sentinel reports of healthcare quality over the last ten years. In Chapter 2, Leon Wyszewianski discusses the fundamental concepts of quality. In Chapter 3, David Ballard and colleagues discuss medical practice variation and provide an updated case study, and Kevin Warren has revised Chapter 4 to reflect the latest quality improvement tools and programs.

In Chapter 5, Robert Lloyd discusses measurement as a building block in quality assessment and improvement. John Byrnes focuses on data collection and its sources in Chapter 6, and Jerod Loeb and colleagues discuss analytic opportunities in quality data in Chapter 7. In Chapter 8, David Nash and colleagues detail a physician profiling system. In Chapter 9, Susan Edgman-Levitan tackles an often discussed but less understood area of patient satisfaction—experiences and perspectives of care—and includes an update on the latest surveys. In Chapter 10, Michael Pugh aggregates data into a management tool called the Balanced Scorecard. Frances Griffin and Carol Haraden in Chapter 11 and

Richard Ward in Chapter 12 dive deeper into two evolving subjects essential to driving performance improvement—patient safety and information technology, respectively. Chapters 13 through 15, by James Reinertsen, A. Al-Assaf, and Scott Ransom and colleagues, provide a triad of keys for change in organizations seeking to become high performers. The triad represents leadership, infrastructure, and strategy for quality improvement. Chapter 16, by Valerie Weber and John Bulger, is a compilation of strategies and tactics necessary to change staff behavior.

Chapter 17, by Jean Johnson and colleagues, a new chapter, provides examples of many of the recent national quality improvement initiatives and an overview of the quality improvement landscape. In Chapter 18, Greg Pawlson and Paul Schyve collaborate to summarize the work of the two major accrediting bodies within healthcare—the National Committee for Quality Assurance and The Joint Commission—and cover the latest changes in the accreditation process. The book concludes with an important chapter by Francois de Brantes on the power of the purchaser to select and pay for quality services, which he has updated to provide the latest information on pay for performance.

Several of these chapters could stand independently. Each represents an important contribution to our understanding of the patient-centered organizations and environment in which healthcare services are delivered. The science and knowledge on which quality measurement is based are changing rapidly. This book provides a timely analysis of extant tools and techniques.

Who should read this book? The editors believe all current stakeholders would benefit from reading this text. The primary audiences for the book are undergraduate and graduate students in healthcare and business administration, public health programs, nursing programs, allied health programs, and programs in medicine. As leadership development and continuing education programs proliferate, this textbook is a resource for executives and practitioners at the front line. We hope this book will break down the educational silos that currently prevent stakeholders from sharing equally in their understanding of patient-centered organizational systems and the environment of healthcare quality.

This textbook and the accompanying instructor manual are designed to facilitate discussion and learning. There are study questions at the end of each chapter in the textbook. The instructor manual contains answers to the study questions and a PowerPoint presentation for each chapter as a teaching aid. For access information, e-mail hap1@ache.org.

Please contact us at doctormaulikjoshi@yahoo.com. Your feedback, your teaching, your learning, and your leadership are essential to raising the bar in healthcare.

Elizabeth R. Ransom
Maulik S. Joshi
David B. Nash
Scott B. Ransom

SCIENCE AND KNOWLEDGE
FOUNDATION

1

HEALTHCARE QUALITY AND THE PATIENT

Maulik S. Joshi and Donald Berwick

Quality in the U.S. healthcare system is not what it should be. People were aware of this issue for years from personal stories and anecdotes. Around the end of the last century, three major reports revealed evidence of this quality deficiency:

- The Institute of Medicine's (IOM) National Roundtable on Health Care Quality report, "The Urgent Need to Improve Health Care Quality" (Chassin and Galvin 1998)
- *To Err Is Human* (Kohn, Corrigan, and Donaldson 2000)
- IOM's *Crossing the Quality Chasm* (IOM 2001)

These three reports made a tremendous statement and called for action on the state of healthcare, its gaps, and the opportunity to improve its quality in the United States to unprecedented levels.

Before we begin discussion of these reports, however, let us begin by defining quality, its evolution, and its implications on our work as healthcare professionals.

Avedis Donabedian, one of the pioneers in understanding approaches to quality, discussed in detail the various definitions of quality in relation to perspective. Among his conceptual constructs of quality, one view of Donabedian's (1990) rang particularly true: "The balance of health benefits and harm is the essential core of a definition of quality." The question of balance between benefit and harm is empirical and points to medicine's essential chimerism: one part science and one part art (Mullan 2001).

The IOM Committee to Design a Strategy for Quality Review and Assurance in Medicare developed an often-cited definition of quality (Lohr 1990):

Quality of care is the degree to which health services for individuals and populations increase the likelihood of desired health outcomes and are consistent with current professional knowledge. . . . How care is provided should reflect appropriate use of the most current knowledge about scientific, clinical, technical, interpersonal, manual, cognitive, and organization and management elements of health care.

In 2001, *Crossing the Quality Chasm* stated powerfully and simply that healthcare should be safe, effective, efficient, timely, patient centered, and equitable. This six-dimensional aim, which will be discussed later in this chapter, provides the best-known and most goal-oriented definition, or at least conceptualization, of the components of quality today.

Important Reports

In 1998, the *Journal of the American Medical Association*'s National Roundtable report included two notable contributions to the industry. The first was its assessment of the state of quality. "Serious and widespread quality problems exist throughout American medicine. These problems . . . occur in small and large communities alike, in all parts of the country, and with approximately equal frequency in managed care and fee-for-service systems of care. Very large numbers of Americans are harmed." The second contribution to the knowledge base of quality was a categorization of defects into three broad categories: overuse, misuse, and underuse. The classification scheme of underuse, overuse, and misuse has become a common nosology for quality defects.

Underuse is evidenced by the fact that many scientifically sound practices are not used as often as they should be. For example, biannual mammography screening in women ages 40 to 69 has been proven beneficial and yet is performed less than 75 percent of the time.

Overuse can be seen in areas such as imaging studies for diagnosis in acute asymptomatic low back pain or the prescription of antibiotics when not indicated for infections, such as viral upper respiratory infections.

Misuse is the term applied when the proper clinical care process is not executed appropriately, such as giving the wrong drug to a patient or incorrectly administering the correct drug.

Many reports have identified the gap between current and optimal healthcare practice. The studies range from evidence of specific processes falling short of the standard (e.g., children not receiving all their immunizations by age two) to overall performance gaps (e.g., risk-adjusted mortality rates in hospitals varying fivefold) (McGlynn et al. 2003).

Although the healthcare community knew of many of these quality-related challenges for years, the 2000 publication *To Err Is Human* exposed the severity of the problems in a way that captured the attention of all key stakeholders for the first time.

The executive summary of *To Err Is Human* began with these headlines (Kohn, Corrigan, and Donaldson 2000):

- Betsy Lehman, a health reporter for the *Boston Globe*, died from an overdose during chemotherapy.
- Ben Kolb, an eight-year-old receiving minor surgery, died due to a drug mix-up.
- As many as 98,000 people die every year in hospitals as a result of injuries from their care.

- Total national costs of preventable adverse events are estimated between $17 billion and $29 billion, of which health care costs are over one-half.

These data points focused on patient safety and medical errors as perhaps the most urgent forms of quality defect. Although many had spoken about improving healthcare, this report spoke about the negative—it framed the problem in a way that everyone could understand and demonstrated that the situation was unacceptable. One of the basic foundations for this report was a Harvard Medical Practice study done more than ten years earlier. For the first time, patient safety (i.e., ensuring safe care and preventing mistakes) became a solidifying force for policymakers, regulators, providers, and consumers.

In March 2001, soon after the release of *To Err Is Human*, IOM released *Crossing the Quality Chasm*, a more comprehensive report offering a new framework for a redesigned U.S. healthcare system. *Crossing the Quality Chasm* provided a blueprint for the future that classified and unified the components of quality through six aims for improvement, chain of effect, and simple rules for redesign of healthcare.

The six aims for improvement, viewed also as six dimensions of quality, are as follows (Berwick 2002):

1. *Safe*: Care should be as safe for patients in healthcare facilities as in their homes.
2. *Effective*: The science and evidence behind healthcare should be applied and serve as the standard in the delivery of care.
3. *Efficient*: Care and service should be cost effective, and waste should be removed from the system.
4. *Timely*: Patients should experience no waits or delays in receiving care and service.
5. *Patient centered*: The system of care should revolve around the patient, respect patient preferences, and put the patient in control.
6. *Equitable*: Unequal treatment should be a fact of the past; disparities in care should be eradicated.

These six aims for improvement can be translated into respective outcome measures and goals. The following points are examples of the types of global measures that can be used to track IOM's six aims.

- Safe care may be measured in terms of the percentage of overall mortality rates or patients experiencing adverse events or harm.
- Effective care may be measured by how well evidenced-based practices are followed, such as the percentage of time diabetic patients receive all recommended care at each doctor visit, the percentage of hospital-acquired infections, or the percentage of patients who develop pressure ulcers (bed sores) while in the nursing home.
- Efficient care may be measured by analyzing the costs of care by patient, by organization, by provider, or by community.

FIGURE 1.1
Four Levels of
the Healthcare
System

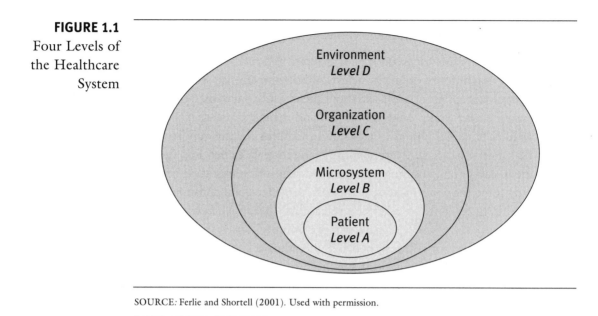

Environment
Level D

Organization
Level C

Microsystem
Level B

Patient
Level A

SOURCE: Ferlie and Shortell (2001). Used with permission.

- Timely care may be measured by waits and delays in receiving needed care, service, and test results.
- Patient-centered measures may include patient or family satisfaction with care and service.
- Equitable care may be viewed by examining differences in quality measures (such as measures of effectiveness and safety) by race, gender, income, or other population-based demographic and socioeconomic factors.

The underlying framework for achieving these aims for improvement depicts the healthcare system in four levels, all of which require changes. *Level A* is what happens with the patient. *Level B* reflects the microsystem where care is delivered by small provider teams. *Level C* is the organizational level—the macrosystem or aggregation of the microsystems and supporting functions. *Level D* is the external environment where payment mechanisms, policy, and regulatory factors reside. Figure 1.1 provides a picture of these four cascading levels. The environment affects how organizations operate, which affects the microsystems housed in them, which in turn affect the patient. "True north" in the model lies at Level A, in the experience of patients, their loved ones, and the communities in which they live (Berwick 2002).

A Focus on the Patient

All healthcare professionals and organizations exist to serve their patients. Technically, medicine has never had more potential to help than it does today. The number of efficacious therapies and life-prolonging pharmaceutical regimens has exploded. Yet, the system falls short of its technical potential. Patients are dissatisfied and frustrated with the care they receive. Providers are overburdened and uninspired by a system that asks too much and makes their work more difficult. Society's attempts to pay for and properly regulate care add complexity and even chaos.

Demands for a fundamental redesign of the U.S. healthcare system are ever increasing. IOM proposed that a laser-like focus on the patient must sit at the center of efforts to improve and restructure healthcare. Patient-centered care is the proper future of medicine, and the current focus on quality and safety is a step on the path to excellence.

Today, patients' perception of the quality of our healthcare system is not favorable. In healthcare, *quality* is a household word that evokes great emotion, including:

- frustration and despair, exhibited by patients who experience healthcare services firsthand or family members who observe the care of their loved ones;
- anxiety over the ever-increasing costs and complexities of care;
- tension between individuals' need for care and the difficulty and inconvenience in obtaining care; and
- alienation from a care system that seems to have little time for understanding, much less meeting, patients' needs.

To illustrate these issues, we will examine in depth the insights and experiences of a patient who has lived with chronic back pain for almost 50 years and use this case study to understand the inadequacies of the current delivery system and the potential for improvement. This case study is representative of the frustrations and challenges of the patients we are trying to serve and reflective of the opportunities that await us to radically improve the healthcare system. (See the section titled "Case Study" later in the chapter.)

Lessons Learned in Quality Improvement

We have noted the chasm in healthcare as it relates to quality. This chasm is wide, and the changes to the system are challenging. An important message is that changes are being made, patient care is improving, and the health of communities is beginning to demonstrate marked improvement. Let us take this opportunity to highlight examples of improvement projects in various settings to provide insight into the progress.

Improvement Project: Improving ICU Care[1]

One improvement project success story took place in 2002 in the intensive care unit (ICU) at Dominican Hospital in Santa Cruz County, California. Dominican, a 379-bed community hospital, is part of the 41-hospital Catholic Healthcare West system.

The staff in Dominican Hospital's ICU learned an important lesson about the power of evidence over intuition. "We used to replace the ventilator circuit for intubated patients daily because we thought this helped to prevent pneumonia," explained Lee Vanderpool, vice president. "But the evidence shows that the more you interfere with that device, the more often you risk introducing infection. It turns out it is often better to leave it alone until it begins to become cloudy, or 'gunky,' as the nonclinicians say."

The importance of using scientific evidence reliably in care was just the sort of lesson that healthcare professionals at Dominican had been learning routinely for more than a decade as they pursued quality improvement throughout the hospital. Dominican's leaders focused on improving critical care processes, and their efforts improved mortality rates, average ventilator days, and other key measures (see Figure 1.2).

FIGURE 1.2

Improving
Critical Care
Processes:
Mortality Rates
and Average
Ventilator Days

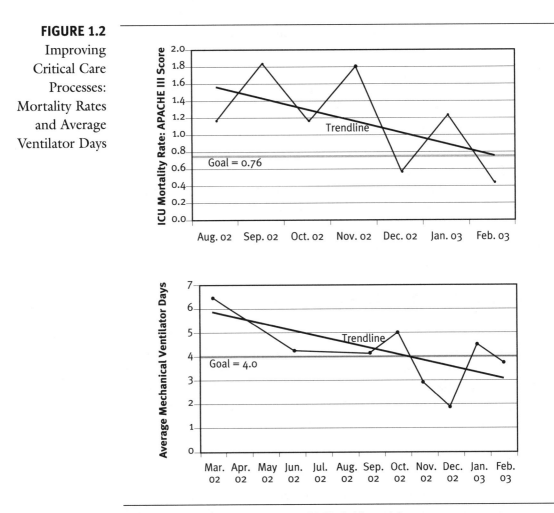

SOURCE: Dominican Hospital, Santa Cruz, CA. Used with permission.

Ventilator Bundling and Glucose Control

After attending a conference in critical care, Dominican staff began to focus on a number of issues in the ICU. "The first thing we tackled was ventilator bundling," said Glenn Robbins, RPh, responsible for the day-to-day process and clinical support of Dominican's critical care improvement team. *Ventilator bundling* refers to a group of five procedures that, performed together, improve outcomes for ventilator patients.[2]

"We were already doing four of the five elements," said Robbins, "but not in a formalized, documented way that we could verify." Ventilator bundling calls for ventilator patients to receive the following: the head of their bed elevated a minimum of 30 degrees; prophylactic care for peptic ulcer disease; prophylactic care for deep vein thrombosis; a "sedation vacation" (a day or two without sedatives); and a formal assessment by a respiratory therapist of readiness to be weaned from the ventilator.

The team tested ideas using Plan-Do-Study-Act (PDSA) cycles, ran various small tests, and then widened implementation of those that worked. Some fixes were complex, and some were simple. To ensure that nurses checked elevation at the head of the bed, for example, Camille Clark, RN, critical care manager, said, "We put a piece of red tape on the bed scales at 30 degrees as a reminder. We started with one nurse, then two, and then it spread. Now when we [perform rounds] in the ICU, we always check to see that the head of the bed is right. It has become an integrated part of the routine."

Another important process change included the use of lists to identify and track therapy goals for each patient. The form went through more than 20 PDSA cycles and 25 different versions before it was used 100 percent of the time for ICU patients. "We got some pushback from the nurses because it felt to them like double-charting," said Clark. "So we kept working on it, and incorporating their suggestions, until it became something that was useful to them rather than simply more paperwork." Getting physicians on board regarding the daily goal list and other aspects of improvement was also a key factor in their project's success.

Next, the team turned its attention to the intravenous insulin infusion protocol used in the ICU and intensified efforts to better control patients' blood sugar. "The literature strongly suggests that controlling hyperglycemia helps reduce mortality in the ICU," said Aaron Morse, MD, critical care medical director. "We initially trialed a more aggressive protocol on about 30 patients, and we've gone through seven or eight PDSA cycles on it. It is now standard protocol, and from the data we have so far, it has been extremely successful. We attribute our very low rate of ventilator-associated pneumonia to changes like the ventilator bundle and glucose control."

Part of introducing a new protocol, or any new idea, involves education. "We worked to educate the staff on the importance of tight glucose control in ICU patients," said Robbins. Equally important is listening to the frontline staff who must implement the new procedures. "The nursing staff provides lots of feedback, which helps us refine our processes. We have vigorous dialogues with both nurses and physicians when we try things."

At Dominican, the culture of improvement was pervasive for more than a decade, so all employees knew that performance improvement was part of their jobs. "We are in our 12th formal year of continuous performance improvement, and most of the people here have been a part of that from the inception," said Vanderpool. As a result of the organization's long-term commitment to quality improvement, Vanderpool said progress was steady on many fronts. "Things that were once barriers to change are not today. People know they have the ability to make changes at the work level and show the trends associated with them. People feel empowered."

"How Did You Get That to Happen?"

Vanderpool said other hospital leaders who were trying to achieve similar improvements as Dominican did in their own quality journeys often asked him the same question: "How did you get that to happen?" He emphasized the value of creating a culture of improvement, which must start at the top of the organization. He demonstrated his commitment to quality by joining clinical staff on rounds in the ICU on a frequent, yet purposefully irregular, basis. "Some organizations overlook the importance of the culture change in performance improvement work," said Sister Julie Hyer, OP, president of Dominican Hospital. "It is fundamental to create a culture that supports and respects improvement efforts."

Robbins cited physician buy-in as another key to successful improvement strategies. "We are lucky to have some very good physician champions here," he said. "They are active, creative, and knowledgeable, and their support makes a huge difference."

Vanderpool, Hyer, and Robbins all acknowledged the value of the collaborative relationships they formed through the IMPACT Network sponsored by the Institute for Healthcare Improvement (IHI). "We are not working just within our institution, but with 40 others," said Robbins. "In between learning sessions, we e-mail each other, talk on the phone, have site visits . . . we have adopted approaches others have used, and others have learned from us."

Vanderpool said that working with outside experts over the past five years breathed new life into the hospital's well-established improvement culture. "After the first four or five years of working doggedly and diligently on our own homegrown improvement projects, we found it got harder to be prophets in our own land. Bringing in expertise from the outside has strengthened our approach and our commitment."

Improvement Project: Redesigning the Clinical Office

The preceding improvement project case exemplified impressive gains in quality in one specific area, the ICU. The project in this section provided evidence of the power of complete redesign of healthcare by addressing multiple parts of the healthcare system and using the six IOM dimensions of quality as a measuring tool.

CareSouth Carolina, which serves 35,000 South Carolina patients in 11 locations, was determined to make significant improvements in office practice in all six of IOM's aims, plus an additional category of equal importance to the organization: vitality, measured by the degree to which stress was minimized in the workplace.

"This work is really a marriage between what we have learned about chronic care management and advanced practice concepts like advanced access," said Ann Lewis, chief executive officer, in 2003. As one of the first participants in the Health Disparities Collaborative, run jointly by IHI and the federal Bureau of Primary Health Care (the Bureau of Primary Health Care provides significant funding for CareSouth and other similar clinics throughout the nation), CareSouth Carolina focused on improving access to quality care for patients with diabetes, asthma, and depression.

The results inspired Lewis to lead her organization into further improvement efforts. "When we started the diabetes collaborative, the average HbA1c of the patients we were tracking was over 13," Lewis recalled. "I didn't even know what that meant. But I learned that every percentage drop in HbA1c represents a 13 percent drop in mortality, and that got my attention. And I would go to group visits where patients with diabetes were practically in tears with gratitude about how much our new approach to care was helping them." Lewis realized that "it's not about the business or economics of healthcare; it's about the outcomes."

The ambitious nature of CareSouth Carolina's goals was testimony to Lewis's success. For example, the clinic aimed to achieve a 7.0 average HbA1c for patients with diabetes, to meet 80 percent of patients' self-management goals, to have 80 percent of each patient's total visit time spent face to face with a provider of care, and to have the third next available appointment (a standard measure of access) be in zero days. "To be truly patient centered," said Lewis, "it's not enough to help patients set goals. It's meeting the goals that puts the rubber to the road. We want the healthiest patients in America," she said. "Why not? The knowledge is there—we know how to make people healthy and how to make care accessible. Let's just do it."

Improvement at CareSouth Carolina Through IOM's Areas of Focus

CareSouth Carolina's work in each of the seven areas of focus reflected creativity, doggedness, and steadfast attention to the voice of the customer, its patients. "We ask the patients all the time what they want, what they think," said Lewis. "They always tell us. But you have to ask."

CareSouth Carolina worked diligently to improve in each of the IOM aim categories. Staff chose to add one more category, vitality, as a measure of staff morale. Although progress toward achieving these ambitious goals varied, the organization remained determined.

Effectiveness

Goal: Asthma patients were to have an average of 10 or more symptom-free days out of 14. Diabetes patients were to have an average HbA1c of 7.0 or less. Figure 1.3 shows CareSouth Carolina's results through July 2003 on these measures.

FIGURE 1.3

Improving Effectiveness: Asthma Symptom-Free Days and Average HbA1c Levels

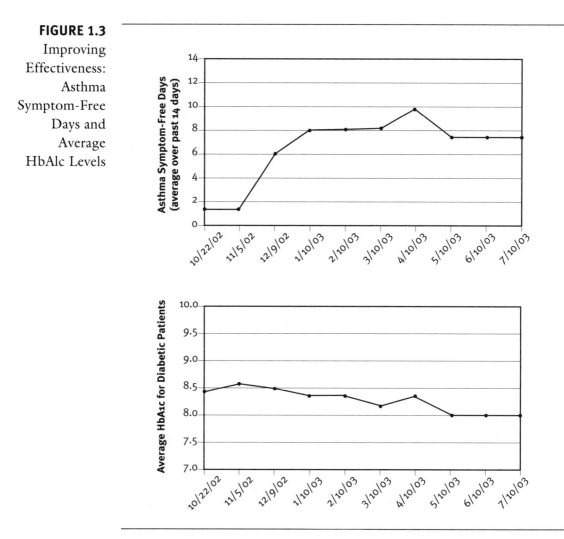

SOURCE: CareSouth, Hartsville, SC. Used with permission.

Action: The experience that CareSouth Carolina staff had already gained in chronic care management through the Health Disparities Collaborative gave them the tools they needed to improve effectiveness of care. "Once you know the model—self-management support, decision support, design of delivery system, clinical information system, community support—you can transfer it from one condition to another pretty smoothly," Lewis said, referring to the Chronic Care Model developed by Ed Wagner, MD, and his colleagues, which is widely regarded as the standard for chronic care management. Wagner, a general internist/epidemiologist, is the director of Improving Chronic Illness Care at the Seattle-based MacColl Institute for Healthcare Innovation at the Center for Health Studies, Group Health Cooperative of Puget Sound.

Patient Safety

Goal: One hundred percent of all medication lists were to be updated at every visit (see Figure 1.4).

Action: "Patients have a hard time remembering what medications they are taking, especially when they take several," said Lewis. "It's best if they bring their medications to each appointment. Patients told us that it would help if they had something to bring them in, so we had very nice cloth medication bags made for everyone on three meds or more. They have our logo on them, and a reminder to bring their medications to each visit. It's a low-tech solution, but it has made a huge difference. We've had some early success in the work, as well as some recent setbacks, but I'm sure we're on the right track."

Patient Centeredness

Goal: Eighty percent of self-management goals set by patients were to be met (see Figure 1.5).

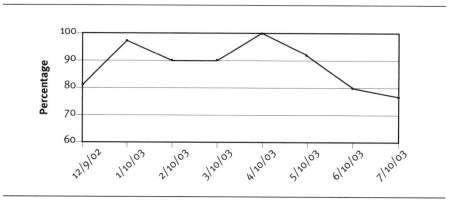

FIGURE 1.4

Improving Patient Safety: Percentage of Medication Lists on All Charts

SOURCE: CareSouth, Hartsville, SC. Used with permission.

FIGURE 1.5
Improving
Patient
Centeredness:
Percentage of
Patients' Self-
Management
Goals Met

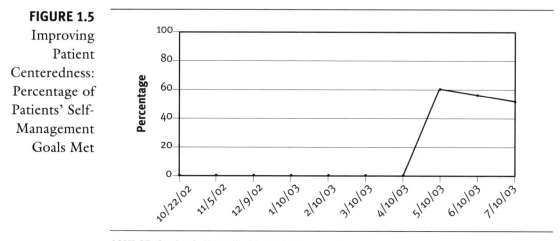

SOURCE: CareSouth, Hartsville, SC. Used with permission.

Action: "One of the biggest challenges the healthcare system faces is to help patients meet their own goals," said Lewis. "We ask our patients in three ways how they want us to help them with self-management: through surveys, in one-on-one patient interviews, and in small focus groups." Through these means, CareSouth Carolina staff members learned how to help patients tailor achievable goals. "Don't tell me to lose 40 pounds," Lewis said, explaining what patients often say. "Tell me how to do it in small steps."

CareSouth Carolina also learned that patients are its best source of guidance regarding what system changes to make. Some of the feedback was surprising, according to Lewis. "Some of our elderly patients say they like it better when they can spend more time here, not less," she said. "And we've learned that centralized appointment scheduling and medical records are not what our patients want. They want to talk with the same person each time they call, someone in their own doctor's practice." Little changes also mean a lot to patients, she said. "They told us to stop weighing them in the hallway where everyone can watch."

Efficiency

Goal: The average amount of time spent with the clinician in an office visit was to be 12 minutes or more (see Figure 1.6).

Action: Working to increase patient time with clinicians and decrease non-value-added time was challenging for the CareSouth Carolina staff, but it made headway. Again, the patients told the organization what they wanted. "They didn't care about the cycle time; they wanted a rich visit, more comprehensive, where they could get more done," said Lewis. Patients liked group visits, time with the nurse as well as the doctor, and opportunities for health education, so the CareSouth Carolina staff worked to organize the delivery system accordingly. The average time patients spend with their doctors also increased.

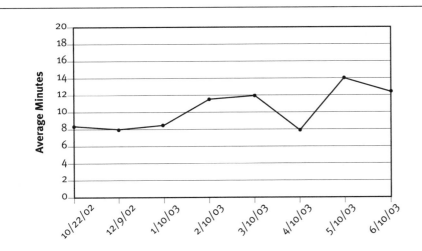

SOURCE: CareSouth, Hartsville, SC. Used with permission.

FIGURE 1.6

Improving Efficiency: Average Minutes Spent with Clinician in an Office Visit

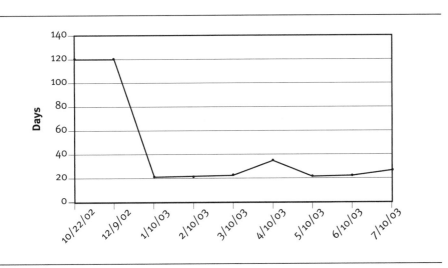

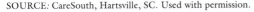

SOURCE: CareSouth, Hartsville, SC. Used with permission.

FIGURE 1.7

Improving Timeliness: Days to Third Next Available Appointment

Timeliness

Goal: The third next available appointment was to be in zero days (see Figure 1.7).

Action: Staff began by combing the schedule for opportunities for more efficient care management of patients, in particular looking for ways to reduce unnecessary follow-up visits, substituting telephone follow-up when appropriate. "Implementing care management and deleting all those short-term return visits from the schedule gave us a big drop in appointment waiting time," said Lewis. Decentralizing appointment tracking was another means of improving timeliness because each microteam was more aware of patients' needs and able to structure providers' schedules in ways that reduced backlog (Murray and Tantau 2000).

Equity

Goal: There was to be zero disparity by race for each key effectiveness measure (see Figure 1.8). (Variation from zero equals disparity.)

Action: With a patient population that was 69 percent nonwhite at the time, CareSouth Carolina took equity very seriously. "This is our strong suit," said Lewis. "It is woven into our very culture." To counter the "clinic mentality" with which community health centers are often wrongly saddled, CareSouth was conscientious not only about providing top-quality care to its patients but also about maintaining the perception of quality. "We look good," she said. "We remodeled, refurnished, repainted, and we say we offer first-class care for first-class people. Disparity is not just about outcomes, it's also about how you treat your patients."

Vitality

Goal: Zero percent of the office team was to report a somewhat or very stressful work environment (currently 20 percent; see Figure 1.9).

Actions: Organizations such as CareSouth Carolina that take on improvement work in multiple categories find that considerable overlap exists in those areas. Lewis said that all the improvements in efficiency and effectiveness

FIGURE 1.8

Improving Equity: Disparity by Race for Key Effectiveness Measures

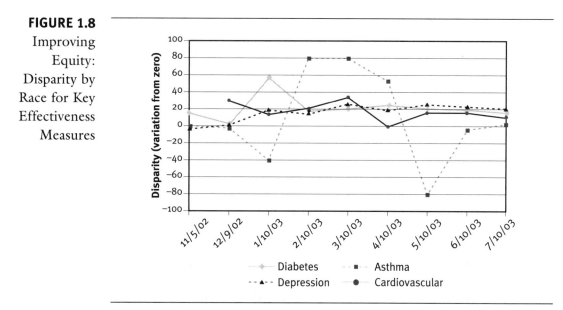

SOURCE: CareSouth, Hartsville, SC. Used with permission.

improved staff morale and "fired everyone up" about the potential for even greater changes. "We have fun here," she claimed, "and we work hard. The one thing providers have told us consistently through the years is that they don't like being stuck in the office later and later each day because patients and paperwork have backed up. They want the workday to go smoothly. And all the changes we are making are addressing that. I'm sure that the stress in our workplace will decrease as these changes take hold."

Lewis was confident that all of these measures would continue to show progress as the improvement programs became fully integrated. She had seen many changes in healthcare, and in her own health center, in her years with the organization. However, this period of growth and change had been unprecedented, she said. "You go home at night dead tired," she admitted, "but knowing you are doing incredible things and providing the best possible care for people who would not have access to it otherwise."

Case Study[3]

This case study was developed after an interview with the patient in 2002.

Mr. Roberts is a 77-year-old gentleman who is retired and living in Florida with his wife. He is an accomplished and affluent person who was a child of the Depression. He worked from the time he was 13 as a long-shoreman and barracks builder. He began experiencing back pain in his early 20s. At that time, he did not receive particularly good medical advice and did not pursue alternative therapies. World War II, 25 years in Asia,

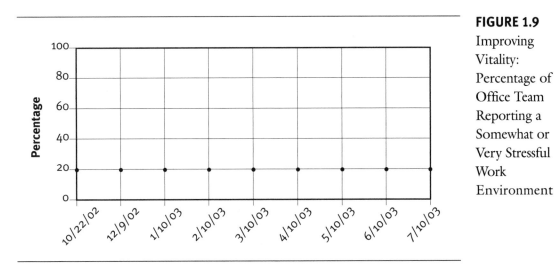

FIGURE 1.9

Improving Vitality: Percentage of Office Team Reporting a Somewhat or Very Stressful Work Environment

SOURCE: CareSouth, Hartsville, SC. Used with permission.

and life as a busy executive took priority, and the pain became a constant but secondary companion.

At age 50, the pain became unbearable. He returned to New York and spent the better part of a year "on his back." In 1980, he underwent the first of four major spine surgeries. Since then, he has had multiple intervertebral discs partially or completely removed. Despite these operations, he still has pain. Over the past two to three years, his pain has been worsening and his functional status has been decreasing.

It is hard to live with pain. Mr. Roberts is not sure he deals with it very well. He does not want to take narcotics because they interfere with his ability to stay sharp and active, and stomach problems prohibit the use of many non-narcotic medications. Most of the time, he has only mild or temporary relief of his pain.

Despite the pain, he is active and gets out as much as he can. Although it has become more difficult, he still takes his wife dancing on Saturday nights. The pain is exhausting, limiting his ability to do what he wants. The worst part about the pain is that it is changing—getting worse—and he is uncertain of its future trajectory. As the pain becomes worse, how will he survive? What are the possibilities for remaining active and independent?

Mr. Roberts states that he has had "reasonably good" doctors. He feels he is privileged because he has connections and acts as his own advocate. These assets have allowed him to expand his healthcare options and seek the best providers and institutions. He is also well informed and assertive and has been an active participant in his healthcare. Although his overall experience in the healthcare system has been favorable, many instances of care have been less than ideal.

Communication Deficits and Lack of a Team Approach

Mr. Roberts has observed that the lack of communication between providers is a huge problem. He has multiple specialists who care for different parts of his body; however, no one person is mindful of how these systems interact to create the whole person or illness. He is never sure whether one physician knows what the other is doing or how one physician's prescriptions might interfere or interact with another's. The physicians never seem inclined to "dig deeply" or communicate as team members treating one person. On many occasions, physicians have recommended therapies that have already been tried and failed. On other occasions, they disagree on an approach to his problem and leave Mr. Roberts to decide which advice to follow. No system is in place to encourage teamwork. "Unless the physician is extremely intelligent, on the ball, or energetic, it just doesn't happen," he says.

Record keeping and transfer of information are also faulty. Despite the fact that physicians take copious notes, the information is not put to use. Mr. Roberts might expend a great deal of time and energy ensuring that his medical records are sent to a new consultant's office. Within a few minutes of the encounter, however, it is apparent that the consultant has not reviewed the chart or absorbed the information. This realization has affected how he uses care. For instance, at one point, Mr. Roberts was experiencing worsening stomach problems. His gastroenterologist was away on vacation for four weeks, and there was no covering physician. The thought of amassing his patient records for transfer to another physician (who likely would not review them and would suggest the same tests and therapies) was so unpleasant that he chose to go without care.

Mr. Roberts states that he spends much of his energy as a patient facilitating communication between providers and transferring information gained from one physician to another. This process is expensive, wasteful, and dangerous. If all the providers could come together and discuss the problem as a group, redundancies and mistakes could be eliminated. Instead, much time and money are wasted reproducing ineffective therapeutic plans and not treating his illness in an efficient, effective, safe, and timely manner.

In addition, effective communication between providers and patients is lacking. Despite the fact that Mr. Roberts has undergone multiple surgeries that have not resolved his pain, many new doctors he sees are quick to offer surgery as the solution to his problem. Seldom do physicians listen to his full story or elicit his thoughts before jumping to conclusions. This problem was painfully illustrated by the recent death of his brother, who died on the operating room table while undergoing a second spinal surgery for similar back problems.

Mr. Roberts suggests that physicians carefully analyze their therapeutic personalities. They cannot assume that all patients are alike or that they will react similarly to a given intervention. Each patient needs to be treated as an individual, and service needs to be respectful of individual choice.

Removing the Question Mark from Patient-Provider Interactions

Mr. Roberts is particularly concerned with the inability of patients to know the true qualifications of their physicians or judge their prescriptions. At one point, he was experiencing severe arm and finger pain. Assuming these symptoms were related to his spine, he sought the advice of a highly recommended chief of neurosurgery at a premier academic center. After eliciting a brief history and performing a short examination, the chief admitted him to the hospital.

The following day, an anesthesiologist came into the room to obtain his consent for surgery. Mr. Roberts had not been told that surgery was under consideration. He asked to speak to the neurosurgeon and insisted on additional consultations. Three days later, a hand surgeon reassured him that his problem was likely self-limiting tendonitis and prescribed conservative therapy. Within a few weeks, his pain had resolved. Mr. Roberts was grateful that he had followed his instinct but concerned for other patients who might not have asserted themselves in this manner.

Mismatch Between Supply and Demand

Mr. Roberts also stated that there is a profound disconnect between supply and demand in the healthcare system. In 1992, his pain had become particularly disabling, and his mobility was extremely restricted. His physicians suggested that he see the only neurosurgeon in the county. Despite his health emergency, he was not able to make an appointment to see this neurosurgeon for more than ten weeks. No other solutions were offered. In pain and unable to walk because of progressively worsening foot drop and muscle weakness, he sought the help of a physician friend. This friend referred him to a "brash, iconoclastic" Harvard-trained neurologist, who, in turn, referred him to a virtuoso neurosurgeon at a county hospital 100 miles away. After only 20 minutes with this neurosurgeon, he was rushed to the operating room and underwent a nine-hour emergency procedure. Apparently, he had severe spinal cord impingement and swelling. He was later told by the neurosurgeon that he would have been a paraplegic or died if he had not received the operation that day.

He subsequently underwent a series of three more spinal operations. Postoperative care was suboptimal; he had to travel 100 miles to see the surgeon for follow-up. Eventually, this surgeon chose to travel to a more centralized location twice per month to accommodate his patients in outlying areas.

Mr. Roberts states that we need to "overcome petty bureaucracies" that do not allow matching of supply with demand. The ready availability of quality care should be patient driven and closely monitored by a third party that does not have a vested interest in the market.

Knowledge-Based Care

Mr. Roberts is concerned about the status of continuing medical education. He guesses that it is probably easy for physicians in large, urban teaching hospitals to keep abreast of the latest diagnostic and therapeutic advances. However, the majority of physicians may not have similar opportunities. The system does not necessarily encourage physicians to keep up to date. This lack of current, in-depth knowledge is particularly important as supply-demand issues force consumers to seek care in "instant med clinics." For example, Mr. Roberts believes emergency care to be an oxymoron. On many occasions, he has gone to the emergency room and has had to wait four to five hours before being treated. This experience is unpleasant and forces people to seek alternative sites of care that may not provide the best care for complex, chronically ill patients.

Mr. Roberts also feels that we need to learn from our errors as well as successes. We should require that groups of physicians regularly review cases and learn how to deliver care in a better way. This analysis needs to occur internally within an institution as well as externally across institutions. Ideally, the analysis would directly involve patients and families to gain their perspectives. In addition, the learning should be contextual; we should not only learn how to do better the next time but also know whether what we are doing makes sense within our overall economic, epidemiological, and societal context.

Mr. Roberts believes that quality healthcare should be knowledge based. This knowledge comes not only from science but also from analysis of mistakes that occur in the process of delivering care. Patients should be involved in the collection and synthesis of these data. The transfer of knowledge among patients, scientists, and practitioners must be emphasized and simplified.

Nonphysician/Nonhospital Care

Mr. Roberts has been impressed with the quality of care provided by people other than physicians, and he believes the growth of alternative healthcare provider models has been a definite advance in the system. As an example, Mr. Roberts cites the effectiveness of his physical therapists as healthcare providers; they are alert, patient conscious, conscientious, and respectful. Mr. Roberts believes that their interventions "guide people to better life," and his functional status has improved because of their assistance. In addition, these providers are careful to maintain close communication with physicians. They function as members of a larger team.

Postoperative care also has improved. At the time of his first surgery more than two decades ago, Mr. Roberts spent two weeks in the hospital. Now, after three days, he is discharged to a rehabilitation facility that is better equipped to help him recuperate and return to full functioning.

Mr. Roberts knows how crucial his family and friends are in his medical care. Without their support, recommendations, constant questioning, and advocacy, his condition would be more precarious. The system needs to acknowledge the patient's other caregivers and involve them in shared decision making and transfer of knowledge.

Conclusion

The previous sections provide a brief insight into some successful improvement projects; it would be even easier to find examples of failures and the subsequent lessons learned. The main message is that, although the information on the gap between current practice and best practice may be daunting, improvement is occurring, albeit in pockets, and the opportunity is before us to continue to make quality a necessity, not just a nicety, in healthcare.

The aim of this textbook is to provide a comprehensive overview of the critical components of the healthcare quality landscape. The case studies highlight the complexity of systems and the interaction of systems that produce the results we achieve in healthcare.

As we improve the quality of healthcare, we will need to improve the multiple systems at every level to truly transform the healthcare system. You, as readers and leaders, should use this text as a resource and framework for understanding the connectivity of multiple aspects of healthcare quality from the bases of science, patient perspective, organizational implications, and environmental effects.

This chapter, specifically, sets the stage by highlighting:

* the current state of healthcare quality;
* the importance of the patient in goals and results;
* promising evidence of the great capacity for significant improvement in systems of care;
* examples of breakthrough improvements happening today; and
* the call to action for all healthcare stakeholders to continue to rethink and redesign our systems to achieve better health for all.

Building on this chapter, this book will outline healthcare quality on the basis of the levels of the healthcare system outlined by IOM.

Study Questions

1. Identify five ways in which you can put patients more in control of their care.
2. Think of an experience you, a family member, or a friend has had with healthcare. Apply IOM's six aims for improvement to the experience, and gauge the experience against the aims and the opportunities for improvement.
3. You are the CEO of your hospital, and the local newspaper has just run a story on "how bad healthcare is." How do you respond to the reporter asking you to comment on the situation? How do you respond to your employees?

Notes

1. Lee Vanderpool (vice president, Dominican Hospital), in discussion with the authors, January 2003.

2. Institute for Healthcare Improvement Innovation Team.
3. This patient story was edited by Matthew Fitzgerald, senior director for science and quality, American College of Cardiology, and originally composed by Heidi Louise Behforouz, MD, assistant professor of medicine, Harvard Medical School; and associate physician and director of the Prevention and Access to Care and Treatment, Division of Social Medicine and Health Inequalities, Brigham and Women's Hospital.

References

Berwick, D. M. 2002. "A User's Manual for the IOM's 'Quality Chasm' Report." *Health Affairs* May/June: 80–90.

Chassin, M. R., and R. H. Galvin. 1998. "The Urgent Need to Improve Health Care Quality. Institute of Medicine National Roundtable on Health Care Quality." *Journal of the American Medical Association* 280: 1000–05.

Donabedian, A. 1990. *The Definition of Quality and Approaches to Its Assessment, Volume I: Explorations in Quality Assessment and Monitoring.* Chicago: Health Administration Press.

Ferlie, E., and S. M. Shortell. 2001. "Improving the Quality of Healthcare in the United Kingdom and the United States: A Framework for Change." *Milbank Quarterly* 79 (2): 281–316.

Institute of Medicine (IOM). 2001. *Crossing the Quality Chasm: A New Health System for the 21st Century.* Washington, DC: National Academies Press.

Kohn, L. T., J. M. Corrigan, and M. S. Donaldson (eds.). 2000. *To Err Is Human: Building a Safer Health System.* Washington, DC: National Academies Press.

Lohr, K. N. (ed.). 1990. *Medicare: A Strategy for Quality Assurance, Volume I.* Washington, DC: Institute of Medicine, National Academies Press.

McGlynn, E. A., S. M. Asch, J. Adams, J. Keesey, J. Hicks, A. DeCristofaro, and E. A. Kerr. 2003. "The Quality of Health Care Delivered to Adults in the United States." *New England Journal of Medicine* 348 (26): 2635–45.

Mullan, F. 2001. "A Founder of Quality Assessment Encounters a Troubled System Firsthand." *Health Affairs* Jan./Feb.: 137–41.

Murray, M., and C. Tantau. 2000. "Same-Day Appointments: Exploding the Access Paradigm." *Family Practice Management* 7 (8): 45–50.

2

BASIC CONCEPTS OF HEALTHCARE QUALITY[1]

Leon Wyszewianski

People perceive the quality of healthcare services in different ways. Consider these two cases.

- The residents of a rural area were shocked to discover that the federal Medicare program had served notice that it would stop doing business with several of the area's physicians because the quality of care they provided was not acceptable. According to Medicare officials, the physicians had a pattern of providing unnecessary and even harmful care to Medicare patients, such as prescribing for patients with heart disease medications that were likely to worsen the patients' condition. These physicians had practiced in the community for at least 25 years each and were known for their dedication and devotion. Their willingness to travel to remote locations without regard to time of day or weather was legendary, as was their generosity toward patients who had fallen on hard times and were unable to pay their medical bills.
- An expert panel of trauma care specialists surveyed and rated hospital emergency departments in a major metropolitan area. The results surprised many of the area's residents. The emergency department rated number one by the panel was known mostly for its crowded conditions, long waits, and harried and often brusque staff.

Several concepts can help make sense of these and similar apparent contradictions and inconsistencies in perceptions of quality of care. This chapter focuses on such concepts, first in relation to the definition of quality of care and second in relation to its measurement.

Definition-Related Concepts

A number of attributes can characterize the quality of healthcare services (Campbell, Roland, and Buetow 2000; Donabedian 2003). As we will see, different groups involved in healthcare, such as physicians, patients, and health insurers, tend to attach different levels of importance to particular attributes and, as a result, define quality of care differently (see Table 2.1).

The Definitional Attributes

The following attributes relevant to the definition of quality of care will be discussed in this chapter:

- Technical performance
- Management of the interpersonal relationship
- Amenities
- Access
- Responsiveness to patient preferences
- Equity
- Efficiency
- Cost-effectiveness

Technical Performance

Quality of technical performance refers to how well current scientific medical knowledge and technology are applied in a given situation. It is usually assessed in terms of the timeliness and accuracy of the diagnosis, appropriateness of therapy, and skill with which procedures and other medical interventions are performed (Donabedian 1980, 1988a).

Management of the Interpersonal Relationship

The quality of the interpersonal relationship refers to how well the clinician relates to the patient on a human level. It is valued foremost for its own sake; by establishing a good interpersonal relationship with the patient, the clinician is able to fully address the patient's concerns, reassure the patient, and, more generally, relieve the patient's suffering, as distinguished from simply curing the patient's disease (Cassell 1982).

The quality of the interpersonal relationship is also important because of how it can affect technical performance (Donabedian 1988a). A clinician who relates well to a patient is better able to elicit from that patient a more complete and accurate medical history (especially with respect to potentially sensitive topics such as use of illicit drugs), which, in turn, can result in a better diagnosis. Similarly, a good relationship with the patient is often crucial in motivating the patient to follow a prescribed regimen of care, such as taking medications or making lifestyle changes.

Amenities

The quality of the amenities of care refers to the characteristics of the setting in which the encounter between patient and clinician takes place, such as comfort, convenience, and privacy (Donabedian 1980). Much like the interpersonal relationship, amenities are valued both in their own right and for their potential effect on the technical and interpersonal aspects of care.

Amenities such as ample and convenient parking, good directional signs, comfortable waiting rooms, and tasty hospital food are all valuable to patients.

In addition, amenities can yield benefits that are more indirect. For example, in a comfortable, private setting that puts the patient at ease, a good interpersonal relationship with the clinician is more easily established, potentially leading to a more complete patient history and, ultimately, a faster and more accurate diagnosis.

Access

The quality of access to care refers to the "degree to which individuals and groups are able to obtain needed services" (IOM 1993). How easily people obtain services depends, in turn, on the extent to which characteristics and expectations of the patient match those of the providers. For example, cost becomes an impediment to access when the amount the provider charges exceeds what the patient is able or willing to pay. Other potential areas in which mismatch between patient and provider creates impediments to receiving care include the provider's location in relation to the patient's capacity to reach it, days and times when care is available in relation to when the patient is able to come in for care, and how well cultural characteristics and expectations of the patient mesh with those of the provider, and vice versa (Penchansky and Thomas 1981; McLaughlin and Wyszewianski 2002).

Responsiveness to Patient Preferences

Although taking into account the wishes and preferences of patients has long been recognized as important to achieving high-quality care, only recently has it been singled out as a factor in its own right. In earlier formulations, responsiveness to patients' preferences was just one of the factors seen as determining the quality of the patient-clinician interpersonal relationship (Donabedian 1980). Now, however, the importance of responsiveness to patients' preferences in the context of quality of care is increasingly being acknowledged, for example, by Donabedian (2003) under the rubric of "acceptability" and by the Institute of Medicine (IOM 2001) as "respect for patients' values, preferences and expressed needs."

Equity

Findings that the amount, type, or quality of healthcare provided can be related systematically to an individual's characteristics, particularly race and ethnicity, rather than to the individual's need for care or healthcare preferences, have heightened concern about equity in health services delivery (Wyszewianski and Donabedian 1981; IOM 2002). Lee and Jones (1933) eloquently described the underlying concept many decades ago: "Good medical care implies the application of all the necessary services of modern, scientific medicine to the needs of all people. Judged from the viewpoint of society as a whole, the qualitative aspects of medical care cannot be dissociated from the quantitative. No matter what the perfection of technique in the treatment of one individual case, medicine does not fulfill its function adequately until the same perfection is within the reach of all individuals."

Efficiency

Efficiency refers to how well resources are used in achieving a given result. Efficiency improves whenever the resources used to produce a given output are reduced. Although economists typically treat efficiency and quality as separate concepts, separating the two in healthcare may not be easy or meaningful. Because inefficient care uses more resources than necessary, it is wasteful care, and care that involves waste is deficient—and therefore of lower quality—no matter how good it may be in other respects. "Wasteful care is either directly harmful to health or is harmful by displacing more useful care" (Donabedian 1988a).

Cost-Effectiveness

The cost-effectiveness of a given healthcare intervention is determined by how much benefit, typically measured in terms of improvement in health status, the intervention yields for a particular level of expenditure (Gold et al. 1996). In general, as the amounts spent on providing services for a particular condition grow, diminishing returns set in, meaning that each unit of expenditure yields ever-smaller benefits until a point where no additional benefits accrue from adding more care (Donabedian, Wheeler, and Wyszewianski 1982).

The maximization perspective on quality is characterized by the expenditure of resources to a point where no additional benefits can be obtained; resources are expended as long as a positive benefit can result, no matter how small. In contrast, the optimization perspective on quality is characterized by halting the expenditure of resources at a point where the additional benefits are considered too small to justify the added costs (Donabedian 1988a; 2003).

The Different Definitions

Although everyone values to some extent the attributes of quality just described, different stakeholders tend to attach different levels of importance to individual attributes (Blumenthal 1996; Harteloh 2004), resulting in differences in how clinicians, patients, managers, payers, and society each tend to define quality of care. Table 2.1 is an attempt to capture the stereotypical differences among these groups on the basis of how much they value individual attributes of care in the context of quality.

TABLE 2.1
Stereotypical Differences in Importance of Selected Aspects of Care to Key Stakeholders' Definitions of Quality

	Technical Performance	Interpersonal Relationship	Amenities	Access	Patient Preferences	Equity	Efficiency	Cost Effectiveness
Clinician	+++	+	+	+	+	+	+	—
Patient	++	+++	+++	++	++	+	+	—
Payer	+	+	+	+	+	+	+++	+++
Manager	++	+	+++	+++	+	++	+++	+++
Society	+++	+	+	+++	++	+++	+++	+++

REPRINTED FROM: *Clinics in Family Practice*, Volume 5 (4), Wyszewianski, L. "Defining, Measuring, and Improving Quality of Care." 807–825, 2003. Used with permission from Elsevier.

Clinicians

Clinicians, such as physicians and others who provide healthcare services, tend to perceive quality of care foremost in terms of technical performance. Within technical performance, clinicians' concerns focus on specific aspects that are well captured by the IOM's (1990) often-quoted definition of quality of care:

> Quality is the degree to which health services for individuals and populations increase the likelihood of desired health outcomes and are consistent with current professional knowledge.

Reference to "current professional knowledge" draws attention to the changing nature of what constitutes good clinical care; clinicians want to emphasize that, because medical knowledge advances rapidly, an assessment of care provided in 2005 in terms of what has been known only since 2007 is neither meaningful nor appropriate. Similarly, mention of the "likelihood of desired health outcomes" corresponds to clinicians' view that, with respect to outcomes, there are only probabilities, not certainties, owing to factors—such as patients' genetically determined physiological resilience—that influence outcomes of care and yet are beyond clinicians' control.

Patients

Clinicians are leery of having quality of care evaluated solely on the basis of health outcomes because some patients view technical performance only on these terms: If the patient did not improve, the physician's competence is called into question (Muir Gray 2001). Other patients recognize that they do not possess the wherewithal to evaluate all technical elements of care. As a result, they tend to defer to others on most matters of technical quality, especially to organizations presumed to have the requisite expertise and insight—such as accrediting bodies, state licensing agencies, and medical specialty boards—and seen as watching over technical quality on the public's behalf (Donabedian 1980).

Patients therefore tend to form their opinions about quality of care on the basis of their assessment of aspects of care they are most readily able to evaluate, chiefly the interpersonal aspects of care and the amenities of care (Cleary and McNeil 1988; Sofaer and Firminger 2005). In fact, because patients' satisfaction is so influenced by their reactions to the interpersonal and amenity aspects of care—rather than to the more indiscernible technical ones—health maintenance organizations, hospitals, and other healthcare delivery organizations have come to view the quality of nontechnical aspects of care as crucial to attracting and retaining patients. This perspective often dismays clinicians, who see it as a slight to technical quality, which is so central to their concept of healthcare quality.

In addition, patients' judgments of quality increasingly reflect the extent to which their preferences are taken into account (Sofaer and Firminger 2005). Although not every patient will have definite preferences in every clinical situation, patients value being consulted about their preferences, especially in situations in which different approaches to diagnosis and treatment involve potential trade-offs, such as between the quality and quantity of life.

Payers

Third-party payers—health insurance companies, government programs like Medicare, and others who pay for care on behalf of the patient—tend to assess quality of care in the context of costs. From their perspective, inefficient care is poor-quality care. Additionally, because payers typically manage a finite pool of resources, they often have to consider whether a potential outcome justifies the associated costs. Payers are therefore more likely to embrace the optimization definition of care, which can put them at odds with individual physicians, who generally take the maximization view on quality. In fact, most physicians consider cost-effectiveness calculations as antithetical to providing high-quality care because they see themselves as duty-bound to do everything possible to help their patients, including advocating for high-cost interventions even when such measures have a small but positive probability of benefiting the patient (Donabedian 1988b). By contrast, third-party payers—especially governmental units that must make multiple trade-offs when allocating resources—are more apt to concur that spending large sums in instances where the odds of a positive result are small does not represent high-quality care but rather a misuse of finite resources. From the third-party payers' point of view, this perspective is reinforced by evidence of the public's growing unwillingness to pay the higher premiums or taxes needed to provide patients with all feasible, potentially beneficial care.

Managers

The primary concern of managers responsible for the operations of hospitals, clinics, and other healthcare delivery organizations is the quality of the nonclinical aspects of care over which they have most control, most visibly amenities and access to care. In addition, the managers' perspective on quality differs markedly from that of clinicians and patients on efficiency, cost-effectiveness, and equity. Because of the manager's role in ensuring that resources are spent where they will do the most good, efficiency and cost-effectiveness are of central concern to managers, as is the equitable distribution of resources. Consequently, managers, like third-party payers, tend to favor an optimization definition of quality, which can put them, too, at odds with clinicians.

Society

At a collective, or societal, level, the definition of quality of care reflects concerns with efficiency and cost-effectiveness similar to those of governmental third-party payers, as well as of managers, and much for the same reasons. In addition, technical aspects of quality loom large at the societal level, where many believe technical care can be assessed and safeguarded more effectively than at the level of individual citizens. Similarly, access to care and equity are important to societal-level concepts of quality to the extent that the collectivity is seen as responsible for ensuring access to care for everyone, including, in particular, disenfranchised groups.

Are the Five Definitions Irreconcilable?

Different though they may seem, the five definitions—the clinician's, the patient's, the payer's, the manager's, and society's—have a great deal in common. Although each definition emphasizes different aspects of care, it does not exclude the other aspects (see Table 2.1). Definitions conflict only in relation to cost-effectiveness. Cost-effectiveness is often central to how payers, managers, and society define quality of care, whereas physicians and patients typically do not recognize cost-effectiveness as a legitimate consideration in the definition of quality. On all other aspects of care, however, no such clash is present; rather, the differences relate to how much each group emphasizes a particular aspect of care.

Strong disagreements do arise, however, among the five parties' definitions, even outside the realm of cost-effectiveness. Conflicts typically arise when one party holds that a particular practitioner or clinic is a high-quality provider by virtue of having high ratings on a single aspect of care, such as the interpersonal. Objections to such a conclusion point out that just because care rates highly on interpersonal quality does not necessarily mean that it rates equally highly on technical, amenity, efficiency, and other aspects (Wyszewianski 1988). Physicians who relate well to their patients, and thus score highly on the interpersonal aspect, nevertheless may have failed to keep up with medical advances and as a result provide care deficient in technical terms. This discrepancy apparently emerged in the case involving Medicare and rural physicians mentioned at the start of the chapter.

Conversely, practitioners who are highly skilled in trauma and other emergency care but who also have a distant, even brusque, manner and work in crowded conditions may rate low on the interpersonal and amenity aspects of care even though, as in the second case described at the start of the chapter, the facility receives top marks from a team of expert clinicians whose primary focus is on technical performance.

Implications

When clinicians, patients, payers, managers, society, and other involved parties refer to quality of care, they each tend to focus on the quality of specific aspects of care, sometimes to the apparent exclusion of other aspects important to other parties. The aspects a party overlooks, however, are seldom in direct conflict with that party's own overall concept of quality (Table 2.1).

Measurement-Related Concepts

Just as the concepts discussed above are useful in advancing our understanding of the definition of quality of care, another set of concepts can help us better understand the measurement of quality of care, particularly with respect to technical care. Consider the following two cases.

- At the urging of the nurses' association, state legislators passed a law that specifies minimum nurse staffing levels for hospitals in the state. The state nurses' association had argued that nurse staffing cutbacks around the state had affected quality of care to the point of endangering patient safety. However, critics of the law charge that legislators passed the law without proof that the staffing levels stipulated in the law are safe. Therefore, in the critics' view, the law has more to do with the state nurses' fear for their jobs than with documented quality-of-care problems.
- Several health plans are competing to be among those offered to the employees of one of the area's newest and largest employers. One of the plans, HealthBest, claims that it provides a higher quality of care than its competitors do. Among the data HealthBest cites to back its claim are statistics showing that, compared to the other plans, HealthBest has 10 to 20 percent higher rates of mammogram screening for breast cancer among its female population ages 52 to 69. One of the other plans, PrimeHealth, disputes that particular inference, arguing that the percentage of women screened through mammography is not a good indicator of quality of care as compared to a plan's success in actually detecting breast cancer at an early stage. On that measure, PrimeHealth claims to do better than HealthBest and the other plans.

The following section introduces several concepts that can help make better sense of the above cases and of similar situations involving the measurement of quality of care.

Structure, Process, and Outcomes

As Donabedian first noted in 1966, all evaluations of quality of care can be classified in terms of one of three aspects of caregiving they measure: structure, process, or outcomes.

Structure

When quality is measured in terms of structure, the focus is on the relatively static characteristics of the individuals who provide care and of the settings where the care is delivered. These characteristics include the education, training, and certification of professionals who provide care and the adequacy of the facility's staffing, equipment, and overall organization.

Evaluations of quality that rely on such structural elements assume that well-qualified people working in well-appointed and well-organized settings will provide high-quality care. However, although good structure makes good quality more likely to ensue, it does not guarantee it (Donabedian 2003). Structure-focused assessments are therefore most revealing when deficiencies are found; good quality is unlikely, if not impossible, if the individuals who provide care are unqualified or if necessary equipment is missing or in disrepair. Licensing and accrediting bodies have relied heavily on structural measures of quality not only because the measures are relatively stable and thus easier to capture but also because they reliably identify providers who demonstrably lack the means to deliver high-quality care.

Process

Process, which refers to what takes place during the delivery of care, also can be the basis for evaluating quality of care. The quality of the process in turn can vary on two aspects: appropriateness, which refers to whether the right actions were taken, and skill, which refers to how well actions were carried out and how timely they were.

Ordering the correct diagnostic procedure for a patient is a measure of appropriateness. When evaluating the process of care, however, appropriateness is only half the story. The other half is in how well and how promptly (i.e., skillfully) the procedure was carried out. Similarly, successful completion of a surgical operation and a good recovery are not enough evidence to conclude that the process of care was high quality. They tell us only that the procedure was accomplished skillfully. For the entire process of care to be judged as high quality, we additionally must ascertain that the operation was indicated (i.e., appropriate) for that patient. Finally, as was the case for structural measures, use of process measures for assessing quality of care rests on a key assumption—in this case, that if the right things are done, and are done right, good results for the patient (i.e., good outcomes of care) are more likely to ensue.

Outcomes

Outcome measures, which capture whether healthcare goals were achieved, are another way of assessing quality of care. Because the goals of care can be defined broadly, outcome measures have come to include the costs of care as well as patients' satisfaction with care (Iezzoni 2003). In formulations that stress the technical aspects of care, however, outcomes typically refer to health status-related indicators such as whether the patient's pain subsided, the condition cleared up, or the patient regained full function (Donabedian 1980).

Clinicians tend to be leery of such outcome measures of quality. As mentioned earlier in relation to how different parties define quality, clinicians are aware that many factors that determine clinical outcomes—including genetic and environmental factors—are not under the clinician's control. Good process only increases the likelihood of good outcomes; it does not guarantee them. Some patients do not improve in spite of the best treatment that medicine can offer, whereas other patients regain full health even though they received inappropriate and potentially harmful care. However, the relation between process and outcomes is not completely random and unpredictable. We know, in particular, that the likelihood that a specific set of clinical activities—a given process—will result in desirable outcomes depends on how efficacious that process has been.

Efficacy

A clinical intervention is efficacious if it has been shown to produce a given outcome reliably when other, potentially confounding factors are held constant. Formal clinical trials or similarly systematic, controlled studies typically establish the efficacy of a clinical intervention. Knowledge about efficacy is crucial to making valid judgments about quality of care using either process or outcome measures. If we know that a given clinical intervention was undertaken in circumstances that match those under which the intervention has been shown to be efficacious, we can be confident that the care was appropriate and, to that extent, of good quality. Conversely, if we know that the outcome of a particular episode of care was poor, we can find out whether it resulted from an inappropriate clinical intervention by determining whether the interventions that took place conformed to what is known about those interventions' efficacy.

Which Is Best?

Of structure, process, and outcome, which is the best measure of quality of care? The answer—that none of them is inherently better and that all depend on the circumstances (Donabedian 1988a, 2003)—often does not satisfy those who are inclined to believe that outcome measures are the superior measure. After all, they reason, outcomes address the ultimate purpose, the bottom line, of all caregiving: Was the condition cured? Did the patient improve?

As previously mentioned, however, good outcomes can result even when the care (i.e., process) was clearly deficient. The reverse is also possible: Although the care was excellent, the outcome may not be good. In addition to the care provided, a number of other factors not within the control of clinicians—such as how frail a patient is—can affect outcomes and must be accounted for through risk-adjustment calculations that are seldom straightforward (Iezzoni 2003).

What a particular outcome ultimately tells us about quality of care depends crucially on whether the outcome can be attributed to the care provided. In other words, we have to examine the link between the outcome and the antecedent process and determine—on the basis of efficacy—whether the care was appropriate and was provided skillfully. Outcomes are therefore useful in identifying possible problems of quality (fingering the suspects) but not in ascertaining whether poor care was actually provided (determining guilt). The latter determination requires delving into the antecedent process of care to establish whether the care provided was the likely cause of the observed outcome.

Criteria and Standards

To assess quality using structure, process, or outcome measures, we need to know what constitutes good structure, good process, and good outcomes. In other words, we need criteria and standards we can apply to those measures of care.

Definitions

Criteria refer to specific attributes that are the basis for assessing quality. *Standards* express quantitatively what level the attributes must reach to satisfy preexisting expectations about quality. An example unrelated to healthcare may help clarify the difference between criteria and standards. Universities often evaluate applicants for admission on the basis of, among other things, the applicants' scores on standardized tests. The scores are thus one of the criteria by which programs judge the quality of their applicants. However, although two programs may use the same criterion—scores on a specific standardized examination—to evaluate applicants, the programs may differ markedly on standards: One program may consider applicants acceptable if they have scores above the 50th percentile, whereas scores above the 90th percentile may be the standard of acceptability for the other program. Table 2.2 provides illustrative healthcare examples of criteria and standards for structure, process, and outcome measures.

Sources

A shift in the way criteria and standards are derived has been occurring in the healthcare field. Before the 1970s, formally derived criteria and standards for quality-of-care evaluations relied on consensus opinions of groups

Type of Measure	Focus of Assessment	Criterion	Standard
Structure	Primary care group practice	Percentage of board-certified physicians in internal or family medicine	100% of physicians in the practice must be board certified in internal or family medicine
Process	Treatment of patients hospitalized for heart attack	Percentage of post-heart attack patients prescribed beta-blockers on discharge	At least 96% of heart attack patients receive a beta-blocker prescription on discharge
Outcome	Blood pressure of patients with diabetes	Percentage of patients with diabetes whose blood pressure is at or below 130/85	At least 50% of patients with diabetes have blood pressure at or below 130/85

TABLE 2.2
Illustrative Examples of Criteria and Standards

REPRINTED FROM: *Clinics in Family Practice*, Volume 5 (4), Wyszewianski, L. "Defining, Measuring, and Improving Quality of Care." 807–825, 2003. Used with permission from Elsevier.

of clinicians selected for their clinical knowledge and experience and the respect they commanded among their colleagues (Donabedian 1982). This approach to formulating criteria took for granted that in their deliberations, the experts would incorporate the latest scientific knowledge relevant to the topic under consideration, but formal requirements that they do so seldom existed.

Toward the mid-1970s, however, the importance of scientific literature in relation to criteria and standards gained considerable visibility, notably through the work of Cochrane (1973) and Williamson (1977). At about the same time, Brook and his colleagues at RAND began to use systematic reviews and evaluations of scientific literature as the starting point for the deliberations of panels charged with defining criteria and standards for studies of quality (Brook et al. 1977). The evidence-based medicine movement of the 1990s, which sought to put into practice what the best evidence showed to be efficacious under a given set of clinical circumstances (Evidence-Based Medicine Working Group 1992; Straus et al. 2005), reinforced this focus on the literature, especially the validity of the studies within that literature. As a result, criteria and standards have come to revolve increasingly around the strength and validity of scientific evidence and much less around the unaided consensus of experts (Eddy 1996, 2005).

Levels

When formulating standards, a critical decision that must be made is the level at which the standards should be set: minimal, optimal, achievable, or something in between (Muir Gray 2001). Minimal standards specify what level must be met for quality to be considered acceptable. The implication is that if care does not meet a minimal standard, remedial action is needed. Optimal standards denote the level of quality that can be reached under the best conditions, typically conditions similar to those under which efficacy is determined. Optimal standards are especially useful as a reference point for setting achievable standards, the level of performance that everyone being evaluated should set as a benchmark. One way to define achievable standards is in relation to the performance of the top quartile of providers of care. The reasoning is that if the top quartile can perform at that level, the other three quartiles should be able to reach it (Muir Gray 2001). Other approaches to setting standards have been proposed for evaluating, for example, access to care (Bower et al. 2003). Because there is no a priori level at which a particular standard should be set, a sensible and frequently adopted approach is to choose the level according to the goals of the underlying evaluation effort.

Utility of Measurement-Related Concepts

How does understanding structure, process, outcomes, efficacy, criteria, and standards give us insight into quality-of-care measurement issues? The two cases cited at the beginning of this section provide some illustrations.

The first case specifies minimum standards of quality in terms of nurse staffing levels, a structural measure of quality. The critics are not questioning the choice of that measure, nor should they; structural measures are well suited to detecting lack of capacity to deliver care of acceptable quality. In this case, hospitals that do not meet minimum staffing levels by definition cannot deliver care of acceptable quality (safe care). However, critics contend that the law's standards specifying minimum staffing levels are not evidence based but instead are set at levels intended to minimize job loss among members of the state nurses' association. An effective rebuttal of the critics' charge would require evidence supporting the law's staffing standards. The evidence would have to come from properly controlled studies showing that quality of care can no longer be considered safe when nurse staffing ratios fall below a specific level, holding all else constant. In other words, silencing the critics requires evidence from the kind of studies on which efficacy determinations are based.

In the second case, both measures under discussion are process measures. However, mammograms belong to a subset of process measures that represent a kind of resting point along the continuum of the activities that make up the process of care. These kinds of resting points share with most outcomes the characteristic of being discrete events that are relatively easily counted; hence, the label *procedural endpoints* has been applied to them (Donabedian 1980).

PrimeHealth's challenge stresses that mammograms are not an outcome (i.e., they are not an end in themselves but rather the means for the early detection of breast cancer). Because performing mammograms is certainly the right thing to do for the target population, appropriateness is not in question. However, PrimeHealth's challenge reminds us that the skill with which the mammograms are performed matters just as much as the number performed. If, because of deficiencies in skill, mammograms are performed incorrectly, resulting in incorrect interpretations, or if they are done correctly but read incorrectly, the mammograms may fail as a means for early detection of breast cancer. Early detection of breast cancer therefore can be claimed to be the better alternative measure of quality; it reflects not just whether mammograms were performed when indicated (appropriateness) but also how well they were performed and interpreted (skill).

Implications

The main insight that can be drawn from a deeper understanding of the concepts related to the measurement of healthcare quality is that the type of measure used—structure, process, or outcome—matters less than what we know about that measure's link to the others. Structural measures are only as good and useful as the strength of their relation to desired processes and outcomes. Accordingly, process and outcome measures also must relate to each other in measurable and reproducible ways—as demonstrated by efficacy studies—to be truly valid measures of quality.

To evaluate structure, process, and outcomes, criteria and standards are essential. Whereas the formulation of criteria is expected to be evidence driven—and thus based on considerations of efficacy—the setting of standards is not similarly tied to scientific literature. Instead, the decision to set standards at a minimal, ideal, or achievable level is most meaningful if driven by the goals behind the specific quality-of-care evaluation for which the standards are to be used.

Study Questions

1. An article in *Consumer Reports on Health* offered the following advice on how to find a new personal physician (Lipman 1997):

   There's no sure way to find a new personal physician who will meet all your needs. . . . Many people simply ask a satisfied friend or relative. A better approach . . . is to ask a healthcare professional—a physician, nurse, therapist, technician, or social worker—who has seen many doctors in action. Almost anyone who works in a hospital can tell you which doctors are regarded highly by their patients and colleagues.

In terms of the attributes of care that typically enter into the definition of quality, what does it mean that it would be preferable to rely on a healthcare professional's opinion—rather than that of a friend or relative who is not a healthcare professional—when choosing a personal physician?

2. Describe an instance in which outcomes would not be a good measure of healthcare quality. Explain why outcomes would not be a good indicator of quality in that instance.

3. The physicians at the Internal Medicine Group (IMG), a group practice, are thinking about how best to assess, for their own internal purposes, their collective and individual performance in preventing and treating osteoporosis. A senior IMG physician has recommended adopting an approach to evaluating osteoporosis care currently used by a large group in California. She points out that it would spare IMG physicians from having to come up with their own criteria and standards for evaluating osteoporosis care.

Almost everyone in the group supports the suggestion and likes the idea of not reinventing the wheel. However, several physicians in the group want to make sure that the California group's approach is actually sound and applicable to IMG physicians. What aspects of the "California approach" should these skeptical physicians examine most closely to achieve their objective? Why?

Note

1. Portions of this chapter include, in modified form, material reprinted from *Clinics in Family Practice* 5 (4), Wyszewianski, L: "Defining, Measuring and Improving Quality of Care," 807–12, 2003. Used with permission from Elsevier.

References

Blumenthal, D. 1996. "Quality of Care—What Is It?" *New England Journal of Medicine* 335 (12): 891–94.

Bower, P., M. Roland, J. Campbell, and N. Mead. 2003. "Setting Standards Based on Patients' Views on Access and Continuity." *British Medical Journal* 326: 258–62.

Brook, R. H., A. Davies-Avery, S. Greenfield, L. J. Harris, T. Lelah, N. E. Solomon, and J. E. Ware, Jr. 1977. "Assessing the Quality of Medical Care Using Outcome Measures: An Overview of the Method." *Medical Care* 15 (9, Suppl.): 1–165.

Campbell, S. M., M. O. Roland, and S. A. Buetow. 2000. "Defining Quality of Care." *Social Science and Medicine* 51: 1611–25.

Cassell, E. J. 1982. "The Nature of Suffering and the Goals of Medicine." *New England Journal of Medicine* 306 (11): 639–45.

Cleary, P. D., and B. J. McNeil. 1988. "Patient Satisfaction as an Indicator of Quality Care." *Inquiry* 25 (1): 25–36.

Cochrane, A. L. 1973. *Effectiveness and Efficiency: Random Reflections on Health Services.* London: Nuffield Provincial Hospitals Trust.

Donabedian, A. 1966. "Evaluating the Quality of Medical Care." *Milbank Quarterly* 44: 166–203.

———. 1980. *Explorations in Quality Assessment and Monitoring. Volume I: The Definition of Quality and Approaches to Its Assessment.* Chicago: Health Administration Press.

———. 1982. *Explorations in Quality Assessment and Monitoring. Volume II: The Criteria and Standards of Quality.* Chicago: Health Administration Press.

———. 1988a. "The Quality of Care: How Can It Be Assessed?" *Journal of the American Medical Association* 260 (12): 1743–48.

———. 1988b. "Quality and Cost: Choices and Responsibilities." *Inquiry* 25 (1): 90–99.

———. 2003. *An Introduction to Quality Assurance in Health Care.* New York: Oxford University Press.

Donabedian, A., J. R. C. Wheeler, and L. Wyszewianski. 1982. "Quality, Cost, and Health: An Integrative Model." *Medical Care* 20 (10): 975–92.

Eddy, D. M. 1996. *Clinical Decision Making: From Theory to Practice.* Sudbury, MA: Jones and Bartlett.

———. 2005. "Evidence-Based Medicine: A Unified Approach." *Health Affairs* 24 (1): 9–17.

Evidence-Based Medicine Working Group. 1992. "Evidence-Based Medicine. A New Approach to Teaching the Practice of Medicine." *Journal of the American Medical Association* 268: 2420–25.

Gold, M. R., J. E. Siegel, L. B. Russell, and M. C. Weinstein (eds.). 1996. *Cost-Effectiveness in Health and Medicine.* New York: Oxford University Press.

Harteloh, P. P. M. 2004. "Understanding the Quality Concept in Health Care." *Accreditation and Quality Assurance* 9: 92–95.

Iezzoni, L. I. (ed.). 2003. *Risk Adjustment for Measuring Healthcare Outcomes*, 3rd ed. Chicago: Health Administration Press.

Institute of Medicine (IOM). 1990. *Medicare: A Strategy for Quality Assurance*. Washington, DC: National Academies Press.

———. 1993. *Access to Health Care in America*. Washington, DC: National Academies Press.

———. 2001. *Crossing the Quality Chasm: A New Health System for the 21st Century*. Washington, DC: National Academies Press.

———. 2002. *Unequal Treatment: Confronting Racial and Ethnic Disparities in Healthcare*. Washington, DC: National Academies Press.

Lee, R. I., and L. W. Jones. 1933. "The Fundamentals of Good Medical Care." *Publications of the Committee on the Costs of Medical Care*, no. 22. Chicago: University of Chicago Press.

Lipman, M. M. 1997. "When to Fire Your Doctor—and How to Find Another." *Consumer Reports on Health* 9 (3): 35.

McLaughlin, C. G., and L. Wyszewianski. 2002. "Access to Care: Remembering Old Lessons." *Health Services Research* 37 (6): 1441–43.

Muir Gray, J. A. 2001. *Evidence-Based Healthcare*, 2nd ed. Edinburgh: Churchill Livingstone.

Penchansky, R., and J. W. Thomas. 1981. "The Concept of Access: Definition and Relationship to Consumer Satisfaction." *Medical Care* 19 (2): 127–40.

Sofaer, S., and K. Firminger. 2005. "Patient Perceptions of the Quality of Health Services." *Annual Review of Public Health* 26: 513–59.

Straus, S. E., W. S. Richardson, P. Glasziou, and R. B. Haynes. 2005. *Evidence-Based Medicine: How to Practice and Teach EBM*, 3rd ed. Edinburgh: Churchill Livingstone.

Williamson, J. W. 1977. *Improving Medical Practice and Health Care: A Bibliographic Guide to Information Management in Quality Assurance and Continuing Education*. Cambridge, MA: Ballinger.

Wyszewianski, L. 1988. "Quality of Care: Past Achievements and Future Challenges." *Inquiry* 25 (1): 13–22.

Wyszewianski, L., and A. Donabedian. 1981. "Equity in the Distribution of Quality of Care." *Medical Care* 19 (12, Suppl.): 28–56.

VARIATION IN MEDICAL PRACTICE AND IMPLICATIONS FOR QUALITY

David J. Ballard, Robert S. Hopkins III, and
David Nicewander

Despite the growing interest in and use of evidence-based medicine, the art of medical practice remains empirical and is subject to considerable differences in process and outcome, even among the finest medical centers (Reinertsen 2003). In examining the 50 best hospitals noted for their "compassionate geriatric and palliative care," the *Dartmouth Atlas of Health Care* project found that the percentage of patients admitted one or more times to an intensive care unit (ICU) during the last six months of life differed widely by region, from 23 percent to 45 percent (Wennberg and McAndrew Cooper 1999; Wennberg 2002) (see Figure 3.1).

To suggest that this variation is important and has profound consequences on quality of care is tempting. This suggestion, however, presumes that variation exists in the observed data and that variation is undesirable. More recent studies have demonstrated the fallacy of such assumptions through further examination of variation, outcomes, and associated measures. For example, Fisher and colleagues (2003a, 2003b) conducted a detailed investigation on the implications of regional variations in Medicare spending on the content, quality, and accessibility of care, and on health outcomes and patients' satisfaction with care. Medicare spending per capita was found to vary widely between regions in the United States. Residents of the highest-spending regions received approximately 60 percent more care than did residents of the lowest-spending regions (Fisher et al. 2003b), had more frequent tests and minor procedures done, and used specialists and hospitals more frequently (Fisher et al. 2003a).

One would expect greater healthcare spending and utilization to be associated with better quality of care and better outcomes. However, further investigation showed that after adjustment for baseline differences, for patients who were similarly ill across regions, there was no statistically significant difference in quality of care. These findings were based on measurements of the acute myocardial infarction (AMI) cohort by receipt of reperfusion within 12 hours, receipt of aspirin and beta-blockers (in the hospital and at discharge), and receipt of angiotensin converting enzyme inhibitors at discharge, as well as of the Medicare Current Beneficiary Survey (MCBS) cohort by receipt of appropriate preventive services (influenza

FIGURE 3.1

Percentage of Medicare Enrollees Admitted to Intensive Care During the Last Six Months of Life, by Hospital Referral Regions (1995–96)

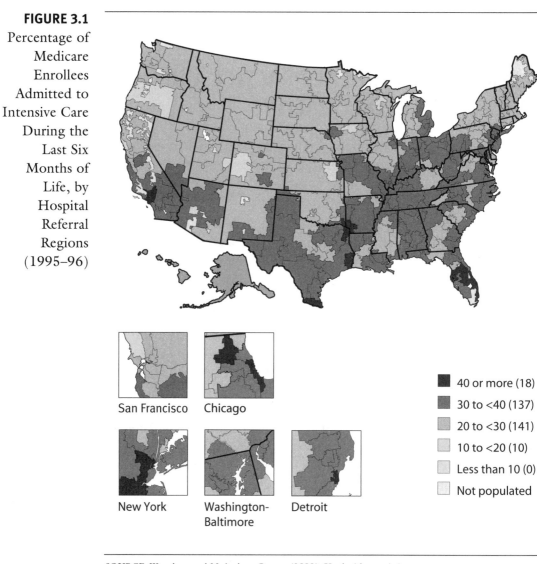

San Francisco   Chicago

New York   Washington-Baltimore   Detroit

■ 40 or more (18)
■ 30 to <40 (137)
▨ 20 to <30 (141)
□ 10 to <20 (10)
□ Less than 10 (0)
□ Not populated

SOURCE: Wennberg and McAndrew Cooper (1999). Used with permission.

vaccine, pneumonia vaccine, Papanicolaou smear, mammography). There also was no statistically significant difference in access to care (e.g., angiography, coronary bypass surgery, and physician office visits after discharge for the AMI cohort; usual source of care; emergency department/outpatient department/physician office visits; and wait times for the MCBS cohort) (Fisher et al. 2003a). Similarly, the examination of outcome measures revealed no significant differences (following adjustment for patient and hospital characteristics) in five-year mortality, functional status changes, or patient satisfaction with differing Medicare expenditure (Fisher et al. 2003b).

This chapter will discuss the application of several distinct types of variation to studies of medical processes and outcomes. Variation can be just as illuminating for what it offers in terms of innovation and improvement as it is instructive for what it can reveal in terms of irregularity and incompatibility (Wheeler 2000).

Background and Terminology

Statisticians, medical researchers and practitioners, and hospital administrators use and understand variation in ways that are sometimes compatible and sometimes mutually exclusive. Each definition is valuable in its particular application, so no one should be considered correct at the expense of another. For purposes of the present discussion, *variation* is the difference between an observed event and a standard or norm. Without this standard, or *best practice*, measurement of variation offers little beyond a description of the observations, with minimal, if any, analysis of what they mean (Gelbach 1993; Katz 2003; Wheeler 2000). Consequently, measurement of variation in healthcare and its application to quality improvement must begin with the identification and articulation of what is to be measured and the standard against which it is to be compared, a process based on extensive research, trial and error, and collaborative discussion.

Random Versus Assignable Variation

Variation can be either random or assignable (Wheeler 2000). *Random variation* is a physical attribute of the event or process, adheres to the laws of probability, and cannot be traced to a root cause. Traditionally, it is considered "background noise" or "expected variation," and it is usually not worth studying in detail. *Assignable variation* arises from a single or small set of causes that are not part of the event or process and therefore can be traced, identified, and implemented or eliminated. In general, researchers are interested in assignable variation because they can link—or assign—variation to a single specific cause and act accordingly. This type of variation is generally easy to measure given the widespread training of healthcare quality researchers in statistical methods, breadth of tests and criteria for determining whether variation is assignable or random, and increasing sensitivity and power of numerical analysis. Measurement of assignable variation, however, is subject to potential misunderstanding because of complexity of design and interpretation, particularly in understanding true variation versus artifact or statistical error (Powell, Davies, and Thomson 2003; Samsa et al. 2002).

Process Variation

Our discussion uses three different categories of variation of quality in medical practice. The first category is *process variation,* which is the difference in procedure throughout an organization (e.g., measurement of physicians' use of various screening methods for colorectal cancer). Some physicians may prefer fecal occult blood testing, others may elect to use sigmoidoscopy or colonoscopy, and another group may prescribe a combination of these tests. An understanding of the difference between process and technique is essential, however; *technique* is the multitude of ways in which a procedure can be performed within the realm of acceptable medical practice (Mottur-Pilson, Snow, and Bartlett 2001).

Outcome Variation

Another category is *outcome variation,* which is the difference in the results of a single process. Most healthcare quality researchers and medical practitioners focus on this measure—the process yielding optimal results (Samsa et al. 2002). When the results of a particular process can be observed in relatively short order or procedural changes can be undertaken in a timely fashion, this optimality is easily determined. Unfortunately, genuine outcome variation requires study over an extended period, often years or decades, and many studies labeled as *outcome research* are actually *process research.*

Performance Variation

The third category, and arguably the most important, is *performance variation,* which is the difference between any given result and the optimal or ideal result (Ballard 2003). This threshold, or best practice, is the standard against which all other measurements of variation are compared, although some key analytical tools, such as statistical process control, do not directly address performance relative to a standard. "From the perspective of the quality of care," argues one physician, "the variation that is the greatest cause for concern is that between actual practice and evidence-based 'best practice,'" which ultimately is what performance variation measures (Steinberg 2003). Assignable variation is merely descriptive and of little value if optimal practice is not defined. Without some concept of a best practice, process variation offers little beyond an enumeration of methods to fulfill some task. Without a threshold value, outcome variation reveals only what happened over time, not the desirability of a particular outcome. Performance variation tells us where we are and how far we are from where want to be, and suggests ways to achieve the desired goal.

Variation in Medical Practice

The language of quality improvement in medical practice suggests a subjective and occasionally pejorative view of variation. Standard procedures, operating protocols, flowcharts, prescriptive guidelines, handbooks, and checklists are all intended to reduce or eliminate variation and hence the potential for error or excessive costs (Mottur-Pilson, Snow, and Bartlett 2001). There is also a widespread tendency to assume that variation implies ranking—that "measures reflect quality and that variations in the measures reflect variations in quality" (Powell, Davies, and Thomson 2003). This interpretation results from causally linking the processes of care provided and the observed quality measures—high measured performance reflects good actual performance, and low measured performance reflects poor actual performance. In many cases, this link between variation and quality is valid, but often the link is tenuous, subjective, and not supportable by research focused on the relationship between processes and outcomes of care.

Variation can be desirable. A successful procedure that differs from other, less successful procedures is by definition a variation. The objective, then, for quality improvement researchers is not simply to identify variation but to determine its value. If variation reveals a suboptimal process, the task is to identify how the variation can be reduced or eliminated in ways that focus on the variation rather than on the people involved. If the variation is good or desirable, understanding how it can be applied across an organization to improve quality more broadly is essential. In other words, understanding the implications for quality of variation in medical practice is not simply learning how to eliminate variation but learning how to improve performance by identifying and accommodating good or suboptimal variation from a predefined best practice.

Scope and Use of Variation in Healthcare

The origins of quality assessment in healthcare in the United States can be traced to the pioneering work of Ernest A. Codman and the Mayo brothers during the early 20th century (Codman 1984, 1996; Mallon 2000). By 1990, the National Academy of Sciences' Institute of Medicine (IOM) (1990) defined quality of care as the "degree to which health services for individuals and populations increase the likelihood of desired health outcomes and are consistent with current professional knowledge." A decade later, IOM (2000, 2001a, 2001b) further articulated the healthcare quality improvement challenge for the United States in three seminal reports. Over the next ten years, The Joint Commission (2003), U.S. Preventive Services Task Force (2003), National Quality Forum (2002), and Centers for Medicare & Medicaid Services (CMS) (2003a) produced explicit indicators for quality measures.

Quality researchers use a variety of categories to measure improvements and detect variation in quality of care, including fiscal, service, and clinical indicators. Hospital-based clinical indicators, for example, are derived from the CMS "Seventh Scope of Work" measures and other advisory directives and include indicators pertaining to AMI, community-acquired pneumonia, and congestive heart failure (CMS 2003a). For each case, organizations may define a threshold that indicates satisfactory compliance with acceptable standards of care (Ballard 2003). One example of a process-of-care measure for AMI is the administration of beta-blockers within 24 hours of admission. The threshold is 90 percent. In other words, on the basis of the total number of AMI admissions at any one hospital or clinic or across any healthcare delivery system, at least 90 percent of admitted patients are afforded the preferred process of care.

Quality in healthcare is measured by its ability to satisfy qualitative standards as well as quantitative thresholds. IOM (2001a) has established six aims for healthcare improvement to ensure that medical care is safe, timely, effective, efficient, equitable, and patient centered (Ballard 2003). As such, clinical indicators that address timeliness of care, for example, from several clinical domains—AMI, surgical infection prevention, and community-acquired pneumonia—are aggregated to assess the appropriate level of time-dependent quality of care at a medical facility.

Variability plays an obvious role in identifying, measuring, and reporting these quality indicators and process-of-care improvements (Goldberg et al. 1994). For example, patient mix may make it difficult to compare process-of-care measures across multiple hospitals in the same system, creating the appearance of variation among facilities' services. Consequently, some healthcare services administrators are reluctant to use quality improvement measures and indicators because they perceive them as biased toward academic medical research centers or large healthcare organizations, which are seen as not subject to broad variation (Miller et al. 2001). This assumption is unfortunate and false because quality improvement efforts can be and have been successfully applied to small organizations and practices, including single-physician practices (Geyman 1998; Miller et al. 2001).

Clinical and Operational Issues

Implementing best practices, establishing clinical indicators, and measuring and interpreting variation involve considerable effort to create and sustain an environment conducive to sustaining them. An organization's size and complexity create functional, geographical, and other systemic constraints to success. The ability to collect appropriate and accurate data that can be rigorously analyzed requires diligent planning (Ballard 2003). Patient demographics and physician case mix affect the data to be studied and can arbitrarily skew the conclusions.

Organizational Size

The size of an organization also affects the ability to disseminate best practices. One group of physicians in a large healthcare delivery system may have developed an effective method to achieve high levels of colorectal cancer screening (Stroud, Felton, and Spreadbury 2003), but the opportunity to describe, champion, and implement such process redesign across dozens of other groups within the system is much more challenging and typically requires incremental resource commitment. Large organizations tend to have rigid frameworks or bureaucracies; change is slow and requires perseverance and the ability to make clear to skeptics and enthusiasts the value of the new procedure in their group and across the system. Small practices may be equally difficult to convert, especially if only one or two physicians or decision makers are involved and unwilling or uninterested in pursuing quality improvements. Irrespective of organizational size, there is often a complex matrix of demands for quality improvement and change agents, so simply changing one process in one location will not necessarily result in quality improvement, especially throughout an organization.

Large organizations also create the potential for multiple layers of quality assessment. The Baylor Health Care System (BHCS) is a not-for-profit healthcare system serving patients throughout North Texas and beyond. It is an integrated healthcare delivery system, including 15 hospitals; over 100 primary care, specialty care, and senior health centers; approximately 450 physicians employed by Health Texas Provider Network; and more than 3,000 affiliated physicians. Consequently, BHCS evaluates its quality improvement efforts at both the hospital and outpatient levels. Obviously, inpatient and outpatient processes of care differ; quality improvement efforts may be applicable to inpatient services at all hospitals, but such process redesign may not be applicable to the outpatient clinics and senior centers.

Organizational Commitment

An organization's commitment to paying for quality improvement studies and implementation is equally affected by its size and infrastructure. Value-based purchasing is increasing; consumers and insurers are using healthcare facilities that embrace quality improvement efforts and hence provide better processes of care and, arguably, outcomes. The Joint Commission, CMS, and Medicare have established minimum standard levels of quality and linked reimbursement schemes to achieving these goals. Although all healthcare organizations are obligated to meet these standards, a number of hospitals and delivery systems chose to use these standards before they were mandatory or have set higher threshold levels because of the compelling business case to do so. Increasing numbers of healthcare organizations fund these efforts internally, both for inpatients and outpatients, because it makes sense in terms of outcomes, patient satisfaction, and their long-term financial picture (happy patients return for additional care or recommend that friends and relatives use the same services) (Ballard 2003; Leatherman et al. 2003; Stroud, Felton, and Spreadbury 2003).

Planning the collection and analysis of suitable data for quality measures requires significant forethought, particularly when considering strategies to assess true variation and minimize false variation, and includes using appropriate measures, controlling case mix and other variables, minimizing chance variability, and using high-quality data (Powell, Davies, and Thomson 2003).

The initial results of a study that compared generalists' and endocrinologists' treatment of patients with diabetes showed what most people would expect—that specialists provided better care. Adjustment for patient case-mix bias and clustering (physician-level variation) substantially altered the results; there was no difference between generalists' and endocrinologists' treatment of diabetes patients. Studies must be designed with sufficient power and sophistication to account for a variety of confounding factors and require sufficient numbers of physicians and patients per physician to prevent the distortion of differences in quality of care between physician groups (Greenfield et al. 2002). Another study evaluated the relationship of complication rates of carotid endarterectomy to processes of care and reported findings similar to the original diabetes survey. Initial analysis showed that facilities with high complication rates likely had substandard processes of care. By repeating the study at the same location but at a different time, researchers found substantially different complication rates and concluded that the "inability, in practice, to estimate complication rates at a high degree of precision is a fundamental difficulty for clinical policy making" (Samsa et al. 2002).

Strength of Data

Moreover, the data must be a representative sample. Physicians and administrators alike may challenge results they do not like because they consider the data suspect for reasons of collection errors or other inaccuracies. For example, despite the impartiality of external record abstractors in gathering data from patient medical charts, critics may claim that these independent abstractors lack an insider's understanding or that they select data to fit an agenda, affecting the results unpredictably. Patient socioeconomic status, age, gender, and ethnicity also influence physician profiles in medical practice variation and analysis efforts (Franks and Fiscella 2002).

Keys to Successful Implementation and Lessons Learned from Failures

Despite the appeal of quality improvement projects, considerable limits and barriers to their successful implementation exist. These barriers are subject to or the result of variation in culture, infrastructure, and economic influences across an organization, and overcoming them requires a stable infrastructure, sustained funding, and the testing of sequential hypotheses on how to improve care.

Administrative and Physician Views

Quality improvement efforts must consider organizational mind-set, administrative and physician worldviews, and patient knowledge and expectations. Their pace is subject to considerable variability in relation to an organization's propensity to change. One example from a primary care setting demonstrated that screening for colorectal cancer improved steadily from 47 percent to 86 percent over a two-year period (Stroud, Felton, and Spreadbury 2003). This evolutionary change minimized the barriers of revolutionary change, especially physician and administrator resistance, as well as other personal issues that are difficult to identify and alter (Eisenberg 2002). Successful conversion of daily practice into an environment that embraces quality improvement requires patience and a long-term vision. Many decision makers expect immediate and significant results and are sensitive to short-term variation in results that suggest the improvements may be inappropriate or not cost-effective. A monthly drop in screening rates, for example, could be viewed as an indication that the screening protocol is not working and should be modified or abandoned altogether to conserve scarce resources. The observed decrease also could be random variation and no cause for alarm or change (Wheeler 2000). Cultural tolerance to variation and change is a critical issue in the successful implementation of quality improvement efforts and can be addressed by systemic adjustments and educational and motivational interventions (Donabedian and Bashur 2003; Palmer, Donabedian, and Povar 1991).

Physicians often think in terms of treating disease on an individual basis rather than in terms of population-based preventive care. As such, physician buy-in is critical to reducing undesired variation or creating new and successful preventive systems of clinical care (Stroud, Felton, and Spreadbury 2003). The process includes training physician champions and inciting them to serve as models, mentors, and motivators, and it reduces the risk of alienating the key participants in quality improvement efforts. Physicians' failure—or refusal—to follow best practices is often inextricably linked to the presence—or absence—of adequate physician champions who have both the subject matter expertise and professional respect of their peers (Mottur-Pilson, Snow, and Bartlett 2001).

Patient Knowledge

Patient education in quality of care is equally subject to variation. Increasingly, patients are aware of the status of their healthcare providers in terms of national rankings, public news of quality successes (and failures), and participation in reimbursement schemes (e.g., insurance, Medicare) favoring healthcare delivery systems that embrace quality improvement efforts. Participation in public awareness efforts such as the CMS Public Domain program, which makes variation and process-of-care measures available to the public (both consumers and researchers), is another opportunity to educate patients about a healthcare organization and its commitment to quality (CMS 2003b; Hibbard, Stockard, and Tisler 2003; Lamb et al. 2003; Shaller et al. 2003).

Organizational Mind-Set

Organizational infrastructure is an essential component in minimizing variation, disseminating best practices, and supporting a research agenda associated with quality improvements. Electronic medical records (EMRs), computerized physician order entry systems, and clinical decision support tools may reduce errors, allow sharing of specific best practices across large organizations, and enable the widespread automated collection of data to support quality improvement research (Bates and Gawande 2003; Bero et al. 1998; Casalino et al. 2003; Hunt et al. 1998). Healthcare organizations therefore are addressing the challenge to articulate and implement a long-term strategy to employ EMR resources. Unfortunately, the economic implications of both short- and long-term infrastructure investments undermine these efforts. Working in an environment that embraces short-term financial gain (in the form of either the quarterly report to stockholders or the report to the chairman of the board), physicians and hospital administrators "often face an outright disincentive to invest in an infrastructure that will improve compliance with best practices" (Leatherman et al. 2003).

Those same economic incentives may be effective in addressing variation in healthcare by awarding financial bonuses to physicians and administrators who meet quality targets or withholding bonuses from those who do not. This economic incentive communicates that future success within an organization is dependent on participating in quality improvement efforts, reducing undesirable variation in processes of care, and encouraging an environment conducive to quality research and improvement. The goals of such incentives are to help people understand that their organization is serious about implementing quality changes and minimizing unwanted variation to ensure alignment with national standards and directions in quality of care, and to encourage them to use an organization's resources to achieve this alignment (Casalino et al. 2003).

Case Study

American College of Cardiology and American Heart Association guidelines recommend prompt percutaneous coronary artery intervention (PCI) for patients with ST-segment elevation myocardial infarction (STEMI) because it significantly reduces mortality and morbidity. Specifically, the guidelines state that no more than 90 minutes should elapse from patient arrival at the hospital to first coronary balloon inflation. From April 2004 to March 2005, the median monthly average door-to-balloon time at Baylor Regional Medical Center at Grapevine, Texas, was 108.75 minutes.

With the launch of the Institute for Healthcare Improvement's 100,000 Lives Campaign in January 2005, AMI care became an area of increased focus for quality improvement within BHCS. Grapevine sought to reduce morbidity and mortality for AMI patients through the development of a STEMI team (incorporating members from the cath lab, radiology, laboratory, and pharmacy; a nursing supervisor; and an ICU charge nurse) and the collective effort of Emergency Medical Services (EMS), the emergency department, and the cath lab staff to initiate a rapid STEMI team call at the first indication of AMI. Since Grapevine implemented the STEMI team in March 2005, average door-to-balloon times have been below the recommended 90 minutes and frequently approach the 60-minute "stretch goal."

In addition to developing the STEMI team, Grapevine encouraged emergency department physicians to accept 12-lead electrocardiograms faxed from the field by emergency medical technicians (EMTs) (allowing notification of an interventional cardiologist and the STEMI team before patient arrival) and visited area EMS/fire stations to emphasize their critical role in caring for STEMI patients. Grapevine also added a tour of the cath lab to orientation for new EMTs and firefighters to provide them with an overall picture of the pathway of care for STEMI patients.

To avoid certain distributional assumptions related to parametric control charts and to address the problem of small subgroup sizes, Grapevine used an individual measure chart based on average moving range to display average monthly door-to-balloon times for April 2004 through March 2007 (see Figure 3.2). Data points are missing for months in which no patients received PCI. From the chart, there is clear evidence of a shift in the process mean; nine or more consecutive points fall below the center line (Western Electric, Test 2) immediately following STEMI team implementation.

An individual measure phase chart was used to compare the process before and after STEMI team implementation (see Figure 3.3). Here, decreased variability and a change in the mean further confirm change in

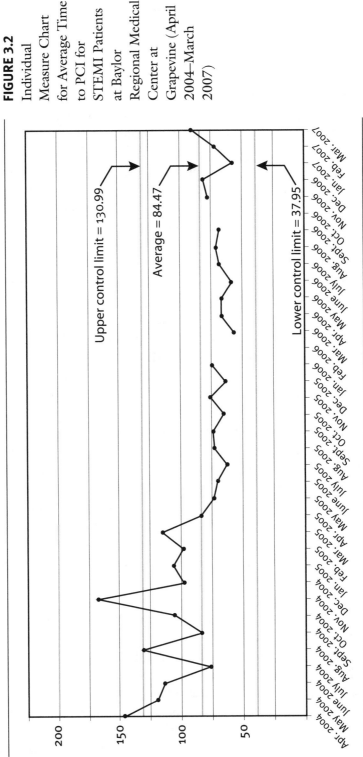

FIGURE 3.2
Individual Measure Chart for Average Time to PCI for STEMI Patients at Baylor Regional Medical Center at Grapevine (April 2004–March 2007)

SOURCE: Baylor Health Care System, Dallas, TX. Used with permission.

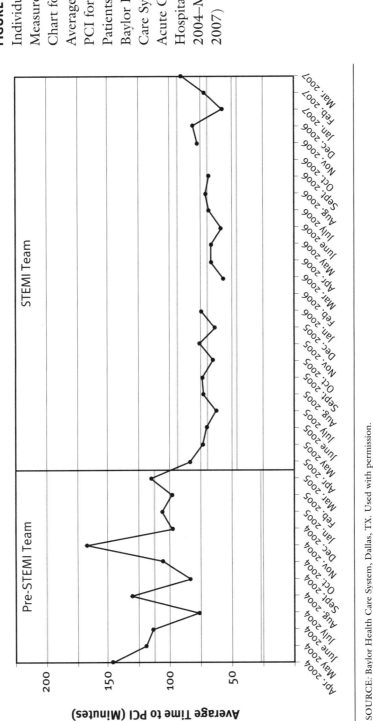

FIGURE 3.3

Individual Measure Phase Chart for Average Time to PCI for STEMI Patients at Five Baylor Health Care System Acute Care Hospitals (April 2004–March 2007)

SOURCE: Baylor Health Care System, Dallas, TX. Used with permission.

the time to PCI process. The lack of evidence for special cause variation during the post-intervention phase indicates that the process change caused by the STEMI team implementation has been sustained.

A similar approach was taken to monitor the time to PCI process with respect to clinical guidelines. Figures 3.4 and 3.5 show the p-chart and phase p-chart, respectively, for the proportion of PCI patients who received treatment within 90 minutes. As with the control charts for the monthly average times, a shift in the process mean at the time of STEMI team implementation is evident from the p-chart and phase p-chart associated with receiving timely reperfusion. Because a p-chart may not be reliable with small subgroup sizes, an individual measure and individual measure phase chart also were produced for the monthly proportion of patients receiving PCI within 90 minutes. The conclusions from these charts are identical to those from the p-charts. The p-charts are displayed here because the control limits more accurately reflect what is possible with this measure (i.e., the proportion of patients receiving PCI within 90 minutes can fall only between 0 and 1).

Conclusion

Contemporary industrial and commercial methods to improve quality, such as Six Sigma and ISO 9000, emphasize the need to minimize variation, if not eliminate it altogether. Although appropriate in a setting that requires the repetitive manufacturing of mass quantities of identical products, these tools may unnecessarily mask variation in the healthcare environment and consequently obscure opportunities to change or improve essential processes of care. The keys to successful management—rather than elimination—of variation in pursuit of quality healthcare are to be able to identify variation; distinguish between random and assignable variation; determine the meaning, importance, or value of the observed variation relative to some standard; and implement methods that will take advantage of or rectify what the variation reveals. Ultimately, variation tells us what is working and what is not, and how far from optimal our healthcare processes are. Rather than avoiding variation in pursuit of quality healthcare, we are better off embracing it as an essential measure of our progress toward success.

Study Questions

1. While exploring opportunities to improve processes of care for a group practice, you find no variability across physicians over time for colorectal cancer screening based on the recommendation of the U.S. Preventive Services Task Force. Is this absence of variation optimal? Why or why not?

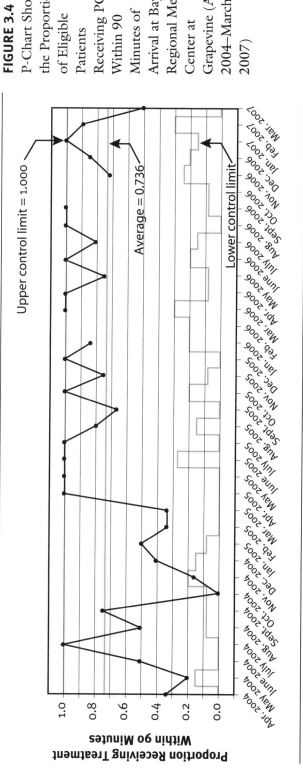

FIGURE 3.4
P-Chart Showing the Proportion of Eligible Patients Receiving PCI Within 90 Minutes of Arrival at Baylor Regional Medical Center at Grapevine (April 2004–March 2007)

SOURCE: Baylor Health Care System, Dallas, TX. Used with permission.

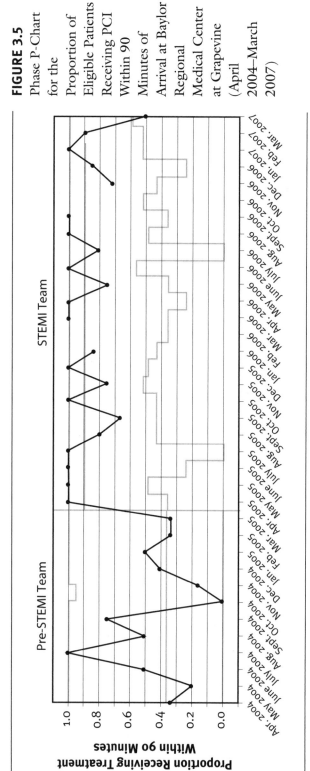

FIGURE 3.5
Phase P-Chart for the Proportion of Eligible Patients Receiving PCI Within 90 Minutes of Arrival at Baylor Regional Medical Center at Grapevine (April 2004–March 2007)

SOURCE: Baylor Health Care System, Dallas, TX. Used with permission.

2. Discuss the role of financial compensation strategies as part of the process to reduce variation in medical practice. How effective are these financial incentives, especially in terms of timing or use with other strategies?
3. Identify ways to distinguish between random and assignable variation. Be sure to assess the strengths and weaknesses of each method.
4. In many cases, improvements in healthcare quality are incremental (evolutionary) changes and not necessarily breakthrough (revolutionary) changes. Discuss the value of multiple small variations in effecting long-term, sustained improvement.

References

Ballard, D. J. 2003. "Indicators to Improve Clinical Quality Across an Integrated Health Care System." *International Journal of Quality in Health Care* 15 (6, Suppl.): 1–11.

Bates, D. W., and A. A. Gawande. 2003. "Improving Safety with Information Technology." *New England Journal of Medicine* 348: 2526–34.

Bero, L. A., R. Grilli, J. M. Grimshaw, E. Harvey, A. D. Oxman, and M. A. Thomson. 1998. "Closing the Gap Between Research and Practice: An Overview of Systematic Reviews of Interventions to Promote the Implementation of Research Findings." *British Medical Journal* 317: 465–68.

Casalino, L., R. R. Gillies, S. M. Shortell, J. A. Schmittdiel, T. Bodenheimer, J. C. Robinson, T. Rundall, N. Oswald, H. Schauffler, and M. C. Wang. 2003. "External Incentives, Information Technology, and Organized Processes to Improve Health Care Quality for Patients with Chronic Diseases." *Journal of the American Medical Association* 289 (4): 434–41.

Centers for Medicare & Medicaid Services (CMS). 2003a. "Quality Improvement Organizations (QIOs) Statement of Work." [Online information; retrieved 9/22/03.] http://cms.hhs.gov/qio/2.asp.

———. 2003b. "Overview of Hospital CAHPS." [Online information; retrieved 9/22/03.] www.cms.hhs.gov/quality/hospital/HCAHPSqanda3.pdf.

Codman, E. A. 1934, reprinted 1984. *The Shoulder: Rupture of the Supraspinatus Tendon and Other Lesions in or About the Subacromial Bursa.* Malabar, FL: Krieger Publishing.

———. 1917, reprinted 1996. *A Study in Hospital Efficiency as Demonstrated by the Case Report of the First Five Years of a Private Hospital.* Oakbrook Terrace, IL: The Joint Commission.

Donabedian, A., and R. Bashur (eds.). 2003. *An Introduction to Quality Assurance in Health Care.* New York: Oxford University Press.

Eisenberg, J. M. 2002. "Measuring Quality: Are We Ready to Compare the Quality of Care Among Physician Groups?" *Annals of Internal Medicine* 136: 153–54.

Fisher, E. S., D. E. Wennberg, T. A. Stukel, D. J. Gottlieb, F. L. Lucas, and E. L. Pinder. 2003a. "The Implications of Regional Variations in Medicare Spending. Part 1: The Content, Quality, and Accessibility of Care." *Annals of Internal Medicine* 138 (4): 273–87.

Fisher, E. S., D. E. Wennberg, T. A. Stukel, D. J. Gottlieb, F. L. Lucas, and E. L. Pinder. 2003b. "The Implications of Regional Variations in Medicare Spending. Part 2: Health Outcomes and Satisfaction with Care." *Annals of Internal Medicine* 138 (4): 288–98.

Franks, P., and K. Fiscella. 2002. "Effect of Patient Socioeconomic Status on Physician Profiles for Prevention, Disease Management, and Diagnostic Testing Costs." *Medical Care* 40 (8): 717–24.

Gelbach, S. H. 1993. "Study Design: The Experimental Approach." In *Interpreting the Medical Literature,* 3rd ed., 78–108. New York: McGraw-Hill.

Geyman, J. P. 1998. "Evidence-Based Medicine in Primary Care: An Overview." *Journal of the American Board of Family Practice* 11 (1): 46–56.

Goldberg, H. I., M. A. Cummings, E. P. Steinberg, E. M. Ricci, T. Shannon, S. B. Soumerai, B. S. Mittman, J. Eisenberg, D. A. Heck, S. Kaplan, J. E. Kenzora, A. M. Vargus, A. G. Mulley, Jr., and B. K. Rimer. 1994. "Deliberations on the Dissemination of PORT Products: Translating Research Findings Into Improved Patient Outcomes." *Medical Care* 32 (7, Suppl.): JS90–110.

Greenfield, S., S. H. Kaplan, R. Kahn, J. Ninomiya, and J. L. Griffith. 2002. "Profiling Care Provided by Different Groups of Physicians: Effects of Patient Case-Mix (Bias) and Physician-Level Clustering on Quality Assessment Results." *Annals of Internal Medicine* 136: 111–21.

Hibbard, J. H., J. Stockard, and M. Tisler. 2003. "Does Publicizing Hospital Performance Stimulate Quality Improvement Efforts?" *Health Affairs* 22 (2): 84–94.

Hunt, D. L., R. B. Haynes, S. E. Hanna, and K. Smith. 1998. "Effects of Computer-Based Clinical Decision Support Systems on Physician Performance and Patient Outcomes: A Systematic Review." *Journal of the American Medical Association* 280: 1339–46.

Institute of Medicine (IOM). 1990. *Medicare: A Strategy for Quality Assurance.* Vol. 1, p. 4. Washington, DC: National Academies Press.

———. 2000. *To Err Is Human: Building a Safer Health System.* Washington, DC: National Academies Press.

———. 2001a. *Crossing the Quality Chasm: A New Health System for the 21st Century.* Washington, DC: National Academies Press.

———. 2001b. *Envisioning the National Health Care Quality Report.* Washington, DC: National Academies Press.

The Joint Commission. 2003. "A Comprehensive Review of Development and Testing for National Implementation of Hospital Core Measures." [Online information; retrieved 9/10/03.] www.jcaho.org/pms/core+measures/cr_hos_cm.htm.

Katz, M. H. 2003. "Multivariable Analysis: A Primer for Readers of Medical Research." *Annals of Internal Medicine* 138: 644–50.

Lamb, R. M., D. M. Studdert, R. M. J. Bohmer, D. M. Berwick, and T. A. Brennan. 2003. "Hospital Disclosure Practices: Results of a National Survey." *Health Affairs* 22 (2): 73–83.

Leatherman, S., D. Berwick, D. Iles, L. S. Lewin, F. Davidoff, T. Nolan, and M. Bisognano. 2003. "The Business Case for Quality: Case Studies and an Analysis." *Health Affairs (Millwood)* 22 (2): 17–30.

Mallon, W. J. 2000. *Ernest Amory Codman: The End Result of a Life in Medicine.* Philadelphia: W. B. Saunders.

Miller, W. L., R. R. McDaniel, B. F. Crabtree, and K. C. Stange. 2001. "Practice Jazz: Understanding Variation in Family Practices Using Complexity Science." *Journal of Family Practice* 50 (10): 872–78.

Mottur-Pilson, C., V. Snow, and K. Bartlett. 2001. "Physician Explanations for Failing to Comply with 'Best Practices'." *Effective Clinical Practice* 4: 207–13.

National Quality Forum. 2002. "National Consensus Standards Endorsed for Monitoring the Quality of Care for Diabetes." [Online press release; retrieved 9/22/03.] www.qualityforum.org/prdiabetes10-01-02FINAL.pdf.

Palmer, R. H., A. Donabedian, and G. J. Povar. 1991. *Striving for Quality in Health Care: An Inquiry into Practice and Policy.* Chicago: Health Administration Press.

Powell, A. E., H. T. O. Davies, and R. G. Thomson. 2003. "Using Routine Comparative Data to Assess the Quality of Health Care: Understanding and Avoiding Common Pitfalls." *Quality and Safety in Health Care* 12: 122–28.

Reinertsen, J. L. 2003. "Zen and the Art of Physician Autonomy Maintenance." *Annals of Internal Medicine* 138: 992–95.

Samsa, G., E. Z. Oddone, R. Horner, J. Daley, W. Henderson, and D. B. Matchar. 2002. "To What Extent Should Quality of Care Decisions Be Based on Health Outcomes? Application to Carotid Endarterectomy." *Stroke* 33: 2944–49.

Shaller, D., S. Sofaer, S. D. Findlay, J. H. Hibbard, D. Lansky, and S. Delbanco. 2003. "Consumers and Quality-Driven Health Care: A Call to Action." *Health Affairs* 22 (2): 95–101.

Steinberg, E. P. 2003. "Improving the Quality of Care—Can We Practice What We Preach?" *New England Journal of Medicine* 348: 2681–83.

Stroud, J., C. Felton, and B. Spreadbury. 2003. "Collaborative Colorectal Cancer Screening: A Successful Quality Improvement Initiative." *BUMC Proceedings* 16: 341–44.

U.S. Preventive Services Task Force. 2003. "Guide to Clinical Preventive Services, 3rd ed., 2000–2002." [Online information; retrieved 9/22/03.] www.ahrq.gov/clinic/cps3dix.htm.

Wennberg, J. E. 2002. "Unwarranted Variations in Healthcare Delivery: Implications for Academic Medical Centres." *British Medical Journal* 325 (26 Oct.): 961–64.

Wennberg, J. E., and M. McAndrew Cooper. 1999. *The Dartmouth Atlas of Health Care.* Chicago: American Hospital Association.

Wheeler, D. J. 2000. *Understanding Variation: The Key to Managing Chaos,* 2nd ed. Knoxville, TN: SPC Press.

4

QUALITY IMPROVEMENT: THE FOUNDATION, PROCESSES, TOOLS, AND KNOWLEDGE TRANSFER TECHNIQUES

Kevin Warren[1]

This chapter describes some of the tools and methods that can be used to improve the quality of healthcare and provides case study examples of some knowledge transfer concepts that promote adoption and sustainability. Included are a number of different approaches to quality improvement. Although they may have different names and categories, you will recognize core commonalities in methods across these approaches.

The Quality Foundation

The strength and principles of the foundation of a product, belief, or concept can define the sustainability of that product, belief, or concept. To better understand and appreciate quality improvement systems and theories used today, you should be familiar with the origin of these principles and the foundation that has shaped their current existence. This chapter discusses some of those influential contributors and thought leaders of quality improvement systems and theories intent on improving process and producing sustainable quality results at highly productive levels. These leaders include:

- Walter Shewhart;
- W. Edwards Deming;
- Joseph M. Juran;
- Taiichi Ohno;
- Kaoru Ishikawa;
- Armand V. Feigenbaum; and
- Philip B. Crosby.

Walter Shewhart (1891–1967)

Dr. Walter A. Shewhart earned his doctorate in physics from the universities of Illinois and California. Shewhart used his understanding of statistics to design tools to respond to variation. Following his arrival at Western

Electric Co. in 1924, Shewhart introduced the concepts of common cause, special cause variation, and statistical control. He designed these concepts to assist Bell Telephone in its efforts to improve reliability and reduce the frequency of repairs within its transmission systems (Cutler 2001). Before Shewhart introduced these concepts, workers reacted to each new data point to improve future output. This tampering actually made matters worse.

Shewhart felt that his most important contribution was not the control chart but rather his work on operational definitions, which ensured that people used common language to define what they measured (Kilian 1988). In his book *Economic Control of Quality of Manufactured Product*, Shewhart introduced the concept of statistical process control (SPC), which has since become the cornerstone for process control in industry (Cutler 2001). These efforts and Shewhart's emphasis on the importance of precise measurement were part of the founding principles that ultimately led to Motorola's development of the Six Sigma approach in the mid-1980s.

W. Edwards Deming (1900–1993)

Many consider Dr. Deming to be the father of quality. A statistics professor and physicist by trade, Deming combined what he learned from Walter Shewhart and taught that by adopting appropriate principles of data-based management, organizations can increase quality and customer loyalty and simultaneously decrease costs by reducing waste, rework, and staff attrition. One of several statisticians and advisers who provided guidance at the request of Japanese industry leaders in the 1950s, he taught top management how to improve design (and thus service), product quality, testing, and sales (the latter through global markets). Deming stressed the importance of practicing continual improvement and thinking of manufacturing as a system (Deming 1986). In the 1970s, Deming developed his *14 Points for Western Management* in response to requests from U.S. managers for the secret to the radical improvement that Japanese companies were achieving in a number of industries. Deming's 14 points represented a unified body of knowledge that ran counter to the conventional wisdom of most U.S. managers (Neave 1990).

As part of his "system of profound knowledge," Deming (2000) promoted that "around 15% of poor quality was because of workers, and the rest of 85% was due to bad management, improper systems and processes." The "system" is based on four parts:

1. Appreciation for a system
2. Knowledge about variation
3. Theory of knowledge
4. Psychology

Deming described the Plan-Do-Study-Act (PDSA) cycle, which can be traced to Shewhart. Deming referred to PDSA as a cycle for learning and improvement. Some have changed the "S" to "C" (Plan-Do-Check-Act [PDCA] cycle), but Deming preferred to use *study* instead of *check* (Neave 1990).

Joseph M. Juran (1904–2008)

After receiving a BS in electrical engineering from the University of Minnesota, Joseph Juran joined Western Electric's inspection department and ultimately became the head of the industrial engineering department. As an internal consultant to Deming on ideas of industrial engineering, Juran began to formulate ideas that resulted in the creation of the concept now known as the Pareto principle (80/20 rule).

Juran, specializing in quality management, is the coauthor of *Juran's Quality Control Handbook* (Juran and Gryna 1951) and also consulted with Japanese companies in the 1950s. Juran defined quality as consisting of two different but related concepts. The first form of quality is income oriented and includes features of the product that meet customer needs and thereby produce income (i.e., higher quality costs more). The second form of quality is cost oriented and emphasizes freedom from failures and deficiencies (i.e., higher quality usually costs less) (American Society for Quality 2007).

Another of Juran's (1989) more notable contributions to the quality movement is known as the "Juran Trilogy." The trilogy describes three interrelated processes: quality planning, quality control, and quality improvement. See Figure 4.1.

FIGURE 4.1
Juran's Quality Trilogy

Quality Planning	• Identify who the customers are. • Determine the needs of those customers. • Translate those needs into our language. • Develop a product that can respond to those needs. • Optimize the product features to meet our needs and customer needs.
Quality Improvement	• Develop a process that is able to produce the product. • Optimize the process.
Quality Control	• Prove that the process can produce the product under operating conditions with minimal inspection. • Transfer the process to operations.

SOURCE: Brown (2003). Used with permission.

Taiichi Ohno (1912–1990)

Taiichi Ohno is generally credited with developing the Toyota Production System (TPS). Ohno's development of TPS and the concept of continuous (one-piece) flow began in 1948, after he was promoted to manage Toyota's Engine Manufacturing Department. Known for saying, "Common sense is always wrong," Ohno began to express concern about poor productivity and perceived waste in operations' "batch and queue" (grouping of individual component development) process. He identified this waste (*muda* in Japanese) within the system and categorized the types of waste (activities that do not add value to the process) (Womack and Jones 2003):

- Overproduction
- Inventory
- Repairs/rejects
- Motion
- Processing
- Waiting
- Transport

In contrast to the batch and queue process, Ohno created a standardized process in which products are produced through one continuous system that completes one product at a time, ultimately producing less waste, greater efficiency, and higher output.

Kaoru Ishikawa (1915–1989)

Kaoru Ishikawa was a student of Deming and a member of the Union of Japanese Scientists and Engineers. Known for study of scientific analysis of causes of industrial process problems, one of his most noted contributions to the quality movement was the creation of the Ishikawa diagram (fishbone diagram) (Hungarian Public Employment Service 2006). Ishikawa's discussions of total quality control (TQC) focused on the importance of participation of all levels of an organization in quality improvement initiatives and use of statistical and precise measurement in the decision-making process.

Professor Ishikawa obtained his doctorate in engineering from Tokyo University. In 1968, building on a series of articles discussing quality control, he authored a textbook that became the *Guide to Quality Control*. Although the concept of quality circles can be traced to the United States, Professor Ishikawa is noted for introducing the concept to Japan as part of his TQC efforts to ensure participation and understanding of quality control at all levels of an organization.

Armand V. Feigenbaum (1922–)

The concept of TQC originated in a 1951 book by Armand V. Feigenbaum. He approached quality as a strategic business tool that requires awareness by everyone in the company, in the same manner that most companies view cost and revenue. He felt that quality reaches beyond managing defects in production and should be a philosophy and a commitment to excellence. Feigenbaum defined TQC as excellence driven rather than defect driven—a system that integrates quality development, quality improvement, and quality maintenance (American Society for Quality, Quality Management Division 1999). The book *Total Quality Control* (1951), originally published as *Quality Control: Principles, Practice, and Administration*, outlines his approach to quality (American Society for Quality 2007). Feigenbaum is known as a leader in quality cost management and for defining quality costs as the costs of prevention, appraisal, and internal and external failure (American Society for Quality 2007).

Philip B. Crosby (1926–2001)

Philip B. Crosby introduced the idea of zero defects in 1961. He defined quality as "conformance to requirements" and measured quality as the "price of nonconformance" (Crosby 1996). Crosby equated quality management with prevention, believing that inspecting, checking, and other nonpreventive techniques have no place in quality management. Crosby taught that quality improvement is a process and not a temporary program or project. Crosby's quality improvement process is based on the Four Absolutes of Quality Management (Crosby 1996).

- Quality is defined as conformance to requirements, not as goodness or elegance.
- The system for causing quality is prevention, not appraisal.
- The performance standard must be zero defects, not "that's close enough."
- The measurement of quality is the price of nonconformance, not indices.

Crosby also felt that statistical levels of compliance tend to program people for failure and that there is absolutely no reason for having errors or defects in a product or service. He felt that companies should adopt a quality "vaccine" to prevent nonconformance, with three ingredients: determination, education, and implementation (American Society for Quality 2007).

Quality Improvement Processes and Approaches

"Form follows function," a concept founded in the field of architecture, describes the importance of understanding what you want to do before you determine how you are going to do it. The premise behind the principle also applies when an organization is deciding what quality improvement process or approach to adopt. This section describes some of the many systems and processes that guide quality improvement efforts today. These quality improvement approaches are derivatives and models of the ideas and theories developed by thought leaders and include:

- PDCA/PDSA;
- Associates for Process Improvement's (API) Model for Improvement;
- FOCUS PDCA;
- Baldrige Criteria;
- ISO 9000;
- Lean; and
- Six Sigma.

Shewhart Cycle/PDCA or PDSA Cycle

As discussed earlier, in the 1920s, Walter Shewhart developed the PDCA cycle used as the basis for planning and directing performance improvement efforts. Since the creation of the PDCA/PDSA cycle, most of the formally recognized performance improvement models have some basis or relation to this original quality improvement model.

Plan:

- Objective: What are you trying to accomplish? What is the goal?
- Questions and predictions: What do you think will happen?
- Plan to carry out the cycle: Who? What? When? Where?

Do:

- Educate and train staff.
- Carry out the plan (e.g., try out the change on a small scale).
- Document the problems and unexpected observations.
- Begin analysis of the data.

Study/Check:

- Assess the effect of the change and determine the level of success as compared to the goal/objective.
- Compare results to predictions.
- Summarize the lessons learned.
- Determine what changes need to be made and what actions will be taken next.

Act:

- Act on what you have learned.
- Determine whether the plan should be repeated with modification or a new plan should be created.
- Perform necessary changes.
- Identify remaining gaps in process or performance.
- Carry out additional PDCA/PDSA cycles until the agreed-upon goal/objective is met.

FIGURE 4.2
API Model for
Improvement

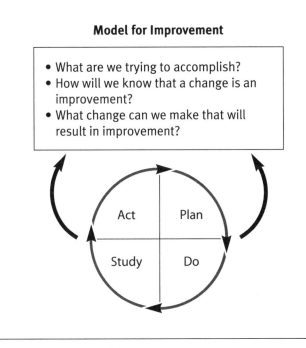

Model for Improvement

- What are we trying to accomplish?
- How will we know that a change is an improvement?
- What change can we make that will result in improvement?

Act | Plan
Study | Do

SOURCE: Langley et al. (1996). Used with permission.

API Improvement Model

Tom Nolan and Lloyd Provost, cofounders of API, developed a simple model for improvement based on Deming's PDSA cycle. The model (see Figure 4.2) contains three fundamental questions that form the basis of improvement: What are we trying to accomplish? How will we know that a change is an improvement? What change can we make that will result in improvement? Focus on the three questions and the PDSA cycle allows the model's application to be as simple or sophisticated as necessary (Langley et al. 1996). The effort required to bring about improvement may vary on the basis of the problem's complexity, whether the focus is on a new or an old design, or the number of people involved in the process (Langley et al. 1996).

FOCUS PDCA Model

Building on the PDSA cycle, the Hospital Corporation of America designed the FOCUS PDCA model to create a more specific and defined approach to process improvement. The key feature of FOCUS PDCA is the preexistence of a process that needs improvement. The intent of this model is to maximize the performance of a preexisting process, although the inclusion of PDCA provides the option of using this model for new or redesign projects (Brown 2003). The acronym FOCUS is broken down as follows:

F = FIND a process to improve.
O = ORGANIZE a team that knows the process.
C = CLARIFY current knowledge of the existing or redesigned process.
U = UNDERSTAND the variables and causes of process variation within the chosen process.
S = SELECT the process improvement and identify the potential action for improvement.

Baldrige Criteria and Related Systems

The Malcolm Baldrige National Quality Award (www.quality.nist.gov)— named for Malcolm Baldrige, who served as secretary of commerce from 1981 until his death in 1987—was created by Public Law 100-107, signed in 1987 (National Institute of Standards and Technology 2003). This law led to the creation of a new public-private partnership to improve the United States' competitiveness.

The Baldrige criteria were originally developed and applied to businesses; however, in 1997, healthcare-specific criteria were created to help healthcare organizations address challenges such as focusing on core competencies, introducing new technologies, reducing costs, communicating and sharing information electronically, establishing new alliances with healthcare providers, and maintaining market advantage. The criteria can be used to assess performance on a wide range of key indicators: healthcare outcomes; patient satisfaction; and operational, staff, and financial indicators. Similar models are in place in Europe and in individual U.S. states.

The Baldrige healthcare criteria are built on the following set of interrelated core values and concepts:

- Visionary leadership
- Patient-focused excellence
- Organizational and personal learning
- Valuing of staff and partners
- Agility
- Focus on the future
- Managing for innovation
- Management by fact
- Social responsibility and community health
- Creating value and results
- Systems perspective

The criteria are organized into seven interdependent categories (National Institute of Standards and Technology 2003):

1. Leadership
2. Strategic planning
3. Focus on patients, other customers, and markets
4. Measurement, analysis, and knowledge management
5. Staff focus
6. Process management
7. Organizational performance results

Baldrige's scoring system is based on a 1,000-point scale. Each of the seven criteria is assigned a maximum value ranging from 85 to 450 maximum points. The most heavily weighted criterion is the results category (450 possible points). The weight of this category is based on an emphasis Baldrige places on results and an organization's ability to demonstrate performance and improvement in the following areas:

- Product and service outcomes
- Customer-focused outcomes
- Financial and market outcomes
- Workforce-focused outcomes
- Process effectiveness outcomes
- Leadership outcomes

ISO 9000

Founded in 1947 as a nongovernmental entity, the International Organization for Standardization (ISO) issued the original 9000 series of voluntary technical standards in 1987 to facilitate the development and maintenance of quality control programs in the manufacturing industry. Its intent was to provide consensus for an approved methodology that would ensure consistency in manufacturing through standardization of processes and services to conform with and fulfill world-market customer requirements.

In 1994, ISO made additional changes to the standards, acknowledging the delineation of services provided by varying industries and product sectors. In 2000, ISO made major changes to the standards to make them more relevant to service and healthcare settings, eliminating ISO 9002 and 9003 and releasing ISO 9001:2000 (Dillon 2002).

Focused more on quality management systems, process approach, and the role of top management, the most recent standards include eight common quality management principles (Cianfrani, Tsiakals, and West 2002):

Principle 1: Customer-Focused Organization
Principle 2: Leadership
Principle 3: Involvement of People
Principle 4: Process Approach
Principle 5: Systems Approach to Management

Principle 6: Continual Improvement

Principle 7: Factual Approach to Decision Making

Principle 8: Mutually Beneficial Supplier Relationships

ISO 9000 has been more widely accepted and applied in countries other than the United States but appears to be the focus of increased interest as a model for organizing quality improvement activities (Cianfrani, Tsiakals, and West 2002).

Lean Thinking

The Massachusetts Institute of Technology developed the term *Lean* in 1987 to describe production methods and product development that, when compared to traditional mass production processes, produce more products, with fewer defects, in a shorter time. The goal was to develop a way to specify value, line up value to create actions in the best sequence, conduct these activities without interruption whenever someone requests them, and perform them more effectively (Womack and Jones 2003). Lean thinking, sometimes called *Lean manufacturing* or *TPS*, focuses on the removal of waste (*muda*), which is defined as anything unnecessary to produce the product or service.

The focus of Lean methodology is a "back to basics" approach that places the needs of the customer first through the following five steps.

1. Define *value* as determined by the customer, identified by the provider's ability to deliver the right product or service at an appropriate price.
2. Identify the *value stream*: the set of specific actions required to bring a specific product or service from concept to completion.
3. Make value-added steps *flow* from beginning to end.
4. Let the customer *pull* the product from the supplier, rather than push products.
5. Pursue *perfection* of the process.

Although Lean focuses on removing waste and improving flow, it also has some secondary effects. Quality is improved. The product spends less time in process, reducing the chances of damage or obsolescence. Simplification of processes results in less variation, more uniform output, and less inventory (Heim 1999).

Six Sigma

Six Sigma (3.4 defects per million) is a system for improvement developed over time by Hewlett-Packard, Motorola, General Electric, and others in the 1980s and 1990s (Pande, Neuman, and Cavanagh 2000). The tools used in Six Sigma are not new. The thinking behind this system came from the foundations of quality improvement from the 1930s through the 1950s.

What makes Six Sigma appear new is the rigor of tying improvement projects to key business processes and clear roles and responsibilities for Executives, Champions, Master Black Belts, Black Belts, and Green Belts.

The aim of Six Sigma is to reduce variation (eliminate defects) in key business processes. By using a set of statistical tools to understand the fluctuation of a process, management can predict the expected outcome of that process. If the outcome is not satisfactory, management can use associated tools to further understand the elements influencing that process. Six Sigma includes five steps—define, measure, analyze, improve, and control—commonly known as DMAIC.

- *Define*: Identify the customers and their problems. Determine the key characteristics important to the customer along with the processes that support those key characteristics. Identify existing output conditions along with process elements.
- *Measure*: Categorize key characteristics, verify measurement systems, and collect data.
- *Analyze*: Convert raw data into information that provides insights into the process. These insights include identifying the fundamental and most important causes of the defects or problems.
- *Improve*: Develop solutions to the problem, and make changes to the process. Measure process changes and judge whether the changes are beneficial or another set of changes is necessary.
- *Control*: If the process is performing at a desired and predictable level, monitor the process to ensure that no unexpected changes occur.

The primary theory of Six Sigma is that focus on variation reduction will lead to more uniform process output. Secondary effects include less waste, less throughput time, and less inventory (Heim 1999).

Quality Tools

One of the difficult things about quality is explaining how a *tool* is different from a *process* or *system*. We can observe people using tools and methods for improvement. We can see them making a flowchart, plotting a control chart, or using a checklist. These tools and procedures are the logical results of systems and models that people put in place (knowingly and unknowingly). People may use several tools and procedures to make improvements, and these tools may form one part of an improvement system. Although we can observe people using the tools of the system, the system (e.g., Six Sigma, ISO 9000) itself is invisible and cannot be observed. There are well over 50 quality tools, many of which were developed to "see" the quality system in which they are designed to support. The American Society for Quality (2007) has formed six categories of quality tools:

1. Cause analysis
2. Evaluation and decision making
3. Process analysis
4. Data collection and analysis
5. Idea creation
6. Project planning and implementation

This section is not intended to be an all-inclusive reference for quality tools and techniques but rather a highlight of some of more widely used tools. The tools are organized in three categories:

1. Basic quality tools
2. Management and planning tools
3. Other quality tools

Basic Quality Tools

Basic quality tools are used to define and analyze discrete processes that usually produce quantitative data. These tools primarily are used to explain the process, identify potential causes for process performance problems, and collect and display data indicating which causes are most prevalent.

Control Chart

A control chart consists of chronological data along with upper and lower control boundaries that define the limits of common cause variation. A control chart is used to monitor and analyze variation from a process to determine whether that process is stable and predictable (results from common cause variation) or unstable and not predictable (shows signs of special cause variation).

Histogram

A histogram is a graphical display of the frequency distribution of the quality characteristic of interest. A histogram makes variation in a group of data apparent and aids analysis of how data are distributed around an average or median value.

Cause-and-Effect/Fishbone Diagram

Cause-and-effect analysis is sometimes referred to as the Ishikawa, or fishbone, diagram. In a cause-and-effect diagram, the problem (effect) is stated in a box on the right side of the chart, and likely causes are listed around major headings (bones) that lead to the effect. Cause-and-effect diagrams can help organize the causes contributing to a complex problem (American Society for Quality 2007).

Pareto Chart

Vilfredo Pareto, an Italian economist in the 1880s, observed that 80 percent of the wealth in Italy was held by 20 percent of the population. Juran later applied this Pareto principle to other applications and found that 80 percent of the variation of any characteristic is caused by only 20 percent of the possible variables. A Pareto chart is a display of occurrence frequency that shows this small number of major contributors to a problem so that management can concentrate resources on correcting them (American Society for Quality 2007).

Management and Planning Tools

Management uses management and planning tools to organize the decision-making process and create a hierarchy when faced with competing priorities. These tools also are useful for dealing with issues involving multiple departments within an organization and for creating an organization-wide quality culture.

Affinity Diagram

The affinity diagram can encourage people to develop creative solutions to problems. A list of ideas is created, and then individual ideas are written on small note cards. Team members study the cards and group the ideas into common categories. The affinity diagram is a way to create order out of a brainstorming session (American Society for Quality 2007).

Matrix Diagram

The matrix diagram helps us to answer two important questions when sets of data are compared: Are the data related? How strong is the relationship? The quality function deployment House of Quality is an example of a matrix diagram. It lists customer needs on one axis and the in-house standards on the second axis. A second matrix diagram is added to show the in-house requirements on one axis and the responsible departments on the other. The matrix diagram can identify patterns in relationships and serves as a useful checklist for ensuring that tasks are being completed (American Society for Quality 2007).

Priorities Matrix

The priorities matrix uses a series of planning tools built around the matrix chart. This matrix helps when there are more tasks than available resources and management needs to prioritize on the basis of data rather than emotion. Groups can use priorities matrices to systematically discuss, identify, and prioritize the criteria that have the most influence on the decision and study the possibilities (American Society for Quality 2007).

Other Quality Tools

Benchmarking

Benchmarking compares the processes and successes of your competitors or of similar top-performing organizations to your current processes to define, through gap analysis, process variation and organizational opportunities for improvement. Benchmarking defines not only organizations that perform better but also how they perform better.

Failure Mode and Effects Analysis

Failure mode and effects analysis (FMEA) examines potential problems and their causes and predicts undesired results. FMEA normally is used to predict product failure from past part failure, but it also can be used to analyze future system failures. This method of failure analysis generally is performed for design and process. By basing their activities on FMEA, organizations can focus their efforts on steps in a process that have the greatest potential for failure before failure actually occurs. Prioritization of failure modes is based on the severity, likelihood of occurrence, and ability to detect the potential failure.

5S

A Japanese tool called 5S (each step starts with the letter "S") is a systematic program that helps workers take control of their workspace so that it actually works for them (and their customers) instead of being a neutral or, as is quite common, competing factor. *Seiri* (Sort) means to keep only necessary items. *Seiton* (Straighten) means to arrange and identify items so they can be easily retrieved when needed. *Seiso* (Shine) means to keep items and workspaces clean and in working order. *Seiketsu* (Standardize) means to use best practices consistently. *Shitsuke* (Sustain) means to maintain the gains and make a commitment to continue the first four Ss.

Knowledge Transfer and Spread Techniques

A key element or measure of any quality improvement effort is the ability to transfer the knowledge learned and replicate the successes in similar areas of the organization. Within any unit, organization, or system, there will be barriers to spread and adoption (e.g., organizational culture, communication, leadership support). However, failure to transfer knowledge effectively may result in unnecessary waste, inconsistency in organizational performance, and missed opportunities to achieve benchmark levels of operational performance.

The Theory of Transfer of Learning, developed in 1901, explored how individuals could transfer learning in one context to another context that shared similar characteristics. The theory relied on the notion that characteristics in the new setting were similar enough to the previous knowledge center to replicate processes, disseminate information, and gain efficiencies from lessons learned (Thorndike and Woodworth 1901).

In 1999, the Institute for Healthcare Improvement (IHI) chartered a team to develop a "Framework for Spread." The stated aim of the team was to "develop, test, and implement a system for accelerating improvement by spreading change ideas within and between organizations" (Massoud et al. 2006). Further findings from the study and team research noted the following questions as important to address when attempting to spread ideas to the target population (Massoud et al. 2006).

1. Can the organization or community structure be used to facilitate spread?
2. How are decisions made about the adoption of improvements?
3. What infrastructure enhancements will facilitate spread?
4. What transition issues need to be addressed?
5. How will the spread efforts be transitioned to operational responsibilities?

Below is a sample list of some of the techniques that can be used to facilitate spread within a department, across an organization, or throughout a system. As with the aforementioned quality improvement systems and tools, the list of knowledge transfer techniques below is not exhaustive but a representative sample of techniques for consideration based on the goals and complexity of the changes being disseminated.

Rapid Cycle Testing/Improvement

Two important characteristics of an effective spread model are staff buy-in and proof that the change will improve performance. Developed by IHI, rapid cycle testing (or improvement) was designed to create various small tests involving small sample sizes and using multiple PDSA cycles that build on the lessons learned in a short period while gaining buy-in from staff involved in the change (Figure 4.3). Successful tests are applied to other units in the organization, whereas unsuccessful tests continue to be revised for potential spread and further implementation. Rapid cycle testing is designed to reduce the cycle time of new process implementation from months to days. To prevent unnecessary delays in testing or implementation, teams or units using rapid cycle testing must remain focused on the testing of solutions and avoid overanalysis. Rapid cycle testing can be

FIGURE 4.3

Example of
Rapid Cycle
Testing

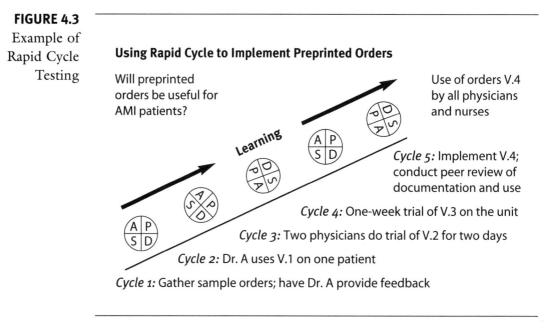

Using Rapid Cycle to Implement Preprinted Orders

Will preprinted orders be useful for AMI patients?

Learning

Use of orders V.4 by all physicians and nurses

Cycle 5: Implement V.4; conduct peer review of documentation and use

Cycle 4: One-week trial of V.3 on the unit

Cycle 3: Two physicians do trial of V.2 for two days

Cycle 2: Dr. A uses V.1 on one patient

Cycle 1: Gather sample orders; have Dr. A provide feedback

SOURCE: Warren (2005). Used with permission.

resource intensive (focuses increased resources into a short period) and therefore may require top-level leadership support.

IHI Breakthrough Series (BTS) Model

IHI has designed a model to support its breakthrough collaborative series. A collaborative consists of 20 to 40 healthcare organizations working together for six to eight months to improve a specific clinical or operational area. Under the guidance of an IHI panel of national experts, team members study, test, and implement the latest available knowledge to produce rapid improvements in their organizations. A key component of the collaborative model is the ability of participants to work with other organizations to discuss similar problems, lessons learned, and barriers to improvement. This framework allows participating teams to build on their existing efforts and modify their approach on the basis of feedback from expert faculty and peers from other participating organizations. A collaborative represents the intensive efforts of healthcare professionals to make significant changes that improve clinical outcomes and reduce costs (IHI 2003).

Case Study: Using the IHI BTS Collaborative Model in Combination with Rapid Cycle Testing to Improve Processes for Surgical Infection Prevention

In summer 2003, the Texas quality improvement organization, TMF Health Quality Institute (formerly Texas Medical Foundation), initiated the 13-

month Surgical Infection Prevention (SIP) Collaborative. The goal of the collaborative was to improve the quality of care for patients admitted to the hospital for surgical treatment. The improvements targeted the application of evidence-based care through system redesign.

The process measures for the collaborative were the Centers for Medicare & Medicaid Services and The Joint Commission national quality indicators/core measures for surgical infection prevention. These indicators (with the exception of supplemental oxygen) became part of The Joint Commission's core measure set for SIP in 2004. The quality indicators were as follows:

- Prophylactic antibiotic selection administered within one hour before surgical incision
- Prophylactic antibiotics consistent with current recommendations
- Prophylactic antibiotics discontinued within 24 hours of the surgery end time
- Maintaining normothermia (optional measure)
- Providing supplemental oxygen (optional measure)
- Avoiding shaving the operative site (optional measure)

The collaborative included 50 hospitals (only 42 hospitals completed the collaborative) that participated in two IHI BTS-like collaborative learning sessions that included rapid cycle quality improvement model methods and one outcomes congress. To facilitate learning during the collaborative, hospitals were asked to identify a pilot population that yielded at least 30 surgeries per month or 100 percent of surgical cases from selected surgical procedures listed below (TMF 2003):

- Coronary artery bypass grafts
- Cardiac surgery
- Colon surgery
- Hip arthroplasty
- Knee arthroplasty
- Abdominal and vaginal hysterectomies
- Vascular surgery

Participation in the SIP Collaborative required participating hospitals to make the following commitments (TMF 2003):

- Form a multidisciplinary team from their hospital of people who were actively involved in the care processes of surgery (team included a senior-level leader, a clinical champion, and a day-to-day leader)
- Complete prework activities (develop an aim statement, identify the population, define measures, collect baseline data)
- Attend two one-day learning sessions (August and November 2003)
- Attend an outcomes congress (summer 2004) to present the hospital team's achievements

- Participate in regular teleconferences to interact with peers and learn about successful care processes
- Share hospital team progress through monthly status and data reports
- Use e-mail lists to share success stories and ask questions

The learning sessions, led by TMF staff and expert physician faculty (infectious disease, surgery, and process improvement), were designed to build on the lessons learned from fellow collaborative participants and, more importantly, to allow team members representing the 50 hospitals to apply the knowledge learned, make modifications to individual project plans, and apply rapid cycle testing between learning sessions.

Many participants made modifications to project plans on the basis of interactions with other participating hospitals. Through the application of consistent processes in participant institutions, the learning sessions allowed participants to develop reasonable and measurable interim process measures to determine the effectiveness of each plan stage. The results of the collaborative (Figure 4.4) identified that although the coordination and participation of a large number of hospitals in a collaborative initiative is an exhaustive task, obstacle avoidance and the support of a shared learning environment to identify lessons learned can shorten the learning cycle, accelerate the quality improvement process, and boost improvement results. Awareness of other individual and organizational efforts and successes in overcoming similar impediments to improvement and collective problem solving produced a more rapid application of evidence-based care practices and the use of process redesign methods.

FIGURE 4.4
Overall Surgical Infection Prevention Collaborative Project Results

Required Measures	Baseline Average %	Final %	Change %	Reduction in Failure Rate	# of Teams
Timely antibiotic administration	61.6	84.7	23.1	60.2	34
Use of recommended antibiotics	81.5	85.0	3.5	18.9	34
Discontinue antibiotics within 24 hours	38.0	62.9	24.9	40.2	34
Optional Measures					
Normothermia	50.0	71.0	21.0	42.0	14
Supplemental oxygen	22.5	72.9	50.4	65.0	5
Avoid shaving	64.2	81.0	16.8	46.9	18

SOURCE: Warren (2005). Used with permission.

Quality Circles

Influenced by W. E. Deming, Kaoru Ishikawa pioneered the development of quality circles. Quality circles are groups of five to ten employees, with management support, who meet to solve problems and implement new procedures. Employees involved in quality circles are encouraged to develop ideas for improvement or request management efforts to propose solutions for adoption. The aims of the quality circle activities are to (Hungarian Public Employment Service 2006):

- contribute to the improvement and development of the enterprise;
- respect human relations and build a workshop offering job satisfaction; and
- deploy human capabilities fully and draw out infinite potential.

Conclusion

The continued success of an organization depends on the strength of the foundation on which it was built and the systems, processes, tools, and methods it uses to sustain benchmark levels of performance. Although quality improvement theory and methodology have been available since the early 1900s, their widespread acceptance and application by the healthcare industry have not occurred as rapidly and effectively as in other industries (e.g., manufacturing). The release of two Institute of Medicine publications (*Crossing the Quality Chasm* [2001] and *To Err Is Human* [2000]) describing significant concerns about the U.S. healthcare system incited a movement toward improvement that significantly increased healthcare institutions' focus on better care and patient safety (Berwick and Leape 2005). However, because of a combination of technical complexity, system fragmentation, a tradition of autonomy, and hierarchical authority structures, overcoming the "daunting barrier to creating the habits and beliefs of common purpose, teamwork and individual accountability" (Berwick and Leape 2005) necessary for spread and sustainability will require continual focus and commitment. The principles described in this chapter have demonstrated success in many healthcare organizations. Healthcare will continue to build on these principles as it strives to maintain benchmark levels of performance by working to provide the right care for every patient at the right time, every time.

Study Questions

1. How would you select and implement one or more of these approaches in your own institution?

2. What are some of the challenges to spreading change? Provide two key questions/issues that need to be considered when applying change concepts in an organization or system.
3. What are some of the key common elements to the different tools discussed in this chapter?
4. What is the difference between a quality improvement system and a tool? Provide examples of each.

Note

1. Chapter 4 of the first edition of this book was written by Mike Stoecklein and has been revised for this edition by Kevin Warren.

References

American Society for Quality. 2007. "Armand V. Feigenbaum Biography." [Online information; retrieved 3/23/07.] www.asq.org/about-asq/who-we-are/bio_feigen.html.

American Society for Quality, Quality Management Division. 1999. *Certified Quality Manager Handbook.* Milwaukee, WI: ASQ Quality Press.

Berwick, D. A., and L. L. Leape. 2005. "Five Years After *To Err Is Human*: What Have We Learned?" *Journal of the American Medical Association* 293 (19): 2384–90.

Brown, J. A. 2003. *The Healthcare Quality Handbook: A Professional Resource and Study Guide.* Pasadena, CA: JB Enterprises.

Cianfrani, C. A., J. J. Tsiakals, and J. E. West. 2002. *The ASQ ISO 9000: 2000 Handbook.* Milwaukee, WI: ASQ Quality Press.

Crosby, Philip B. 1996. *Quality Is Still Free.* New York: McGraw-Hill.

Cutler, A. N. 2001. "Biography of Walter A. Shewhart." [Online information; retrieved 3/23/07.] www.sigma-engineering.co.uk/light/shewhartbiog.htm.

Deming, W. E. 1986. "Principles for Transformation of Western Management." In *Out of the Crisis*, by W. E. Deming, 18–96. Cambridge, MA: MIT Press.

———. 2000. *The New Economics for Industry, Government, Education*, 2nd ed. Cambridge, MA: MIT Press.

Dillon, R. 2002. "Health Care and ISO 9000: An Interview with Dr. Michael Crago." *Infusion* 8 (4): 43–47.

Feigenbaum, A. V. 1951. *Total Quality Control.* New York: McGraw-Hill.

Heim, K. 1999. "Creating Continuous Improvement Synergy with Lean and TOC." Paper presented at the American Society for Quality Annual Quality Congress, Anaheim, California, May.

Hungarian Public Employment Service. 2006. "The Fathers of Quality Systems." [Online information; retrieved 4/5/07.] http://en.afsz. hu/resource.aspx?resourceID=en_vp_2005-008_annex.

Institute for Healthcare Improvement (IHI). 2003. Home page. [Online information; retrieved 3/23/07.] www.ihi.org.

Institute of Medicine (IOM). 2000. *To Err Is Human: Building a Safer Health System.* Washington, DC: National Academies Press.

————. 2001. *Crossing the Quality Chasm: A New Health System for the 21st Century.* Washington, DC: National Academies Press.

Juran, J. M. 1989. *Juran on Leadership for Quality.* New York: Free Press.

Juran, J. M., and F. M. Gryna (eds.). 1951. *Juran's Quality Control Handbook.* New York: McGraw-Hill.

Kilian, C. 1988. *The World of W. Edwards Deming.* Knoxville, TN: SPC Press.

Langley, G., K. Nolan, T. Nolan, C. Norman, and L. Provost. 1996. *The Improvement Guide: A Practical Approach to Enhancing Organizational Performance.* San Francisco: Jossey-Bass.

Massoud, M. R., G. A. Nielson, K. Nolan, T. Nolan, M. W. Schall, and C. Sevin. 2006. *A Framework for Spread: From Local Improvements to System Wide Change.* IHI Innovation Series white paper. Cambridge, MA: Institute for Healthcare Improvement.

National Institute of Standards and Technology. 2003. "Getting Started with the Baldrige Criteria for Performance Excellence: A Guide to Self-Assessment and Action." [Online information; retrieved 3/23/07.] http://baldrige.nist.gov/Getting_Started.htm.

Neave, H. R. 1990. *The Deming Dimension.* Knoxville, TN: SPC Press.

Pande, P. S., R. P. Neuman, and R. R. Cavanagh. 2000. *The Six Sigma Way: How GE, Motorola, and Other Top Companies Are Honing Their Performance.* New York: McGraw-Hill.

Texas Medical Foundation (TMF). 2003. *Surgical Infection Prevention Collaborative Handbook.* Austin, TX: TMF Health Quality Institute.

Thorndike, E. L., and R. S. Woodworth. 1901. "The Influence of Improvement in One Mental Function Upon the Efficiency of Other Functions." *Psychological Review* 8: 247–61.

Warren, K. 2005. "Structure + Process = Outcomes (Donabedian)." Presented at the University of Texas Graduate School of Nursing, Austin, Texas, March 15.

Womack, J. P., and D. T. Jones. 2003. *Lean Thinking: Banish Waste and Create Wealth in Your Corporation.* New York: Free Press.

ORGANIZATION AND MICROSYSTEM

MILESTONES IN THE QUALITY MEASUREMENT JOURNEY

5

Robert C. Lloyd

I dentifying and developing appropriate quality measurements are essential aspects of quality management. Many healthcare professionals use Shewhart control charts to analyze the variation in their data, but they often struggle to find the appropriate measures to place on the control charts. Control charts based on inappropriate or poorly developed measures are of no value. This chapter provides a template and practical recommendations for selecting and developing measures. The text discusses seven milestones in the quality measurement journey and offers recommendations for avoiding pitfalls along the way.

There was a time when only providers cared about measuring the efficiency and effectiveness of healthcare services. Today, although providers are more focused than ever on performance measurement, they must balance their own measurement needs against rising demands from external groups and organizations, including:

- purchasers of care (individuals and companies);
- business coalitions (representing companies within defined geographical areas);
- insurance companies interested in structuring contractual agreements around quality outcomes and service;
- regulatory organizations, state data commissions, and departments of health and welfare;
- Centers for Medicare & Medicaid Services (CMS); and
- the media (especially newspapers, television, and healthcare magazines).

Not only are more organizations demanding healthcare data; they also are making a strong argument for the release of these data to the public, which is a fundamental switch from how healthcare data historically have been treated. Before the early 1980s, one could obtain data on hospitals or physicians only through the subpoena process. Today, the public release of provider data is quite common. Internet sites, state data commissions, CMS, and proprietary vendors make these data available. The basic theory behind such releases is that they will make providers more accountable for the outcomes they produce, improve quality and safety, and help to contain costs. Consistent support of this theory remains elusive, however.

The Measurement Challenge

This increased focus on and mandate for healthcare data place healthcare providers in a different situation than they have known in the past. Providers are being asked to document what they do, evaluate the outcomes of their efforts, and be prepared to share their results with the public. Unfortunately, many providers struggle to address the measurement mandate proactively, which leads organizations to assume a defensive posture when external organizations release the data. In such cases, the provider usually responds in one of the following ways.

- The data are old (typically one to two years) and do not reflect our current performance.
- The data are not stratified and do not represent appropriate comparisons.
- Our patients are sicker than those at the other hospitals in our comparison group (i.e., no risk adjustments were made to the data).

Although these responses frequently have some credibility, they are generally regarded, especially by organizations that release the data, to be feeble excuses and attempts by providers to justify their current ways of delivering care. A more proactive posture would be to develop an organization-wide approach to quality measurement that meets both internal and external demands. This approach is not a task to be completed once, but rather a journey that has many potential pitfalls and detours. As on any worthwhile journey, key milestones exist that mark your progress and chart your direction. The remainder of this chapter outlines seven major milestones that will aid in your search for a few good measures.

Milestones Along the Quality Measurement Journey

Seven key milestones are summarized in Table 5.1. Because of space limitations, all the details associated with each milestone are not provided. Some of the detail is presented in other chapters of this book, and additional detail can be found in references that address quality measurement topics (Caldwell 1995; Carey 2003; Carey and Lloyd 2001; Gaucher and Coffey 1993; Langley et al. 1996; Lloyd 2004; Provost and Murray 2007).

Milestone 1

The first step in the quality measurement journey is strategic. It is achieved by engaging in serious dialogue within the organization on the role of performance measurement. Many organizations do not know their measurement objectives. Usually, the organization either takes a defensive posture

Milestone	Activities Performed at This Milestone
1	Develop a measurement philosophy
2	Identify the concepts to be measured (types and categories of measures)
3	Select specific measures
4	Develop operational definitions for each measure
5	Develop a data collection plan and gather the data (giving special consideration to stratification and sampling)
6	Analyze the data using statistical process control methods (especially run and control charts)
7	Use the analytic results (data) to take action (implement cycles of change, test theories, and make improvements)

TABLE 5.1
Quality Measurement Journey Milestones and Their Related Activities

toward data (as discussed above) or waits to see what it is asked to provide. Is measurement a part of your organization's day-to-day functioning, or is it something done periodically to prepare reports for board meetings or respond to external requirements? Does everyone in the organization understand the critical role of performance measurement, or do employees think that the development of measures is something only management does?

The first step toward this milestone should be the creation of an organizational statement on the role of measurement. Another way to view this step is to consider developing a measurement philosophy. Three simple questions should be explored when developing a measurement philosophy.

- Do we know our data better than anyone else does?
- Do we have a balanced set of measures that encompasses clinical, operational, customer service, and resource allocations?
- Do we have a plan for using the data to make improvements?

A good test of whether you have reached this initial milestone is to ask the members of an improvement team about their measurement objectives. If they say they are gathering data because their manager told them to, you have not reached this milestone. If, on the other hand, the team members indicate that they want to learn more about the variation in their processes in order to improve performance, this milestone is well in sight.

Milestone 2

The second milestone is both strategic and operational. It consists of deciding which concepts (sometimes called types or categories of measures) the organization wishes to monitor. Donabedian (1980, 1982) provided a simple and clear approach to organizing a measurement journey. He proposed three basic categories of measures: structures (S), processes (P), and outcomes (O). The relationship between these three categories usually is shown as follows:

$$S + P = O.$$

Structures represent the physical and organizational aspects of the organization (e.g., design of the outpatient testing area, hiring practices, tuition reimbursement policies). As Deming (1995) constantly pointed out, "Every activity, every job, is part of a process." Management creates *processes*, and workers refine them. Structures combine with processes to produce *outcomes* (results).

Donabedian's model has served as a general rubric for many organizations. Frequently, however, organizations need to be more specific than structures, processes, and outcomes. In this case, most organizations turn to either their strategic plan or literature. One of the more frequently referenced sources is the Institute of Medicine's (2001) report *Crossing the Quality Chasm*, which identifies the following six aims for improvement. Healthcare should be:

1. safe;
2. effective;
3. patient centered;
4. timely;
5. efficient; and
6. equitable.

The Joint Commission (1993) also has identified the following dimensions of clinical performance to categorize measures:

• Appropriateness
• Availability
• Continuity
• Effectiveness
• Efficacy
• Efficiency
• Respect and caring
• Safety
• Timeliness

Rather than use externally derived categories to structure measures, most healthcare organizations prefer to build their measurement system around their strategic objectives. One way to test how well this approach has been deployed throughout the organization is to ask a team which of the organization's strategic objectives it is meeting through its improvement work. If the team members look at you with bewilderment, you can assume that they are not clear on how their work fits into the bigger picture.

Regardless of the method used, an organization must decide which concepts, types, or categories of measures it wishes to track. If it does not reach consensus on this issue, the rest of the journey will be a random walk through the data.

Milestone 3

Once an organization has decided on the types of measures it wishes to track, the next step in the journey is to identify specific measures. Many people do not understand how this step differs from milestone 2. Consider trying to find your seat at a baseball game. Milestone 2 identifies the section in which you are sitting (e.g., Section 110). Milestone 3 focuses on the specific row and seat you have been assigned (e.g., Row N, Seat 21).

A healthcare example should provide further clarification. Imagine your organization has identified patient safety as one of its strategic objectives. Safety seems like a good thing to monitor, but you cannot measure patient safety directly because it is a concept. Concepts are vague. You need to specify (1) what aspect of patient safety you intend to measure and (2) the actual measures. Table 5.2 shows how this cascading process works. Note that even within the broad category of patient safety, you need to identify the aspect (i.e., which section in the ballpark) you will measure. Within patient safety, for example, you could focus on medication errors, patient falls, wrong-site surgeries, missed/delayed diagnoses, or blood product errors.

This example selects medication errors as the aspect of patient safety to be measured. Within the medication error area, many things could be

---

Concept: *Patient safety*	**TABLE 5.2** The Relationship Between a Concept and Specific Measures
What **aspect** of patient safety do we want to measure? *Medication errors*	
What **specific measures** could we track?	
• *Number of medication orders that had an error* • *Total number of errors caught each day* • *Percentage of orders with an error* • *Medication error rate* • *Number of wasted IVs* • *Percentage of administration errors*	
Which **specific indicator** will you select?	

measured, so you need to choose a more specific indicator. A quality improvement team bases its selection (from Table 5.2 or any list it develops) on the questions it wishes to answer. If you are interested in tracking the absolute volume of an activity, a simple count of the number of medication errors may be sufficient. If, on the other hand, you are interested in a relative measure, you would be better off measuring the percentage of medication errors or the measure most frequently used—the medication error rate (i.e., number of medication errors per 1,000 doses dispensed). In measure selection, there are more options than most people realize. The challenge is to be specific about which section, row, and seat you have selected.

Milestone 4

Development of operational definitions of specific measures begins at milestone 4. This activity requires inquisitive minds (left-brained people often are good at developing operational definitions) and patience.

Every day, we are challenged to think about operational definitions. They are essential to good measurement and critical to successful communication between individuals. For example, a neighbor of mine just returned from vacation. I asked whether he had a good vacation. He responded, "It was better than good; it was great!" When I asked him where he went, he said that he had gone away for a week with four of his friends (all male) and played golf all day and cards all night and smoked cigars. These activities may not meet everyone's definition of a good vacation, but for my neighbor, they met all the criteria of his operational definition.

Basically, an *operational definition* is a description, in quantifiable terms, of what to measure and the specific steps needed to measure it consistently. A good operational definition:

• gives communicable meaning to a concept or an idea;
• is clear and unambiguous;
• specifies the measurement method, procedures, and equipment;
• provides decision-making criteria when necessary; and
• enables consistency in data collection.

Remember, however, that operational definitions are not universal truths. They can be debated and argued ad nauseam. A good operational definition represents, therefore, a statement of consensus by individuals responsible for tracking the measure. Note also that the operational definition may need to be modified at some future point, which is not unusual. The date of a modification must be noted because it could have a dramatic effect on the results.[1]

In healthcare, many terms call for more precise operational definitions. How does your organization define the following terms?

- A patient fall (a partial fall, a fall with injuries, or an assisted fall)
- A complete history and physical
- A successful physical therapy session
- Restraint (physical versus chemical restraint)
- A prompt response to a call button
- A good employee performance review
- Surgical start time
- An accurate patient bill
- Quick turnaround time
- A clean patient room
- A quick admission
- A readmission
- Hand hygiene compliance
- A successful quality measurement journey

The problem created by poor operational definitions should be obvious. If you do not use the same operational definition each time you record and plot data on a chart, you will either miss a true change in the data or think a change has occurred when in fact one has not. Using the same operational definition becomes even more critical if you are trying to compare several hospitals or clinics in a system. When national comparisons are made, the operational definition challenge becomes extremely complex. All good measurement begins and ends with operational definitions.

Milestone 5

Data collection is the billboard for milestone 5. Unfortunately, many teams begin their quality measurement journey at this marker. Faced with the challenge of presenting data, teams' first reaction is to go find some. This orientation typically directs teams toward convenient data that are readily available and familiar to everyone. It also can cause teams to collect the wrong data in the wrong amounts (too little or too much).

The problem with using readily available, convenient data is that the data usually do a poor job of answering the questions necessary to assess performance. For example, quality improvement teams commonly use average length of stay and average cost (or charges) per discharge as proxy measures for quality. Both average length of stay and average cost are gross outcome measures (the O part of the Donabedian model). What is the team doing to measure the structures or processes of care? When asked this question, teams frequently respond, "Well, we currently don't collect data on these components, and it's easier for us to go with what we have always used and what is available. It's good enough, isn't it?"

Ten years ago, the "good enough" approach to data collection might have been acceptable. Today, however, because of the increasing demand to demonstrate effectiveness of care and efficiency of healthcare processes, this mind-set is not acceptable. Performance quality and excellence do not occur because organizations do what they have always done or what is convenient. Most healthcare observers agree that the industry does not need perpetuation of the status quo.

The data collection phase of the journey consists of two parts: (1) planning for data collection and (2) the actual data gathering. A well-designed data collection strategy should address the following questions.

Planning for data collection:

- What process(es) will be monitored?
- What specific measures will be collected?
- What are the operational definitions of the measures?
- Why are you collecting these data? What is the rationale for collecting these data rather than other types of data?
- Will the data add value to your quality improvement efforts?
- Have you discussed the effects of stratification on the measures?
- How often (frequency) and for how long (duration) will you collect the data?
- Will you use sampling? If so, what sampling design have you chosen?

Gathering the data:

- How will you collect the data? (Will you use data sheets, surveys, focus group discussions, phone interviews, or some combination of these methods?)
- Will you conduct a pilot study before you collect data for the entire organization?
- Who will collect the data? (Most teams ignore this question.)
- What costs (monetary and time costs) will be incurred by collecting these data?
- Will collecting these data have negative effects on patients or employees?
- Do your data collection efforts need to be taken to your organization's institutional review board for approval?
- What are the current baseline measures?
- Do you have targets and goals for the measures?
- How will the data be coded, edited, and verified?
- Will you tabulate and analyze these data by hand or by computer?
- Are there confidentiality issues related to the use of the results?
- How will these data be used to make a difference?
- What plan do you have for disseminating the results of your data collection efforts?

Once you have resolved these issues, the data collection should go smoothly. Unfortunately, many quality improvement teams do not spend sufficient time discussing their data collection plans; they want to move immediately to the data collection step. This haste usually guarantees that the team will (1) collect too much (or too little) data; (2) collect the wrong data; or (3) become frustrated with the entire measurement journey. When individuals or groups become frustrated with the measurement process, they begin to lose faith in the data and results, which leads to a major detour in the quality measurement journey. As a result, if the team or management collects data that do not reflect its preconceived notions of reality, it tends to (1) distort the data (which is unethical and illegal); (2) distort the process that produced the data; or (3) kill the messenger.[2] A well-designed data collection plan contributes significantly to a team's ability to avoid these data pitfalls.

Two key data collection skills—stratification and sampling—enhance any data collection effort. These skills are based more on logic and clear thinking than on statistics, yet many healthcare professionals have received limited training in both concepts.

Stratification

Stratification is the separation and classification of data into reasonably homogeneous categories. The objective of stratification is to create strata, or categories, within the data that are mutually exclusive and facilitate discovery of patterns that would not be observed if the data were aggregated. Stratification allows understanding of differences in the data caused by:

- day of the week (are Mondays different than Wednesdays?);
- time of day (registration is busier between 9 a.m. and 10 a.m. than between 2 p.m. and 3 p.m.);
- time of year (do we see more of this diagnosis in February than in June?);
- shift (does the process differ for day and night shifts?);
- type of order (stat versus routine);
- experience of the worker;
- type of procedure (nuclear medicine films versus routine X-rays); and
- type of machine (such as ventilators or lab equipment).

If you do not think about how these factors could influence your data before you collect them, you run the risk of (1) making incorrect conclusions about your data and (2) having to filter out the stratification effect manually after you have collected the data. Consider the following example of how stratification could be applied to the pharmacy process. A quality improvement team is interested in determining the percentage of medication orders that are delivered to nurses' stations within one hour of the order's receipt in the pharmacy. Before collecting data on this question, the team should determine whether it believes that this percentage could differ by floor, time of day, day of week, type of medication ordered, pharmacist on duty, or volume of orders received. If the team believes that one or more of these factors will influence the outcome, it should take steps to ensure that it collects the data relevant to these factors each time the pharmacy receives an order.

Stratification is an essential aspect of data collection. If you do not spend time discussing the implications of stratification, you will end up thinking that your data are worse (or better) than they should be.

Sampling

Sampling is the second key skill that healthcare professionals need to develop. If a process does not generate a lot of data, you probably will analyze all the occurrences of an event and not need to consider sampling. Sampling usually is not required when the measure is a percentage or a rate. For example, computation of the percentage of no-shows for magnetic resonance imaging (MRI) typically does not require a sampling plan. When a process generates considerable data, however (e.g., turnaround times for medication orders), a sampling plan is usually appropriate. Sampling is probably the most important thing you can do to reduce the amount of time and resources spent on data collection.

Like stratification, however, many healthcare professionals receive little training in sampling procedures. As a result, they collect either too much or too little data or question the results they obtain, causing issues with the reliability and validity of the data. Ishikawa's classic work *Guide to Quality Control* (1982) identified four conditions for developing a sampling plan: accuracy, reliability, speed, and economy. Samples usually do not meet all four criteria simultaneously. Sampling, therefore, consists of a series of compromises and trade-offs. The key to successful sampling lies in understanding the overall purpose of selecting a sample and then selecting the most appropriate sampling methodology to apply to the data.

The basic purpose of sampling is to be able to draw a limited number of observations and be reasonably confident that they represent the larger population from which they were drawn. What happens, though, when a sample is not representative of the population from which it was drawn? The sample presents a picture that is either more positive than it should be (a positive sampling bias) or more negative than it should be (a negative sampling bias). A well-drawn sample, therefore, should be representative of the larger population. For example, if you are using a survey to gather patient satisfaction feedback by mail, you would not send a survey to every patient.[3] You would start by sending surveys to roughly 50 percent of the patients and see how many are returned. This limited survey allows you to determine the response rate. Assume that 25 percent of these patients return the surveys. The next task is to determine how representative of the total population these respondents are.

		TABLE 5.3
Probability Sampling Techniques	• Systematic sampling • Simple random sampling • Stratified random sampling • Stratified proportional random sampling	Probability and Nonprobability Sampling Techniques
Nonprobability Sampling Techniques	• Convenience sampling • Quota sampling • Judgment sampling	

To test this question, you need to develop a profile of the total population. Typically, this profile is based on standard demographics such as gender, age, type of visit, payer class, and whether the respondent is a new or returning patient. If the distribution of these characteristics in the sample is similar (within 5 percent) to that found in the total population, you can be comfortable that your sample is reasonably representative of the population. If the characteristics of the sample and the population show considerable variation, however, you should adjust your sampling plan.

Inevitably, the number one question asked during a discussion on sampling is, "How much data do I need?" There is no simple answer; the size of the population, importance of the question being asked, and resources available for drawing the sample all influence the volume of data you need. If, for example, you are drawing a single sample at a fixed point in time (what Deming called an enumerative study), a reasonable minimum sample size is between 20 and 30 observations (e.g., selecting the wait times for 20 emergency room patients on Monday of next week). On the other hand, if you are sampling for quality improvement purposes (what Deming called an analytic study), you should take a different approach. Analytic studies are dynamic and monitor a process as it unfolds over time. Sampling for analytic studies therefore requires the selection of fewer observations (e.g., five to ten) drawn at multiple (as opposed to single) points in time.

There are two basic approaches to sampling: *probability* and *nonprobability*. The dominant sampling techniques associated with each approach are shown in Table 5.3 and briefly described below. You can find a more detailed discussion on sampling in any basic text on statistical methods or research design.[4]

Probability sampling is based on a simple principle—statistical probability. In other words, within a known population of size n, there will be a fixed probability of selecting any single element (n_i). The selection of this element (and subsequent elements) must be determined by objective

statistical means if the process is to be truly random (not affected by judgment, purposeful intent, or convenience).

Campbell (1974) lists three characteristics of probability sampling.

1. A specific statistical design is followed.
2. The selection of items from the population is determined solely according to known probabilities by means of a random mechanism, usually
   using a table of random digits.
3. The sampling error (i.e., the difference between results obtained from
   a sample survey and results that would have been obtained from a census of the entire population conducted using the same procedures as in
   the sample survey) can be estimated, and, as a result, the precision of
   the sample result can be evaluated.

There are numerous ways to draw a probability sample. All are variations on the simple random sample. The most frequently used probability sampling methods are summarized below.

- *Systematic sampling* is what most healthcare professionals think is random sampling. Although systematic sampling is a form of random sampling, it is one of the weakest approaches to probability sampling. Its
  chief advantage is that it is easy to do and inexpensive. Systematic sampling (sometimes called mechanical sampling) is achieved by numbering
  or ordering each element in the population (e.g., time order, alphabet-
  ical order, medical record order) and then selecting every kth element.
  The key point that most people ignore when doing a systematic sample
  is that the starting point for selecting every kth element should be generated through a random process and should be equal to or less than k
  but greater than zero. A random starting point is usually selected by
  using a random number table (found in the back of any good statistics
  book) or computer-based random number generator (found in all statistical software programs and spreadsheet packages). For example, if you
  wanted to select a systematic sample of 60 medical records from a total
  of 600, you would pull every tenth record. To determine the starting
  point for the sample, however, you would need to pick a random number between one and ten. Suppose that the random draw produces the
  number eight. To start our systematic sample, we would go to the eighth
  medical record on our list, pick it, and then select every tenth record
  after this starting point. Technically, this method is known as a systematic sample with a random start (Babbie 1979). The problem with systematic sampling is that groups of data that could provide knowledge
  about the process are eliminated. If, for example, you are selecting every
  tenth record, you have automatically eliminated from further consideration records one through nine. If something occurs regularly in the data
  or if something causes your data to be organized into groups of six or
  seven, for example, these records would be eliminated from considera-

tion automatically. The other problem with this form of sampling in healthcare settings is that the people drawing the sample do not base the start on a random process; they merely pick a convenient place to start and then apply the sampling interval they have selected. This method introduces bias and increases the sampling error.

- *Simple random sampling* is drawn in a way that gives every element in the population an equal and independent chance of being included in the sample. As mentioned in the previous section on systematic sampling, a random number table or computer-based random number generator ensures this equanimity. A random sample also can be drawn by placing equally sized pieces of paper with a range of numbers on them (e.g., 1 to 100) in a bowl and picking a predetermined number to be the sample. The problem with simple random samples is that they may over- or underrepresent segments of the population.

- *Stratified random sampling.* Stratifying the population into relatively homogeneous categories before the sample is drawn improves the sample's representation of the population and reduces the sampling error. Once the strata have been identified, a random selection process is applied within each. For example, you might stratify a clinic's appointments into well-baby visits, follow-up visits, and unscheduled visits and then sample randomly within each category. Even though this approach is more precise than simple random sampling, it still could over- or underrepresent one or more of the strata in the sample. Creation of a stratified proportional random sample prevents this issue.

- *Stratified proportional random sampling.* In this case, the approach outlined for stratified random sampling is used, with a twist. The proportion (or percentage) that each stratum represents in the population is determined, and this proportion is replicated in the sample. For example, if we knew that well-baby visits represent 50 percent of the clinic's business, follow-up visits represent 30 percent, and unscheduled visits represent 20 percent, we would draw 50 percent of the sample from well-baby visits, 30 percent from follow-up visits, and 20 percent from unscheduled visits. This draw would produce a sample not only representative but also proportionally representative of the population distribution. This method would further increase the precision of the sample and further reduce the sampling error. The stratified proportional random sample is one of the more sophisticated sampling designs; users require considerable knowledge about the population they are sampling. It also can be more costly in terms of both money and time.

Nonprobability sampling techniques should be used when estimating the reliability of the selected sample or generally applying the results of the sample to a larger population is not the principal concern. The basic objective of nonprobability sampling is to select a sample that the researchers believe is typical of the larger population. The problem is that there is no way to actually measure how typical or representative a nonprobability sample is with respect to the population it supposedly represents. In short, nonprobability samples can be considered as good enough for the people drawing the sample. The problem with nonprobability sampling is that people have a tendency to apply the sample results generally to larger populations, which is completely inappropriate.

For example, a local TV news reporter conducted a survey by approaching ten people as they exited a grocery store. The reporter asked them how they felt about the proposed local tax increase designed to support teacher salary increases. Only eight of the ten people agreed to be interviewed. Of these eight interviews, the reporter selected three interview excerpts not favoring the tax increase. After assembling the footage and her notes, the reporter looked into the camera and said, "There you have it—a unanimous opinion that the tax increase is not warranted." The implication is that there is public consensus against the proposal, when in fact the reporter has selected a limited convenience sample of three cases and jumped to a conclusion. This same situation could happen if you decided to interview ten patients in your emergency room on a given day and drew conclusions about your emergency services from these people. You have taken limited data and made a huge jump in logic. This jump is also known as the *ecological fallacy*—sampling a microcosm and generally applying the results to the entire ecology (i.e., the entire population).

There are three major forms of nonprobability sampling: convenience, quota, and judgment.

- *Convenience sampling* is designed to obtain a small number of observations that are readily available and easy to gather. Convenience sampling is also known as chunk sampling (Hess, Riedel, and Fitzpatrick 1975) or accidental sampling (Maddox 1981; Selltiz et al. 1959). There is no science behind convenience sampling. It produces a biased sample that is basically a collection of anecdotes that cannot be applied generally to larger populations. In convenience sampling, the primary consideration is the importance of whether the sample is representative of the larger population. If the consequences of having a nonrepresentative sample do not matter, the convenience sample may be good enough as a starting point.
- *Quota sampling* was developed in the late 1930s and used extensively by the Gallup Organization. Babbie (1979) describes the steps involved in developing a quota sample.

  1. Develop a matrix describing the characteristics of the target population. This may entail knowing the proportion of male and female; various age, racial, and ethnic proportions; as well as the educational and income levels of the population.

2. Once the matrix has been created and a relative proportion assigned to each cell in the matrix, data are collected from persons having all the characteristics of a given cell.
3. All persons in a given cell are then assigned a weight appropriate to their proportion of the total.
4. When all the sample elements are so weighted, the overall data should provide a reasonable representation of the total population.

Theoretically, an accurate quota sampling design should produce results that are reasonably representative of the larger population. Remember, however, that the actual selection of the elements to fill the quota is left to the individual gathering the data, not to random chance. If the data collectors are not diligent and honest about their work, they will end up obtaining their quotas in a manner more similar to convenience sampling than true quota sampling. Another challenge in quota sampling is the process by which the data collectors actually gather the data. For example, if you established a quota sample to gather data in the emergency room, but only during the day shift, you would run the risk of missing key data points during the afternoon and evening shifts. The final challenge in this sampling design is that people frequently misunderstand the word *quota*. People tend to apply the popular definition of the term (i.e., I need a quota of ten charts) rather than the more statistical definition of the term outlined by Babbie in the preceding list. In this case, quota is seen as something to fill with a minimum number of observations. This approach produces a convenience sample, not a quota sample.

- *Judgment sampling* is driven by the knowledge and experience of the person drawing the sample. No objective mechanical means are used to select the sample. The assumption is that, through experience, good judgment, and appropriate strategy, researchers can select a sample that is acceptable for their objectives. Obviously, the challenge in this form of sampling is people's perception of the knowledge and wisdom of the person making the judgment. If people believe that this person exhibits good wisdom, they will have confidence in the sample the person selects. If people doubt the person's knowledge, they will discredit the sample. Deming (1950, 1960) considered judgment sampling to be the method of choice for quality improvement research. Langley et al. (1996) maintain that "a random selection of units is rarely preferred to a selection made by a subject matter expert." In quality improvement circles, this type of sampling is also known as *expert sampling, acceptance sampling*, or *rational sampling*. Individuals who have expert knowledge of the process decide how to arrange the data into homogeneous subgroups and draw the sample. They can select the subgroups by either random or nonrandom procedures. Deming's (1950, 1960) view also stressed that samples should be selected at regular intervals, not at a single point. Most sampling designs, whether probability or nonprobability, are static. The researcher decides on a time frame and then draws as much data as possible. In contrast, Deming (1950, 1960, 1975) emphasized that sampling should be done in small doses and pulled as a continuous stream of data. The primary criticism of judgment sampling is that the "expert" may not fully understand all facets of the population under investigation and may therefore select a biased sample. Advocates of judgment sampling contend that by selecting multiple samples over time, the potential bias of the expert will be mitigated by the inherent variation in the process.

Building knowledge about the various sampling techniques is one of the best ways to reduce the amount of time and effort spent on collecting data. Done correctly, sampling is also one of the best ways to ensure that the collected data are directly related to the questions at hand. Done incorrectly, sampling inevitably will lead to a debate that challenges the data, the process that produced the data, or the collector's credibility.

Milestone 6

After collecting data, many quality improvement teams think they have completed the majority of their work, when in fact it has just begun. Data do not convert to information magically. In his classic article on the differences between data and information, Austin (1983) states:

> Data refers to the raw facts and figures which are collected as part of the normal functioning of the hospital. Information, on the other hand, is defined as data, which have been processed and analyzed in a formal, intelligent way, so that the results are directly useful to those involved in the operation and management of the hospital.

Data are the bits and pieces we collect to measure the performance of a process. Data are not information. Information, on the other hand, can be produced only by subjecting data to an inquiry process of deductive (general to specific) and inductive (specific to general) thinking. The standard approach to this form of data-based inquiry is the scientific method (Lastrucci 1967).

The analytical and interpretive steps the team must apply to the data are critical to a successful outcome. Often, however, lack of planning for the analytical part of the quality measurement journey causes a team to run into a dead end. Many teams put considerable effort into defining measures and collecting data only to hit a major roadblock because they did not take time to figure out how they would analyze the data or who would interpret the numbers.

A dialogue about reaching this milestone must take place, or all the effort put into the earlier part of the journey will be futile. Table 5.4 provides

TABLE 5.4

Discussion Questions for Developing an Analysis Plan

When data collection begins, how will you respond to the following questions?

- Where will the data be physically stored? Survey data can be problematic and mount up quickly. Will you save the surveys (i.e., the physical surveys), store them on an electronic medium, or recycle them when you are done with your analysis?
- Who will be responsible for receiving the data, logging them into a book, and assigning identification numbers?
- Have you set up a codebook for the data? If not, who will?
- How will you enter the data into a computer (e.g., scan the data, enter them manually, or create an automatic download from an existing database)?
- Who will enter the data? Will you verify the data after they have been entered? Have you considered using a professional data entry service?
- Who will be responsible for analyzing the data? (This question applies whether you are performing manual or automated analysis.)
- What computer software will you use? Will you produce descriptive statistical summaries, cross-tabulations, graphic summaries, or control charts?
- Once you have computer output, who will be responsible for translating the raw data into information for decision making? Will you need to develop a written summary of the results? Are there different audiences that need to receive the results? Have they requested different report formats?

a list of discussion questions that you should consider as you develop an analysis plan. Remember, however, that you must think through the components and specific activities of an analysis plan before you begin to collect data.

If you are engaged in a quality improvement initiative, the best analytic path to follow is one guided by statistical process control methods. This branch of statistics was developed by Dr. Walter Shewhart in the early 1920s while he worked at Western Electric Co. (Schultz 1994). Shewhart's primary analytic tool, the control chart, serves as the cornerstone for all quality improvement work. Statistical analysis conducted with control charts is different from what some consider "traditional research" (e.g., hypothesis testing, development of p-values, design of randomized clinical trials). Traditional research is designed to compare the results at time one (e.g., the cholesterol levels of a group of middle-aged men) with the results at time two (typically months after the initial measure). Research conducted in this manner is referred to as *static group comparisons* (Benneyan, Lloyd, and Plsek 2003). The focus is not on how the data varied over time but rather whether the two sets of results are "statistically different" from each other.

On the other hand, research based on control chart principles takes a different, dynamic view of the data. Control charts approach data as a continuous distribution that has a rhythm and pattern. In this case, control charts are more like electrocardiogram readouts or patterns of vital signs seen on telemetry monitors in intensive care units. Control charts are plots of data arranged in chronological order. The mean or average is plotted through the center of the data, and then the upper control limit and lower control limit are calculated from the inherent variation in the data. The control limits are not set by the individual constructing the chart, and they are properly referred to as sigma limits (not standard deviations). Additional details on control charts can be found in other chapters of this book or in the literature (Benneyan, Lloyd, and Plsek 2003; Carey 2003; Carey and Lloyd 2001; Lloyd 2004; Provost and Murray 2007; Western Electric Co. 1985; Wheeler 1995; Wheeler and Chambers 1992).

Milestone 7

The final leg of the measurement journey involves taking *action* with the data and the conclusion about the inherent variation in the measure you are tracking. Data without a context for action are useless. Unfortunately, a considerable amount of healthcare data are collected, analyzed, and then not used for action.

In 1998, Don Berwick provided a simple formula for quality improvement. During his keynote address at the National Forum on Quality Improvement in Health Care, he stressed that real improvement results from the interaction of three key forces: will, ideas, and execution. Dr. Berwick's reference to execution is essentially the same as taking action. Quality improvement requires action. This tenet is the essence of the Plan-Do-Study-Act (PDSA) cycle described in chapter 4. Without action, the PDSA cycle is nothing more than an academic exploration of interesting stuff. When Shewhart first identified the components of the PDSA cycle (Schultz 1994), he intended to place data completely in a context for action. A team's ultimate goal should not be data collection. The ultimate goal is action, to make things better for those we serve. As an old Palestinian proverb states, you can't fatten a cow by weighing it.

When groups are asked to evaluate how effective they are with respect to will, ideas, and execution, they consistently provide bothersome answers. I have administered the self-assessment shown in Table 5.5 to hundreds of healthcare professionals in the United States and abroad. Most respondents mark high for will, medium to high for ideas, and low for execution. They seem to give themselves high marks for good intentions and desires, moderate to high marks for generating ideas on how they can improve things, and low assessments on being able to act and implement change. For many (both within and outside the healthcare industry), this low level of execution has been a persistent problem. There is hope, however, in the simple fact that learning how to manage and execute change effectively is easier than instilling goodwill in people who have none.

Key Component	Self-Assessment		
Will	High	Medium	Low
Ideas	High	Medium	Low
Execution	High	Medium	Low

All three components MUST be viewed together. Focusing on one or even two of the components will guarantee suboptimal performance. Systems thinking lies at the heart of continuous quality improvement!

TABLE 5.5
A Self-Assessment for Making Quality Improvement a Reality

Conclusion

The milestones reviewed in this chapter and summarized in Table 5.1 can serve as guideposts for your quality measurement journey. However, measures and data serve little purpose unless they are used to test theories and make improvements. You must view them not as isolated tasks but as an integrated way of thinking about how to channel will, ideas, and action into an organization-wide road map for improvement.

Study Questions

1. What are several of the major reasons why more organizations are requiring healthcare providers to provide data on what they do and the outcomes they produce?
2. Why are operational definitions so important to good measurement? Provide an example of a vague operational definition, and then describe what you would do to make the definition more specific and clear.
3. Explain how stratification differs from sampling. Provide an example of when you would use stratification and when it is appropriate to develop a sampling strategy.
4. Name the two basic approaches to sampling. Which approach is better? Why do you make this conclusion? Select one sampling methodology, and describe how you would apply it to a quality improvement initiative.

Notes

1. Several years ago, I had the opportunity to observe a team that forgot to note when it changed the operational definition of a key measure. The team members noticed a dramatic improvement in their measure

and were eager to present their finding to the organization's quality council. The shift in their data was so dramatic that I asked whether they had done something different when they collected their data. Frequently, a change in the operational definition or sampling plan can produce a large shift in the data. They all said no. I continued to ask whether they were doing something differently, however, and I finally found a data analyst who recalled a "slight" modification in the operational definition. Interestingly, this change to the measure's definition coincided with the shift in the results. If the team had applied the former operational definition to the more recent data, the results would not have shown a change. Similarly, if the team had applied the new definition to the previous data, it would have observed this same improved performance.

2. Wheeler (1993) states this conclusion in a slightly different fashion. "When people are pressured to meet a target value, there are three ways they can proceed: (1) they can work to improve the system, (2) they can distort the system, (3) or they can distort the data." Wheeler credits Brian Joiner as the originator of this list.

3. The exception occurs under one or more of the following conditions: (1) low patient volume, (2) low response rate, or (3) short data collection period. For example, if your hospital has an average daily census of 72 patients and you know historically that the average response rate to the survey was only 10 percent, you probably would send a survey to every patient. Similarly, if you were going to survey only one week out of the entire quarter, you would want to send a survey to every patient. Remember that sampling is an extremely useful tool, but it is not always necessary.

4. You do not have to obtain the most recent books on sampling or statistical methods to find more detailed information. The basic principles behind modern sampling techniques have existed since the 1940s. Many of the books I have on this subject, for example, are 20 to 30 years old and are very consistent with more recent books on sampling methodology.

References

Austin, C. 1983. *Information Systems for Hospital Administration*. Chicago: Health Administration Press.

Babbie, E. R. 1979. *The Practice of Social Research*. Belmont, CA: Wadsworth.

Benneyan, J., R. Lloyd, and P. Plsek. 2003. "Statistical Process Control as a Tool for Research and Health Care Improvement." *Journal of Quality and Safety in Healthcare* 12 (6): 458–64.

Berwick, D. 1998. "Eagles and Weasels." Plenary presentation presented at the IHI National Forum on Quality Improvement in Health Care, Orlando, FL.

Caldwell, C. 1995. *Mentoring Strategic Change in Health Care.* Milwaukee, WI: ASQ Quality Press.

Campbell, S. 1974. *Flaws and Fallacies in Statistical Thinking.* Englewood Cliffs, NJ: Prentice-Hall.

Carey, R. 2003. *Improving Healthcare with Control Charts.* Milwaukee, WI: ASQ Quality Press.

Carey, R., and R. Lloyd. 2001. *Measuring Quality Improvement in Healthcare: A Guide to Statistical Process Control Applications.* Milwaukee, WI: ASQ Quality Press.

Deming, W. E. 1950. *Some Theory of Sampling.* New York: John Wiley & Sons.

———. 1960. *Sample Design in Business Research.* New York: John Wiley & Sons.

———. 1975. "On Probability as a Basis for Action." *American Statistician* 29 (4): 146–52.

———. 1995. *Out of the Crisis.* Cambridge, MA: MIT Press.

Donabedian, A. 1980. *Explorations in Quality Assessment and Monitoring. Volume I: The Definition of Quality and Approaches to Its Assessment and Monitoring.* Chicago: Health Administration Press.

———. 1982. *Explorations in Quality Assessment and Monitoring. Volume II: The Criteria and Standards of Quality.* Chicago: Health Administration Press.

Gaucher, E., and R. Coffey. 1993. *Total Quality in Healthcare.* San Francisco: Jossey-Bass.

Hess, I., D. Riedel, and T. Fitzpatrick. 1975. *Probability Sampling of Hospitals and Patients.* Chicago: Health Administration Press.

Institute of Medicine. 2001. *Crossing the Quality Chasm: A New Health System for the 21st Century.* Washington, DC: National Academies Press.

Ishikawa, K. 1982. *Guide to Quality Control.* White Plains, NY: Quality Resources.

The Joint Commission. 1993. *The Measurement Mandate: On the Road to Performance Improvement in Health Care.* Oakbrook Terrace, IL: The Joint Commission.

Langley, G., K. Nolan, T. Nolan, C. Norman, and L. Provost. 1996. *The Improvement Guide.* San Francisco: Jossey-Bass.

Lastrucci, C. 1967. *The Scientific Approach: Basic Principles of the Scientific Method.* Cambridge, MA: Schenkman.

Lloyd, R. 2004. *Quality Health Care: A Guide to Developing and Using Measures.* Sudbury, MA: Jones and Bartlett.

Maddox, B. 1981. "Sampling Concepts, Strategy and Techniques." Technical Report 81-1, July 1. Harrisburg, PA: Pennsylvania Department of Health, State Health Data Center.

Provost, L., and S. Murray. 2007. *The Data Guide*. Austin, TX: Associates in Process Improvement and Corporate Transformation Concepts.

Schultz, L. 1994. *Profiles in Quality*. New York: Quality Resources.

Selltiz, C., M. Jahoda, M. Deutsch, and S. Cook. 1959. *Research Methods in Social Relations*. New York: Holt, Rinehart and Winston.

Western Electric Co. 1985. *Statistical Quality Control Handbook*. Indianapolis, IN: AT&T Technologies.

Wheeler, D. 1993. *Understanding Variation: The Key to Managing Chaos*. Knoxville, TN: SPC Press.

———. 1995. *Advanced Topics in Statistical Process Control*. Knoxville, TN: SPC Press.

Wheeler, D., and D. Chambers. 1992. *Understanding Statistical Process Control*. Knoxville, TN: SPC Press.

DATA COLLECTION

John J. Byrnes

Everywhere you turn, everyone wants data. What do they mean? Where do you find data? Is chart review the gold standard, the best source? Are administrative databases reliable? Can they be the gold standard? What about health plan claim databases—are they accurate? What is the best source for inpatient data that reflect the quality of patient care from both a process and an outcome perspective? When working in the outpatient environment, where and how would you obtain data that reflect the level of quality delivered in physician office practices? These questions challenge many healthcare leaders as they struggle to develop quality improvement and measurement programs. This chapter clarifies these issues and common industry myths and provides a practical framework for obtaining valid, accurate, and useful data for quality improvement work.

Categories of Data

Quality measurements can be grouped into four categories, or domains: clinical quality (including both process and outcome measures), financial performance, patient satisfaction, and functional status. To report on each of these categories, several separate data sources may be required. The challenge is to collect as much data as possible from the fewest sources with the objectives of consistency and continuity in mind. For most large and mature quality improvement projects, teams will want to report their performance in all four domains.

Considerations in Data Collection

The Time and Cost of Data Collection

All data collection efforts take time and money. The key is to balance the cost of data collection and the value of the data to your improvement efforts. In other words, are the cost and time spent collecting data worth the effort? Will the data have the power to drive change and improvement?

Generally, medical record review and prospective data collection are considered the most time-intensive and expensive ways to collect information. Many reserve these methods for highly specialized improvement projects or use them to answer questions that have surfaced following review of administrative data sets. Administrative data[1] are often considered cost-effective, especially since the credibility of administrative databases has improved and continues to improve through the efforts of coding and billing regulations, initiatives,[2] and rule-based software development. Additionally, third-party vendors have emerged that can provide data cleanup and severity adjustment. Successful data collection strategies often combine code- and chart-based sources into a Data collection plan that capitalizes on their respective strengths and cost-effectiveness.

The following example illustrates how an administrative system's cost-effectiveness can be combined with the detailed information in a medical record review. A data analyst, using a clinical decision support system (administrative database), discovered a higher-than-expected incidence of renal failure (a serious complication) following coronary artery bypass surgery. The rate was well above 10 percent for the most recent 12 months (more than 800 patients were included in the data set) and had slowly increased over the last six quarters. However, the clinical decision support system did not contain enough detail to explain whether this complication resulted from the coronary artery bypass graft procedure or was a chronic condition present on admission.

To find the answer, the data analyst used chart review to (1) verify that the rate of renal failure as reported in the administrative data system was correct, (2) isolate cases representing postoperative incidence, (3) identify the root cause(s) of the renal failure, and (4) answer physicians' additional questions about the patient population. In this example, the analyst used the administrative system to identify unwanted complications in a large patient population (a screening or surveillance function) and reserved chart review for a smaller, focused review (80 charts) to validate the incidence and determine why the patients were experiencing the complication. This excellent example shows effective use of two common data sources and demonstrates how the analyst is able to capitalize on the strengths of both while using each most efficiently.

Collecting the Critical Few Rather than Collecting for a Rainy Day

Many quality improvement teams collect all possible data for potential use. Ironically, justification for this approach often is based on time economy—if the chart has been pulled, collection should be thorough; the team may need the data down the road. This syndrome of stockpiling "just in case" versus fulfilling requirements "just in time" has been studied in supply chain management and proven to be ineffective and inefficient; it also creates quality issues (Denison 2002). This approach provides little value to the data collection effort and is one of the biggest mistakes quality improvement teams make. Rather than provide a rich source of information, this approach unnecessarily drives up the cost of data collection, slows the data collection process, creates data management issues, and overwhelms the quality improvement team with too much information.

For all quality improvement projects, teams should collect only the data required to identify and correct quality issues. They should be able to link every data element collected to a report, thereby ensuring that they do not collect useless data (James 2003). In the reporting project discussed above, the hospital team was limited to selecting no more than 15 measures for each clinical condition. It also selected indicators that (1) evidence-based literature has shown to have the greatest effect on patient outcomes (e.g., in congestive heart failure, the use of angiotensin converting enzyme [ACE] inhibitors and beta-blockers, and evaluation of left ventricular ejection fraction); (2) reflect areas where significant improvements are needed; (3) will be reported in the public domain (Joint Commission core measures); and (4) provide a balanced view of the clinical process of care, financial performance, and patient outcomes.

Inpatient Versus Outpatient Data

The distinction between inpatient and outpatient data is an important consideration in planning the data collection process because the data sources and approaches to data collection may be different.

Consider the case of a team working on a diabetes disease management project. Disease management projects tend to focus on the entire continuum of care, so the team first will need to gather data from both inpatient and outpatient settings. Next, the team will need to identify whether patients receive the majority of care in one setting or the other and decide whether data collection priorities should be established with this setting in mind. For diabetes, the outpatient setting has the most influence on patient outcomes, so collection of outpatient data should be a priority. Third, the team must select the measures that reflect the aspects of care that have the most influence on patient outcomes. Remembering to collect the critical few, the team should consult the American Diabetes Association (ADA) guidelines for expert direction. Finally, the team must recognize that the sources of outpatient data are different than the sources of inpatient data, and they tend to be more fragmented and harder to obtain.

To identify outpatient data sources, the team should consider the following questions.

- Are the physicians in organized medical groups that have outpatient electronic medical records, which could be a source of data? Will their financial or billing systems be able to identify all patients with diabetes in their practices? If not, can the health plans in the area supply the data by practice site or individual physician?

- Some of the most important diabetes measures are based on laboratory testing. Do the physicians have their own labs? If so, do they archive the laboratory data for a 12- to 24-month snapshot? If they do not do their own lab testing, do they use a common reference lab that would be able to supply the data?

Sources of Data

The sources of data for quality improvement projects are numerous. Some sources are simple to access, and others are more complex. Some are more expensive. In the average hospital or health system, data sources include medical records, prospective data collection, surveys of various types, telephone interviews, focus groups, administrative databases, health plan claim databases, cost accounting systems, patient registries, stand-alone clinical databases, and lab and pharmacy databases.

The following objectives are essential to a successful quality improvement project and data collection initiative.

1. Identify the purpose of the data measurement activity (for monitoring at regular intervals, investigation over a limited period, or onetime study).
2. Identify the most appropriate data sources.
3. Identify the most important measures for collection (the critical few).
4. Design a commonsense data collection strategy that will provide complete, accurate, and timely information.

Together, these objectives will provide the team with the information required to drive quality improvements.

Medical Record Review (Retrospective)

Retrospective data collection involves identification and selection of a patient's medical record or group of records after the patient has been discharged from the hospital or clinic. Review generally cannot occur until all medical and financial coding functions are complete because these coded criteria are used as a starting point to identify the study cohort. For several reasons, many quality improvement projects depend on medical record review for data collection.

Many proponents of medical record review believe it to be the most accurate method of data collection. They believe that because administrative databases have been designed for financial and administrative purposes rather than quality improvement, they contain inadequate detail, many errors, and "dirty data"—that is, data that make no sense or appear to have come from other sources.

Some database projects rely on medical record review because many of the data are not available in administrative databases. Measures that require a time stamp, such as administration of antibiotics within one hour before surgical incision, are an example of data not available in administrative databases.

Several national quality improvement database projects, including HEDIS, Joint Commission core measures, Leapfrog,[3] and the National Quality Forum's (NQF) Voluntary Consensus Standards for Hospital Care, depend on retrospective medical record review for a significant portion of required data. The records contain not only measures requiring a time stamp but, for some measures, also require the data collector to include or exclude patients on the basis of criteria that administrative databases do not capture consistently.

The percentage of patients with congestive heart failure who are receiving an ACE inhibitor is an example of this type of measure. The use of ACE inhibitors in this population is indicated for all patients with an ejection fraction of less than 40 percent. The ejection fraction is not part of the typical administrative database. Sometimes this information is contained in a stand-alone database in the cardiology department and is generally inaccessible, or it may be contained only in a transcribed report in the patient's medical record. Hence, accurate reporting of this measure, one of the most critical interventions that a patient with congestive heart failure will receive, depends completely on retrospective chart review.

A recent consensus document presented to NQF[4] suggested that clinical importance should rate foremost among criteria for effectiveness and that measures that score poorly on feasibility[5] because of the burden of medical record review should not be excluded solely on that basis if their clinical importance is high (NQF Consumer, Purchaser, and Research Council Members 2002).

Medical record review continues to be a key component of many data collection projects, but it needs to be used judiciously because of the time and cost involved. The approach to medical record review involves a series of well-conceived steps, beginning with the development of a data collection tool and ending with the compilation of collected data elements into a registry or electronic database software for review and analysis.

Prospective Data Collection, Data Collection Forms, and Scanners

Prospective data collection also relies on medical record review, but it is completed during a patient's hospitalization or visit rather than retrospectively. Nursing staff, dedicated research assistants, or full-time data analysts commonly collect the data. The downside to asking nursing staff to perform data collection is that it is a time-consuming task that can distract nurses from their direct patient care responsibilities. A better approach would be to hire research assistants or full-time data analysts who can perform the data collection and be responsible for data entry and analysis. Because this job is their sole responsibility, the accuracy of data collection is greater. If the staff also is responsible for presenting its work to various quality committees, it is likely to review the data more rigorously.

Obviously, this method of data collection is expensive, but if staff can minimize the time required for data entry, it can focus on accurate collection and the analysis/reporting functions. Converting the data collection forms into a format that can be scanned is one way to save time. With this approach, data entry can be as simple as feeding the forms into the scanner and viewing the results on the computer screen. Successful execution hinges on careful design of the forms and careful completion to ensure that the scanner captures all the data.

The most efficient data collection tools follow the actual flow of patient care and medical record documentation, whether the data are collected retrospectively or prospectively. There are numerous advantages to prospective data collection. Detailed information not routinely available in administrative databases can be gathered. Physiologic parameters can be captured, such as the range of blood pressures for a patient on vasoactive infusions or 24-hour intake and output for patients with heart failure. Data requiring a time stamp also can be captured. Timely administration of certain therapies (e.g., antibiotic administration within one hour before surgical incision or within four hours of hospital arrival for patients with pneumonia) has shown to improve patient outcomes. Certain stroke patients' chance of recovery depends on the timing of "clot buster" administration, which in general must occur within three hours of symptom onset. For patients with acute myocardial infarction, the administration of aspirin and beta-blockers within the first 24 hours is critical to survival.

Through prospective chart review, the data collection staff can spot patient trends as they develop rather than receive the information after the patients have been discharged. For instance, the staff may detect an increasing incidence of ventilator-associated pneumonia sooner, or it may spot an increase in the rate of aspiration in stroke patients as it occurs.

Unfortunately, the downside to this data collection approach is cost. Prospective data collection is very costly and time consuming, and it often requires several full-time data analysts.

Administrative Databases

Administrative databases are a common source of data for quality improvement projects. *Administrative data* are information collected, processed, and stored in automated information systems. These data include enrollment or eligibility information, claims information, and managed care encounters. The claims and encounters may be for hospital and other facility services, professional services, prescription drug services, or laboratory services.

Examples of administrative data sources are hospital or physician office billing systems, health plan claim databases, health information management or medical record systems, and registration systems (admission/discharge/transfer). Ideally, a hospital also maintains a cost accounting system that integrates these systems into one database and provides the important data on patient cost. Although each of these sources has its unique characteristics, for the purposes of discussion they will be considered collectively as administrative databases (with the exception of health plan claim databases, which will be covered later in the chapter).

Administrative databases are an excellent source of data for reporting on clinical quality, financial performance, and certain patient outcomes. Use of administrative databases is advantageous for the following reasons.

1. They are a less expensive source of data than other alternatives such as chart review or prospective data collection.
2. They incorporate transaction systems already used in the daily business operations of a healthcare organization (frequently referred to as *legacy systems*).
3. Most of the code sets embedded in administrative databases are standardized,[6] simplifying internal comparison between multi-facility organizations and external benchmarking with purchased or government data sets.
4. Most administrative databases are staffed by individuals who are skilled at sophisticated database queries.
5. Expert database administrators in information technology departments provide database architecture and support.
6. The volume of available indicators is 100 times greater than that available through other data collection techniques.
7. Data reporting tools are available as part of the purchased system or through third-party add-ons or services.
8. Many administrative databases, especially well-managed financial and cost accounting systems, are subject to regular reconciliation, audit, and data cleanup procedures that enhance the integrity of their data.

Consider Spectrum Health's clinical reporting (CR) system, which uses two administrative data systems as the primary source of data for quality improvement projects: the billing system and the medical record system. It extracts information from these sources and subjects it to an extensive data cleanup. It also adjusts for severity, applies statistical analysis, and compares to benchmarks. Spectrum Health updates the database monthly and archives historical data in its data warehouse for future quality improvement projects and clinical studies.

The yearly cost to maintain this system for three of Spectrum Health's hospitals is approximately equal to the combined salaries of four to five data analysts, yet the system's reporting power surpasses anything that five analysts performing chart review could accomplish. This system is a good value proposition because successful implementation of one or two quality improvement projects carefully selected from the many opportunities identified by the system can reimburse its full cost. One of the first projects identified by the system was the need to improve blood product utilization in total joint replacements to avoid wasting money by cross-matching blood that is never used. The savings realized as a result of this project more than covered the cost of the system for the first year.

Some argue that administrative data are less reliable than data gathered by chart review (Iezzoni et al. 1994). However, administrative data can be just as reliable as data from chart review when they are properly cleaned and validated, the indicator definitions are clear and concise, and the limitations of the data are understood. For example, the most common measures from the CR system were validated using four approaches: (1) chart review using an appropriate sampling methodology, (2) chart review performed for the Joint Commission core measures, (3) comparison to similar measures in stand-alone databases that rely on chart abstraction or prospective data collection strategies (e.g., National Registry of Myocardial Infarction), and (4) face validation performed by physicians with expertise in the clinical condition being studied. Results proved the administrative data sources to be just as reliable.

Patient Surveys: Satisfaction and Functional Status

Patient Satisfaction Surveys

Patient satisfaction surveys are a favorite tool of quality improvement professionals, especially teams interested in the perceptions of patients, either in terms of the quality of care or the quality of service provided. However, underestimation of the scientific complexity underlying survey research often leads to undesirable results. There is an art (and science) to constructing surveys that produce valid, reliable, relevant information. Likewise, survey validation itself is a time-consuming and complex undertaking.

A quality improvement team can design the survey itself, hire an outside expert to design the survey, or purchase an existing, well-validated survey or survey service. Usually, the fastest and least expensive approach is to purchase existing, well-validated survey instruments or to hire a survey organization to provide a solution. Press Ganey is one such organization.[7]

The frequency with which surveys are conducted and reported to the organization is also important. When patient satisfaction surveys are conducted on a continual basis using a proper sampling methodology, the organization has the ability to respond rapidly to changes in patients' wants and needs. It also has the ability to respond rapidly to emerging breaks in service.

The ability to report survey results at an actionable level is critical; in most cases, *actionable level* means the nursing unit or location of service. Furthermore, full engagement at the management and staff levels is important to ensure that results are regularly reviewed and action plans are developed.

One of the most successful patient satisfaction survey projects was the "Point of Service Patient Satisfaction Surveys" at Lovelace Health Systems in the late 1990s. In that program, any patient who received care within the system could comment on the quality of the care and service he or she experienced. The survey forms were short (one page), concise, and easy to read, and patients could complete them in a few minutes. The questions assessed the most important determinants of satisfaction (as selected by the survey research staff), and patients could provide comments at the end of the survey. The unit manager collected and reviewed the surveys on a daily or weekly basis to identify emerging trends and quickly correct negative outcomes. Survey results were tabulated monthly and posted in all units where everyone could see them, including patients who visited the clinics and inpatient areas. Senior management also reviewed the results on a unit-by-unit basis each month.

Functional Status Surveys

In general, the purpose of medical treatments and hospital procedures is to improve patients' functional status or quality of life. For example, patients hospitalized for congestive heart failure should be able to walk farther, have more energy, and experience less shortness of breath following hospital treatment. Patients who undergo total knee replacements should have less knee pain when they walk; have a good range of joint motion; and be able to perform activities of daily living such as walking, doing yard work, and performing normal household chores.

Functional status usually is measured before and at several points following the treatment or procedure. For some surgical procedures, such as total joint replacement, a baseline assessment commonly is made before the procedure, and then assessments are made at regular intervals following surgery, often at 1, 3, 6, and 12 months postoperative. The survey can be collected by several means, including mail, telephone, and Internet.

Health Plan Databases

Health plan databases are an excellent source of data for quality improvement projects, particularly projects that have a population health management focus. For many years, health plans have used a variety of means to collect data on their performance, track the management of the care received by their members, and direct programs in disease management and care management. Because of this experience, health plan data have become more and more reliable. Most health plans now have sophisticated data warehouses and a staff of expert data analysts.

Health plan databases are valuable because they contain detailed information on all care received by health plan members. They track care through bills (claims). Bills are generated for all services provided to a patient. When the bill is submitted to the health plan for payment, it is captured in a claim-processing system. As a result of this process, all care received by a population of patients, including hospitalizations, outpatient procedures, physician office visits, lab testing, and prescriptions, is documented in the health plan claim database.

Why is this process so important? From a population management perspective, the health plan claim database is often the only source for all information on the care received by a patient as well as populations of patients. It provides a comprehensive record of patient activity and can be used to identify and select patients for enrollment in disease management programs. Claim databases are excellent tracking tools for examining the continuum of care and are the only available external source of information on physician office practice.

Health plan databases commonly are used to identify patients who have not received preventive services such as mammograms, colon cancer screening, and immunizations. They can identify patients who are not receiving the appropriate medications for many chronic medical conditions, such as heart failure or asthma. They also can be used to support physicians in their office practices. Figure 6.1 is an example of a report developed at Spectrum Health[8] for a systemwide diabetes disease management program. It provides participating physicians with a quarterly snapshot of (1) the percentage of their patients who are receiving all treatments and tests recommended by ADA guidelines, (2) how the physician's performance compares to the performance of his or her peers, and (3) all patients whose treatment has not met ADA standards in the last quarter and who need recommended tests or treatments.

What are the limitations of health plan databases? As with hospital administrative databases, considerations include accuracy, detail, and timeliness. Users of health plan claim databases also must keep in mind that changes in reimbursement rules (and the provider's response to those changes) may affect the integrity of the data over time. Recoding may make some historical data inaccurate, especially as they relate to tracking and trending of complication rates and the categorization of certain types of complications. Finally, health plan databases track events, the type of procedure performed, or completion of a lab test. They do not contain detailed information on the outcomes of care or the results of tests (e.g., lab tests, radiology examinations, biopsies). Nevertheless, health plan claim data are inexpensive to acquire, are available electronically, and encompass large populations across the continuum of care. Used properly, they are a rich source of data for population management, disease management, and quality improvement projects.

FIGURE 6.1

Diabetes
Provider
Support
Report

Rolling Calendar Year July 1, 2001–June 30, 2002   PCP:
Provider Group:

I. Provider-Specific Data

Criteria	ADA Standards	Points	Tested	In Standard	Percentage
Education	1 / 2 year	48	42	42	88
Eye exams	Annual	48	30	30	63
Hemoglobin A,C ordered	Annual	48	45	45	94
Hemoglobin A,C level	≤7.0	48	45	37	82
Microalbumin ordered	Annual	48	31	31	65
Microalbumin >30	Rx filled	10	10	5	50
LDL ordered	Annual	48	42	42	88
LDL level	<100	48	42	31	73

* Patients in this report have had at least two diagnoses of diabetes.

II. Percentage of Patients Within Standard

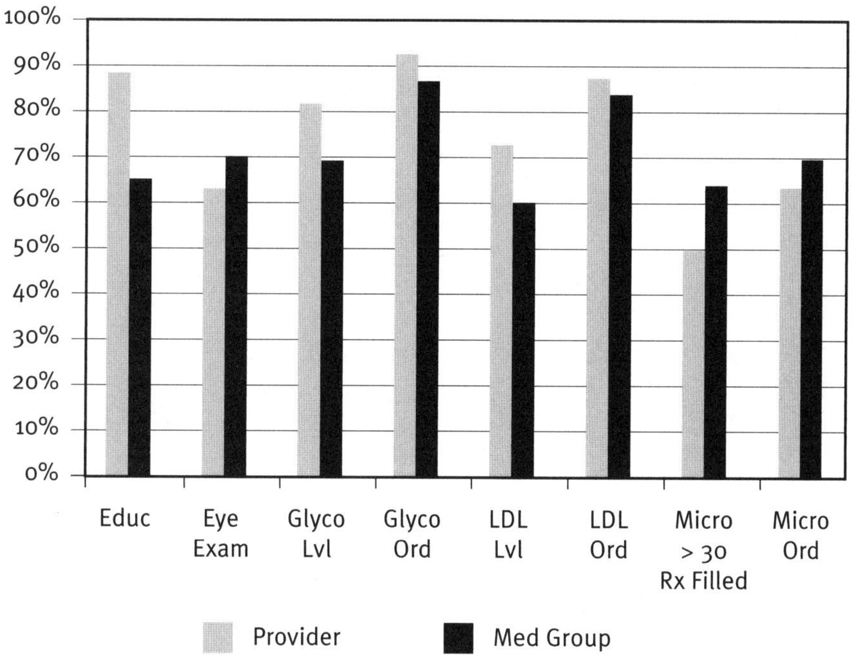

(continued)

FIGURE 6.1
(continued)

III. High-Risk Patient Detail—Patients Outside ADA Standards in Current Quarter

Criteria for inclusion—one or more of the following: (1) no education in last two years; (2) no eye exam in last one year; (3) Hemoglobin A,C > 7.0 or no Hemoglobin A,C ordered in last year; (4) no microalbumin in last one year; (5) microalbumin > 30 and no ACE/ARB filled; or (6) LDL ≥ 100 or no LDL ordered in last year.

Name	MR No.	Education	Eye Exam	Hemoglobin Ordered	Hemoglobin Level	Microalbumin Ordered	Microalbumin > 30, Rx Filled	Lipids Ordered	Lipids Result
Patient	100-319-xxx		7/21/99	7/15/99	6.7	5/28/99	N	2/29/00	120
Patient	100-427-xxx					2/22/00		2/22/00	118
Patient	100-587-xxx								
Patient	100-595-xxx	8/12/99		8/21/99	7.0				
Patient	100-623-xxx			2/2/00	10.8			1/21/00	142
Patient	100-666-xxx	7/14/99		12/15/99	10.7				
Patient	100-782-xxx	2/12/00		11/27/99	11.0				
Patient	100-847-xxx	2/12/00		3/12/99	7.0				
Patient	100-849-xxx	12/27/99		8/1/99	6.1			5/24/99	118
Patient	100-882-xxx	10/15/98		8/31/99	6.8			3/21/00	132
Patient	100-882-xxx	4/25/99		4/23/00	6.3				
Patient	100-893-xxx	7/31/98		9/19/99	12.4			8/25/99	123
Patient	100-901-xxx	6/15/99		6/2/00	6.3				
Patient	100-901-xxx	1/15/00		1/23/00	12.0			9/19/99	98
Patient	100-902-xxx	1/18/00		5/15/99	12.4			7/31/99	92
Patient	100-909-xxx							2/15/00	145
Patient	100-914-xxx	12/27/99		10/10/99	11.9			10/6/99	150
Patient	100-914-xxx			2/4/00	10.8			4/14/00	92
Patient	100-919-xxx			4/29/00	6.2			6/1/00	89
Patient	100-809-xxx	6/13/00	6/15/00	6/2/00	6.9	4/2/00		2/11/00	126
Patient	100-914-xxx	1/15/00	12/20/99	12/12/99	11.2	12/12/99	N	1/16/00	132
Patient	100-917-xxx	1/18/00	2/13/00	1/18/00	6.9	1/15/00	N	11/21/99	160
Patient	100-929-xxx	7/22/99	8/1/99	7/21/99	10.0	7/21/99	N	12/5/99	98

NOTE: ADA = American Diabetes Association.
SOURCE: Spectrum Health, Grand Rapids, MI. Copyright 2008 Spectrum Health. Used with permission.

Patient Registries

Many organizations establish condition-specific patient registries for their more sophisticated quality improvement projects because they do not have a reliable source of clinical information, available data are not timely, or they wish to collect patient outcome information over several months following a hospitalization or procedure. Often, development of a patient registry involves all of the above considerations, and the registry includes data collected through all of the aforementioned approaches.

Because of their detail and straightforward design, patient registries are a powerful source of quality improvement data. Registries usually are specialty or procedure specific. Acute myocardial infarction, total joint replacement, coronary artery bypass graft, and congestive heart failure are common examples of procedure- or condition-specific registries.

The use of patient registries is advantageous for the following reasons.

1. They are a rich source of information because they are customized.
2. They can collect all the data that the physician or health system determines are most important.
3. They can be used for quality improvement and research purposes.
4. They are not subject to the shortcomings of administrative or health plan databases.
5. Myriad data sources and collection techniques can be combined to provide a complete picture of the patient experience, including the quality of care provided and long-term patient outcomes (often up to a year following the procedure).

Patient registries are versatile and flexible because just about any reliable data source or collection methodology can be used to populate the registry, including administrative data, outbound call centers, prospective data collection, retrospective chart review, and a variety of survey instruments, particularly for patient satisfaction and functional status. However, with all customized database projects, the volume of data collected and the insight they will provide or the change they will drive must be weighed against the cost of the data collection. A team overseeing a registry project must collect only data necessary to the success of its project.

Consider the use of an orthopedic patient registry. First, a team including a service line director, a medical director, and physicians was established to oversee the project. The inclusion of physicians from the beginning created a tremendous level of physician involvement, to the point that the physicians felt great pride of ownership in the project. Second, the scope of data collection was narrowed to focus on only total knee and hip replacements. Third, the purpose and use of the registry were clearly outlined; its function was limited to identifying clinical issues and improving the quality of patient care. Fourth, the number of data elements was

TABLE 6.1
Orthopedic
Patient
Registry Data
Elements

Orthopedic Database Characteristics

Total data elements	329
Manual data elements	216
Electronic data elements	113
No. of patients (monthly)	106
Data sources	
• Patient	
• Case managers	
• OR system	
• Billing/cost accounting system	
• Call center	

Number of Data Elements by Category

Patient history	32
Demographic	56
Functional status	42
Procedures/OR	26
Complications	3
Devices/equipment	13
Postoperative	45
Follow-up	28 (× 4) = 112

Number of Data Elements by Source

Patient	35
Case manager	69
OR system	48
Billing/cost accounting system	65
Call center	112

SOURCE: Spectrum Health, Grand Rapids, MI. Copyright 2008 Spectrum Health. Used with permission.

restricted to the critical few—elements most important to assessing patient outcomes and the integrity of the patient care processes—which meant the team would report and review them regularly.

Data collection was accomplished through several means, as illustrated in Table 6.1 and Figure 6.2. Patients were identified through the administrative database. Data collection was completed prospectively during the hospitalization, and missing data were captured by retrospective chart review. To ease the data-entry burden, all data were collected on forms that could be scanned. The outbound call center tracked outcomes over time through a variety of patient interview tools and survey instruments, making calls 1, 3, 6, and 12 months after the primary procedure. Ultimately, the data were combined in a database product available to all and audited for completeness and accuracy.

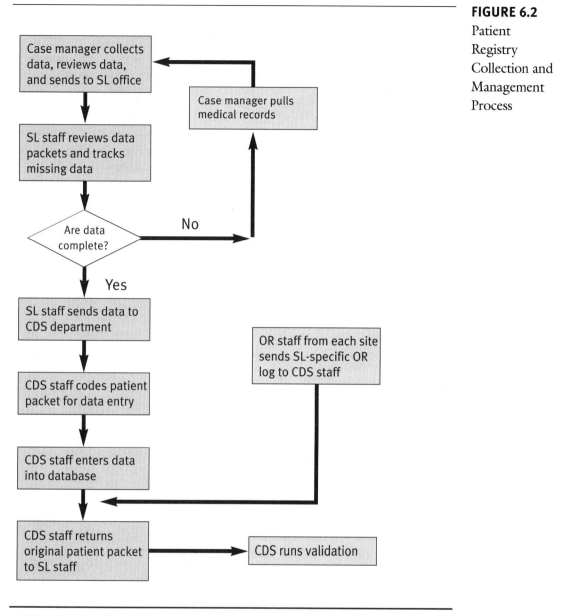

FIGURE 6.2
Patient
Registry
Collection and
Management
Process

NOTE: CDS = clinical decision support; OR = operating room; SL = service line.

Case Study in Clinical Reporting

Spectrum Health's CR system contains many disease-specific dashboards (see Table 6.2) that report performance at the system, hospital, and physician levels. Figure 6.3, a dashboard for total hip replacement, provides examples of clinical quality and financial performance measures. In addition

TABLE 6.2

Clinical Reporting System— Available Disease and Project Reports

1. Chest pain	29. Pediatric asthma
2. Heart attack	30. Very low birth weight neonates
3. PCI	31. Pediatric appendectomy
4. Heart failure	32. RSV/bronchiolitis
5. Pneumonia	33. Pediatric chemotherapy
6. Normal delivery	34. Pediatric VP shunts
7. C-section	35. Pediatric hospitalist conditions
8. Bypass surgery	a. Bronchitis and asthma
9. Valve surgery	b. Esophagitis and
10. Stroke—ischemic	gastroenteritis
11. Total hip replacement	c. Kidney and UTI
12. Total knee replacement	d. Nutritional and
13. Hip fracture	miscellaneous metabolic
14. Abd. hysterectomy—non-CA	disorders
15. Abd. hysterectomy—CA	e. Otitis media and URI
16. Lap hysterectomy	f. Pediatric pneumonia
17. Cholecystectomy—lap	g. Seizure and headache
18. Cholecystectomy—open	h. Fever of unknown origin
19. Lumbar fusion	36. NICU, PICU, and adult ICU
20. Lumbar laminectomy	(medical, surgical, and burn)
21. Bariatric surgery	37. AHRQ patient safety indicators
22. Colon resection	38. Pain management
23. Diabetes and glycemic control	39. Sickle cell
24. DVT	40. Sepsis
25. COPD	41. 100,000 Lives Campaign
26. Upper GI bleed	42. 5 Million Lives Campaign
27. SCIP	43. National patient safety goals
28. Peripheral vascular procedures	44. Rapid response team

to the dashboard's spreadsheet-like display, the CR system shows trends for each measure over the last 24 months (see Figure 6.4).

To produce the CR system, Spectrum Health used a variety of data sources, including extracts from the finance and medical record systems. The decision support department processed the data by applying a series of rigorous data cleanup algorithms, adjusting for severity, and adding industry benchmarks. The resulting report contained measures of clinical processes (antibiotic utilization, deep vein thrombosis [DVT] prophylaxis, beta-blocker administration, autologous blood collection, and blood product administration), financial performance (length of stay, total patient charges, pharmacy charges, lab charges, X-ray charges, and IV therapy charges), and clinical outcomes (DVT, acute myocardial infarction, and readmission within 31 days). From more than 200 indicators available in the database, the total joint quality improvement team selected these measures as the most important in assessing the quality and cost of care delivered. The measures also included some Joint Commission core measures.[9]

FIGURE 6.3

Clinical
Dashboard—
Hip
Replacement

Spectrum Health — Clinical Outcomes Report (COR)–**Hip Replacement**

March 1, 2006 to February 28, 2007

Administrative Data — Process

Name	No. of patients	1st gen. Ceph	Vancomycin	Coumadin	Heparin	Low mol. wt. heparin	Coumadin or LMW heparin	Beta blocker	Autologous blood coll.	Blood prod. given	DVT prophylaxis*	Hip revision
BL	617	95.5%	9.9%	14.6%	23.0%	91.2%	96.6%	39.9%	1.8%	33.2%	99.7%	20.4%
BW	136	90.4%	11.8%	5.9%	5.1%	100.0%	100.0%	41.9%	4.4%	30.9%	100.0%	13.2%
SH-GR	753	94.6%	10.2%	13.0%	19.8%	92.8%	97.2%	40.2%	2.3%	32.8%	99.7%	19.1%

Administrative Data — Outcome | Education

Name	No. of patients	DVT	AccPuncLac	Any 30 days	readmit 2nd DX	AMI Los	Education participation rate*
BL	617	0.6%	0.0%	4.2%	0.0%	3.67	59.3%
BW	136	0.0%	0.0%	4.4%	0.7%	3.78	
SH-GR	753	0.5%	0.0%	4.2%	0.1%	3.69	

** The education rate reflects all total joint replacement patients who had their surgery within the time period stated on this dashboard.

JCAHO SCIP — JCAHO Surgical Care Improvement Project

Name	No. of patients	Preop dose (SCIP-INF-1)*		Antibiotic Selection (SCIP-INF-2)		Postop duration (SCIP-INF-3)*	
SH-GR	Varies	96.0%	n = 75	100.0%	n = 76	97.2%	n = 72

Administrative Data — Direct Costs

Name	No. of patients	ICU cost	Laboratory cost	OR cost	Pharmacy cost	Radiology cost	R&B cost	Supplies cost	Therapy cost	Other cost	Total cost
BL	617	$71	$180	$2,219	$384	$79	$1,460	$1,944	$394	$217	$6,948
BW	136	$101	$127	$1,140	$405	$101	$1,801	$5,062	$389	$285	$9,410
SH-GR	753	$76	$170	$2,024	$388	$83	$1,521	$2,507	$393	$230	$7,393

Administrative Data — Fully Allocated Costs

Name	No. of patients	ICU cost	Laboratory cost	OR cost	Pharmacy cost	Radiology cost	R&B cost	Supplies cost	Therapy cost	Other cost	Total cost
BL	617	$117	$251	$3,711	$492	$162	$3,020	$2,078	$559	$326	$10,715
BW	136	$189	$176	$2,279	$515	$171	$3,215	$5,263	$578	$416	$12,802
SH-GR	753	$130	$237	$3,452	$496	$163	$3,055	$2,653	$562	$342	$11,092

Administrative Data — Potential Direct Cost Savings

Name	No. of patients	DVT		AccPuncLac		AMI 2nd DX		Total cost (Patients above average)	
BL	Varies	$51,618	n = 4	$0	n = 0	$0	n = 0	$679,916	n = 189
BW	Varies	$0	n = 0	$0	n = 0	$9,653	n = 1	$165,825	n = 61
SH-GR	Varies	$49,770	n = 4	$0	n = 0	$11,614	n = 1	$920,655	n = 270

* Denotes indicators selected for "The Joint Commission"

Prepared June 10, 2007 by the Spectrum Health Quality Department.

To obtain patient satisfaction information, the team used the hospital's patient satisfaction surveys. The outbound call center administered these surveys by telephone within one week of a patient's discharge. The results were reported by nursing unit or physician, updated monthly, and charted over the last six to eight quarters.

To complete the measurement set, the team included the results of patients' functional status (following their treatments). A patient who underwent a total knee replacement, for example, should have experienced less knee pain when he or she walked, should have had a good range of joint motion, and should have been able to perform the activities of daily living. For this report, the team examined the patient's functional status before and after hospitalization to demonstrate the treatments were effective.

In summary, data collection in all four categories—clinical quality, financial performance, patient satisfaction, and functional status—is important to maintain a balanced perspective of the process of care. Quality

FIGURE 6.4

Clinical Report: Example of Trended Data Over 24 Months

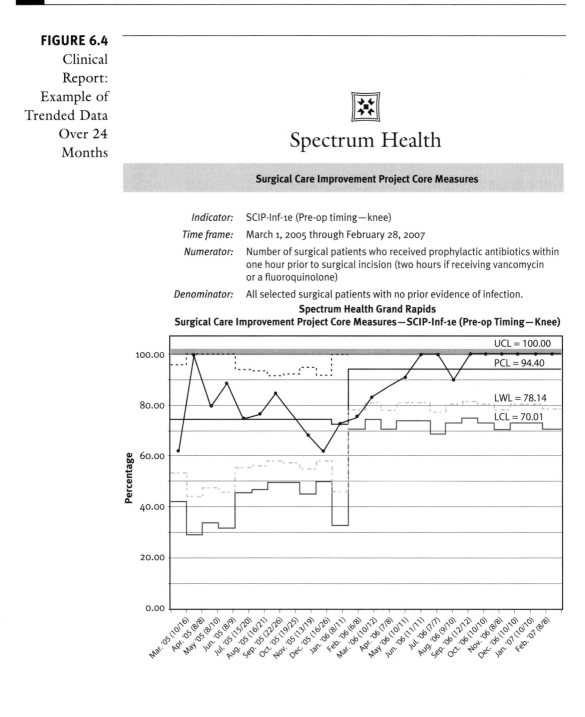

Spectrum Health

Surgical Care Improvement Project Core Measures

Indicator: SCIP-Inf-1e (Pre-op timing—knee)

Time frame: March 1, 2005 through February 28, 2007

Numerator: Number of surgical patients who received prophylactic antibiotics within one hour prior to surgical incision (two hours if receiving vancomycin or a fluoroquinolone)

Denominator: All selected surgical patients with no prior evidence of infection.

Spectrum Health Grand Rapids
Surgical Care Improvement Project Core Measures—SCIP-Inf-1e (Pre-op Timing—Knee)

improvement teams that fail to maintain this balance may experience surprising results. For instance, a health system in the Southwest initially reported on a series of successful quality improvement projects—clinical care had improved, patient satisfaction was at an all-time high, and patient outcomes were at national benchmark levels. However, subsequent review of the projects identified that some of the interventions had a negative effect on financial outcomes. Several interventions significantly decreased revenue, and others increased the cost of care. If financial measures had been included in the reporting process, the negative financial effect could have been minimized and the same outstanding quality improvements would have resulted. In the end, the projects were considered only marginally successful because they lacked a balanced approach to process improvement and measurement.

Conclusion

There are many data sources and data collection approaches from which to choose. Rarely does one method serve all purposes, so it is important to understand the advantages and disadvantages of all methods. For this reason, the case above, like all successful quality improvement initiatives, uses a combination of data and data collection techniques, capitalizing on strengths and minimizing weaknesses. Knowledge of the different sources and techniques will help you to use data more effectively and efficiently in your clinical quality improvement efforts.

Study Questions

1. What are notable advantages and disadvantages of the use of medical records versus administrative sources for collecting quality data?
2. Give two examples of areas in which you can identify a balanced set of measures.
3. Will electronic medical records improve data collection? Why or why not?

Acknowledgments

Special thanks go to Lori Anderson for her diligent review, suggestions, and contributions, as well as to Monica Carpenter for her editorial assistance.

Notes

1. Administrative data generally reflect the content of discharge abstracts (e.g., demographic information on patients such as age, sex, and zip code; information about the episode of care such as admission source, length of stay, charges, and discharge status; diagnostic and procedural codes). The Uniform Hospital Discharge Data Set and the Uniform Bill (UB-92) of the Centers for Medicare & Medicaid Services (CMS), formerly known as the Health Care Financing Administration (HCFA), provide specifications for the abstraction of administrative/billing data.

2. Examples include the Health Insurance Portability and Accountability Act (HIPAA) of 1996 (Public Law 104-191); International Classification of Diseases, Ninth Revision (ICD-9), developed by the World Health Organization (WHO) and transitioned to ICD-10-CM; Systematized Nomenclature of Medicine (SNOMED) project; and Unified Medical Language System (UMLS).

3. The Leapfrog Group is a coalition of more than 140 public and private organizations that provide healthcare benefits. It was created to help save lives and reduce preventable medical mistakes by mobilizing employer purchasing power to initiate breakthrough improvements in the safety of healthcare and by giving consumers information to make more informed hospital choices.

4. NQF is a private, not-for-profit membership organization that was created to develop and implement a national strategy for healthcare quality measurement and reporting. Its mission is to improve U.S. healthcare through endorsement of consensus-based national standards for measurement and public reporting of healthcare performance data that provide meaningful information about whether care is safe, timely, beneficial, patient centered, equitable, and efficient.

5. Feasibility implies that the cost of data collection and reporting is justified by the potential improvements in care and outcomes that result from the act of measurement.

6. The Uniform Hospital Discharge Data Set and UB-92 standardize the abstraction of administrative/billing data, including admission source, charges (national revenue codes), discharge status, and diagnostic and procedural codes (ICD-9, CPT-4, NCD, and HCPCS).

7. For more information, see www.pressganey.com.

8. This report was developed as part of a systemwide Spectrum Health Diabetes Collaborative. Lovelace Health System developed the original design in Albuquerque, New Mexico, as part of the Episode of Care Disease Management Program.

9. Creation of the Joint Commission core measures was an initial attempt to integrate outcomes and other performance measurement into the

accreditation process by requiring hospitals to collect and submit 25 measures distributed across five core measurement areas.

References

Denison, D. C. 2002. "On the Supply Chain, Just-in-Time Enters New Era." *Boston Globe,* May 5.

Iezzoni, L. I., J. Daley, T. Heeren, S. M. Foley, J. S. Hughes, E. S. Fisher, C. C. Duncan, and G. A. Coffman. 1994. "Using Administrative Data to Screen Hospitals for High Complication Risk." *Inquiry* 31 (1): 40–55.

James, B. 2003. *Designing Data Systems. Advanced Training Program in Health Care Delivery Research.* Salt Lake City, UT: Intermountain Healthcare.

National Quality Forum Consumer, Purchaser, and Research Council Members. 2002. "Hospital Performance Measurement Project. Proposal to NQF." Washington, DC: National Quality Forum.

Suggested Reading

American Governance and Leadership Group, LLC. 2001. "The Leader's Perspective: Concepts, Tools and Techniques in Opportunity Analysis." *Disease Management & Quality Improvement Report* 1 (6).

Anderson, L. 2001a. "Using Administrative Data for Quality Improvement." Paper presented at the Second Annual Symposium on Disease Management, American Governance and Leadership Group, La Jolla, CA, May 7–8.

———. 2001b. "A Revolutionary Advance in Disease Management: Combining the Power of Disease Management Programs, Evidence Based Medicine, Electronic Medical Records, and Outcome Reporting Systems to Drive Quality in Health Care." *Disease Management & Quality Improvement Report* 1 (1): 1–9.

Byrnes, J. J., and L. B. Anderson. 2001. "Hardwiring Quality Improvement into the Core of Our Business by Emulating the Financial Model of Accountability and Reporting." *Disease Management & Quality Improvement Report* 1 (4): 1–8.

Carey, R. G., and R. C. Lloyd. 2001. *Measuring Quality Improvement in Healthcare: A Guide to Statistical Process Control Applications.* Milwaukee, WI: ASQ Quality Press.

Eddy, D. M. 1998. "Performance Measurement: Problems and Solutions." *Health Affairs (Millwood)* 17 (4): 7–25.

Fuller, S. 1998. "Practice Brief: Designing a Data Collection Process." *Journal of the American Health Information Management Association* 70 (May): 12–16.

Gunter, M., J. Byrnes, M. Shainline, and J. Lucas. 1996. "Improving Outcomes Through Disease Specific Clinical Practice Improvement Teams: The Lovelace Episodes of Care Disease Management Program." *Journal of Outcomes Management* 3 (3): 10–17.

Iz, P. H., J. Warren, and L. Sokol. 2001. "Data Mining for Healthcare Quality, Efficiency, and Practice Support." Paper presented at the 34th Annual Hawaii International Conference on System Sciences, Wailea, HI, January 3–6.

The Joint Commission. 2003. *2003 Hospital Accreditation Standards.* Oakbrook Terrace, IL: The Joint Commission.

Lucas, J., M. J. Gunter, J. Byrnes, M. Coyle, and N. Friedman. 1995. "Integrating Outcomes Measurement into Clinical Practice Improvement Across the Continuum of Care: A Disease-Specific EPISODES OF CARE Model." *Managed Care Quarterly* 3 (2): 14–22.

Micheletti, J. A., T. J. Shlala, and C. R. Goodall. 1998. "Evaluating Performance Outcomes Measurement Systems: Concerns and Considerations." *Journal of Healthcare Quality* 20 (2): 6–12.

Mulder, C., M. Mycyk, and A. Roberts. 2003. "Data Warehousing and More." *Healthcare Informatics* 1 (March): 6–8.

Reader, L. 2001. "Applications of Computerized Dynamic Health Assessments: The Move from Generic to Specific." *Disease Management & Quality Improvement Report* 1 (8).

STATISTICAL TOOLS FOR QUALITY IMPROVEMENT[1]

Stephen Schmaltz, Jerod M. Loeb, Linda S. Hanold, and Richard G. Koss

Fundamentals of Performance Measurement

Purpose of Measurement

Organizations measure performance to meet multiple internal and external needs and demands. Internal quality improvement literature identifies three fundamental purposes for conducting performance measurement: (1) assessment of current performance; (2) demonstration and verification of performance improvement; and (3) control of performance.

These purposes are designed to complement and support internal performance improvement activities. The first step in a structured performance improvement project is to assess current performance. This assessment helps identify the strengths and weaknesses of the current process, thus identifying areas for intervention. It also provides the baseline data against which the organization will compare future measurement data after it has implemented interventions. The comparison of post-intervention measurement data to baseline data will demonstrate and verify whether the intervention brought about an improvement. Measurement of performance control provides an early warning and correction system that highlights undesirable changes in process operations. This measurement is critical to sustaining improvements realized through process improvement activities.

Organizations also measure performance to meet external needs and demands, including healthcare provider accountability, decision making, public reporting, and organizational evaluation, and to support national performance improvement goals and activities. Healthcare purchasers and payers are demanding that providers demonstrate their ability to provide high-quality patient care at fair prices. Specifically, they are seeking objective evidence that hospitals and other healthcare organizations manage their costs well, satisfy their customers, and have desirable outcomes. Consumers are interested in care-related information for selection purposes. In other words, they use information to identify where they believe they will have the greatest probability of a good outcome for treatment of their condition. Evaluators such as The Joint Commission and the National Committee on

Quality Assurance factor this information into their evaluation and accreditation activities. Performance measurement data can fulfill these needs if the measure construct is sound, the data analyses/data interpretations are scientifically credible, and the data are reported in a useable format that is easy to understand.

Generally, effective performance measurement benefits organizations in the following ways (The Joint Commission 2000):

- Provides factual evidence of performance
- Promotes ongoing organization self-evaluation and improvement
- Illustrates improvement
- Facilitates cost-benefit analysis
- Helps to meet external requirements and demands for performance evaluation
- May facilitate the establishment of long-term relationships with various external stakeholders
- May differentiate the organization from competitors
- May contribute to the awarding of business contracts
- Fosters organizational survival

Framework for Measurement

Performance improvement can be considered a philosophy. The organization-wide application of this philosophy composes the organizational framework for measurement. Healthcare organizations committed to ongoing performance improvement have incorporated this philosophy or framework into their overall strategic planning process. Performance improvement projects are not isolated but rather a part of a cohesive performance improvement program. A cohesive performance improvement program comprises a performance improvement process, a plan, and projects (The Joint Commission 2000).

The performance improvement process is a carefully chosen, strategically driven, values-based, systemic, organization-wide approach to the achievement of specific, meaningful, high-priority organizational improvements. The performance improvement plan is derived from this overall context.

The performance improvement plan consists of a detailed strategy for undertaking specific projects to address improvement opportunities. This plan should include (1) the identified and prioritized opportunities for improvement; (2) the staff needed to coordinate and conduct the improvement project; (3) expected time frames; and (4) needed financial and material resources. An organization should integrate its performance improvement plan with the organization-wide strategic plan so that the performance improvement priorities are viewed as being as important as other organizational priorities and so that they are given equal consideration in the allocation of resources and in the short- and long-term planning processes.

Performance improvement projects evolve from the establishment and articulation of the performance improvement plan. Projects are the diverse, individual, focused initiatives into which hospitals invest to achieve clearly defined, important, measurable improvements.

The following components support successful implementation of performance improvement programs and attainment of project goals and objectives.

- Leadership commitment—Leaders must create the setting that demands and supports continuous improvement. Leaders affect how staff works, which in turn affects how patients experience the care and services delivered. The literature identifies leadership by senior management as the most critical factor in organizational performance improvement success.
- Staff understanding and participation—Another critical component to successful performance improvement is staff involvement. Each employee is responsible for an organization's performance and, therefore, for the improvement of that performance. Employees must understand the healthcare organization's mission, vision, and values and their work's contribution to achieving that vision. They need to understand the value of continuous organizational improvement and their role in this context. They must become familiar with principles, tools, and techniques of improvement and become adept at using these implements to measure, assess, and improve.
- Establishment of partnerships with key stakeholders—Establishment of such partnerships will provide an understanding of each stakeholder's specific and unique performance data and information needs and allow the organization to produce customized, meaningful performance reports that present the information in the most easily understood and informative format for various external audiences.
- Establishment of a performance improvement oversight entity—This group oversees all aspects of the healthcare organization's performance improvement process, including determination of improvement priorities, integration of performance improvement efforts with daily work activities, initiation and facilitation of performance improvement projects, performance improvement education, development of performance improvement protocols, monitoring the progress of improvement efforts, quantification of resource consumption for each project, communication of improvement internally and externally, and assurance that process improvements are sustained.
- Selection and use of a performance improvement methodology—Use of a single improvement methodology across all improvement initiatives is critical to facilitating a cohesive and consistent approach to improvement within the organization. An organization can develop improvement methodologies internally or can adapt or adopt them from external sources

such as The Joint Commission's FOCUS-PDCA method or Ernst and Young's IMPROVE method.

- Development of performance improvement protocols—Performance improvement protocols describe how the organization implements its performance improvement process. They typically describe the purpose and responsibilities of the oversight entity, the process for proposing improvement projects, the process for reviewing and selecting projects, methods for convening project teams, the roles and responsibilities of team members, the selected performance improvement method and how to implement it, and reporting and communication requirements.
- Identification and response to performance improvement resource needs—Performance improvement requires investment and support, including an expert resource person, employees who are allocated dedicated time to work on the project, education, information and knowledge, equipment, and financial resources.
- Recognition and acknowledgment of performance improvement successes and efforts—Acknowledgment of improvement successes builds organizational momentum for future successes, engenders a sense of meaningful contribution in individual employees, and bonds the organization in celebration. In-house or public recognition of improvement successes rewards teams by showing respect and appreciation for their unique talents, skills, and perspectives. In turn, this recognition fosters employee dedication and loyalty.
- Continuous assessment of improvement efforts' effectiveness—Healthcare organizations are not static, and neither are the functions performed in these organizations. Improvement efforts must be reviewed routinely to determine that successes are sustained in the rapidly changing environment of today's healthcare organization (The Joint Commission 2000).

Selecting Performance Measures

Numerous opportunities for improvement exist in every healthcare organization. However, not all improvements are of the same magnitude. Improvements that are powerful and worthy of organization resources include those that will positively affect a large number of patients, eliminate or reduce instability in critical clinical or business processes, decrease risk, and ameliorate serious problems. In short, focus on high-risk, high-volume, problem-prone areas is most appropriate to maximize performance improvement investment.

Because performance measurement lies at the heart of any performance improvement process, performance measures must be selected in a thoughtful and deliberate manner. An organization may develop performance measures internally or adopt them from a multitude of external resources. However, regardless of the source of performance measures, each measure should be evaluated against certain characteristics to ensure a credible and beneficial measurement effort. The following characteristics are critical to performance measures.

- Relevant—Selected measures should relate directly to your organization's improvement goals and should be linked to your organization's mission, vision, values, and strategic goals and objectives.
- Reliable—Reliability refers to data constancy and consistency. Reliable measures accurately and consistently identify the events they were designed to identify across multiple healthcare settings.
- Valid—Valid measures identify opportunities for improvement (i.e., events that merit further review) relative to the services provided and the quality of the healthcare results achieved. Valid measures are measures that raise good questions about current processes and, therefore, underlie the identification of improvement opportunities.
- Cost-effective—Performance measurement requires resource investment and, therefore, implies that the ultimate value of the measurement activity should justify the related resource expenditure. Some measurement activities are not worth the investment necessary to collect and analyze the data. Cost versus benefit (i.e., value) of all measurement activities must be considered.
- Under the control of the provider—There is little value in collecting data on processes or outcomes over which the organization has little or no control. A provider must be able to influence (i.e., implement interventions on) the processes and outcomes tracked by any performance measure it uses.
- Precisely defined and specified—Performance measures and their data elements must be defined and specified precisely to ensure uniform application from measurement period to measurement period and to ensure comparability across organizations. Precisely defined and specified measures ensure that the organization will collect and calculate the measures in the same way each time and that other organizations will do the same.
- Interpretable—*Interpretability* refers to the extent to which users of the data and information understand the measure's rationale and results.
- Risk adjusted or stratified—Adjustment/stratification refers to the extent to which the influences of factors that differ among comparison groups can be controlled or taken into account (The Joint Commission 2000, 1998).

The presence or absence of some of these characteristics may not be obvious before implementation. Pilot testing may help with this determination. Pilot testing may disclose that a particular measure is not appropriate before significant resources have been invested in the activity.

Finally, an organization should consider various types of performance measures in its performance measure selection process. Avedis Donebedian (1980) first described three components of quality: structure, process, and outcomes. An organization can develop meaningful measures for each of these components. *Structures* describe hospital characteristics such as organization structure, specialty services provided, and patient census.

Processes include components of clinical care (i.e., how care and services are provided) such as assessment and evaluation, diagnosis, and therapeutic and palliative interventions. *Clinical outcomes* are multidimensional and describe how delivered care affects the patient's health, health status, functionality, and well-being. Structure, process, and outcome measures can be defined further as *continuous-variable measures* or *rate-based measures.*

- Continuous-variable measures—Each value of a continuous-variable measure is a precise measurement that can fall anywhere along a continuous scale. An example is the number of days from surgery to discharge of patients undergoing coronary artery bypass graft (CABG) procedures.
- Rate-based measures—The value of a rate-based measure reflects the frequency of an event or condition and is expressed as a proportion or ratio. A *proportion* shows the number of occurrences over the entire group within which the occurrence could take place (for example, pneumonia patients with a pneumococcal vaccination over all patients with pneumonia). A ratio shows occurrences compared to a different but related phenomenon (for example, ventilated patients who develop pneumonia over inpatient ventilator days).

Statistical Process Control

Statistical process control (SPC) is the use of numbers and data to study the things we do in order to make them behave the way we want (McNeese and Klein 1991). In other words, SPC is a method of using data to track processes (the things we do) so that we can improve the quality of products and services (make them behave the way we want). SPC uses simple statistical tools to help us understand any process that generates products or services.

Statistical process control evolved from work done by Walter Shewhart in the 1920s at Bell Labs in New York. Developed as a quality control tool in manufacturing, SPC was introduced into healthcare only about 20 years ago. During World War I, Shewhart was directed to design a radio headset for the military. One of the key pieces of information he needed to design a headset was the width of people's heads. Shewhart measured them and discovered not only that head width varied but that it varied according to a pattern. The size of most people's heads fell within a relatively narrow range, but some people had heads that were larger or smaller than the norm, and a few heads were much larger or smaller than average. Shewhart found that this pattern of variation, now know as the normal distribution (or bell-shaped curve), also was present in many manufacturing processes (McNeese and Klein 1991).

Later, Shewhart developed a control chart based on this pattern of variation. Control charts, one of the SPC tools discussed later in this chapter, are used to track and analyze variation in processes over time. They were not widely used until World War II, when control charts assisted in the production of wartime goods.

After World War II, the Japanese began to use SPC extensively to improve the quality of their products as they were rebuilding their economy. Japanese industry underwent massive statistical training as a result of the influence and efforts of Shewhart, W. Edwards Deming, and J. M. Juran. SPC did not catch on in the West until the 1980s, by which time the United States and Europe were scrambling to catch up with the quality standards set by Japanese manufacturers.

The theory behind SPC is straightforward. It requires a change in thinking from error detection to error prevention. In manufacturing, once a product is made, correcting errors is wasteful, time consuming, and expensive. The same is true in healthcare. Making the product or providing the service correctly the first time is better and more cost-effective.

SPC changes the approach toward producing a product or service. The approach moves from inspecting the product or evaluating the service after it is produced to understanding the process itself so that it (the process) can be improved. Problems should be identified and resolved before the product is produced or the service is provided, which requires monitoring how the process is performing through routine, selective measurements.

All processes, whether in manufacturing or healthcare, produce data. SPC uses data generated by the process to improve the process. Process improvement, in turn, leads to improved products and services. Figure 7.1 illustrates how a process that generates a product or service simultaneously generates data that can be analyzed using SPC tools and used to improve that process continuously.

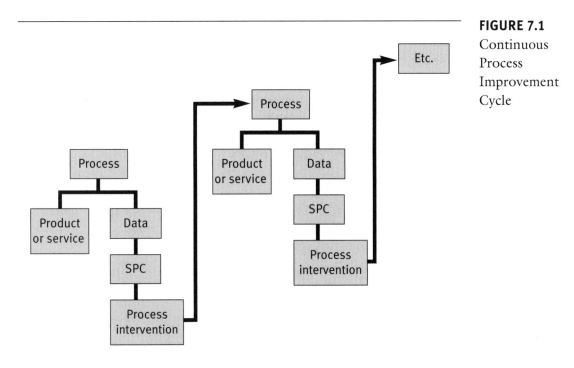

FIGURE 7.1

Continuous Process Improvement Cycle

In summary, the use of SPC in healthcare has a number of benefits, including (1) increased quality awareness on the part of healthcare organizations and practitioners, (2) an increased focus on patients, (3) the ability to base decisions on data, (4) implementation of predictable healthcare processes, (5) cost reduction, (6) fewer errors and increased patient safety, and (7) improved processes that result in improved healthcare outcomes and better quality care.

Control Chart Analysis

Every process varies. For example, a healthcare organization is unlikely to have the same number of patient falls every month. However, not every process will vary in the same way. For example, suppose that in a given year, the number of patient falls averaged 20 per month and ranged between 17 and 23 per month. These data suggest a stable process because the variation is predictable within given limits. In SPC terminology, this type of variation is called *common cause variation*. Common cause variation does not imply that the process is functioning at either a desirable or an undesirable level; it describes only the nature of variation—that it is stable and predicable within given limits.

Next, suppose that during the following year, the average number of falls stayed the same, but in one month, there were 35 falls. This type of variation is called *special cause variation*. The process has changed and is no longer predictable within limits. In this case, the special cause is a negative finding. The healthcare organization should not make changes to its fall prevention protocols until it identifies and eliminates the special cause.

On the other hand, if the observed variation were only common cause variation (as in the first case), introduction of a new fall prevention program to improve the process would be appropriate. After introducing a fall prevention program, if the number of falls in the second year decreased to an average of 17 per month with a range of 14 to 19, this change would be a positive special cause. This special cause would signal the success of the intervention.

In summary, the control chart will tell a healthcare organization whether the observed variation results from common or special causes so that it knows how to approach a process improvement. If there is a special cause, the healthcare organization should investigate and eliminate it, not change the process. If there is common cause variation, implementation of a process change to improve it is appropriate. A control chart will reveal whether the change was effective.

Elements of a Control Chart

A control chart is a line graph with a centerline that represents the overall process average (or mean). It shows the flow of a process over time, as

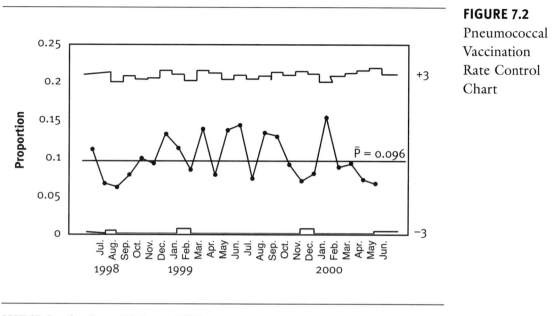

FIGURE 7.2

Pneumococcal
Vaccination
Rate Control
Chart

SOURCE: Data from Lee and McGreevey (2000).

distinguished from a distribution, which is a collection of data not necessarily organized in the order they were collected. A control chart is a dynamic presentation of data; a distribution is a static presentation. The measure of the process being monitored or evaluated appears on the vertical axis.

A control chart also has an upper and lower control limit. The control limits are not the same as the confidence limits of a distribution. The *control limits* describe the variability of a process over time and usually are set at three standard deviations (or sigmas), whereas the *confidence limits* of a distribution describe the degree of certainty that a given point is different from the average score—in other words, an "outlier." Data falling outside the three-sigma limits are a signal that the process has changed significantly. This data point is properly referred to as a special cause, not an outlier. However, the three-sigma rule is only one test to detect special cause variation. See Figure 7.2 for an example of a control chart.

Tests for a Special Cause

There are two errors (or mistakes) that we can make in trying to detect a special cause. First, we can conclude that there is a special cause when one is not present (Type I error). Second, we can conclude that there is no special cause when in fact one is present (Type II error). Walter Shewhart, who developed the control chart, recommended that using three-sigma control limits offered the best balance between making either the first or the second mistake.

FIGURE 7.3
Control
Chart Tests
for Special
Cause
Variation

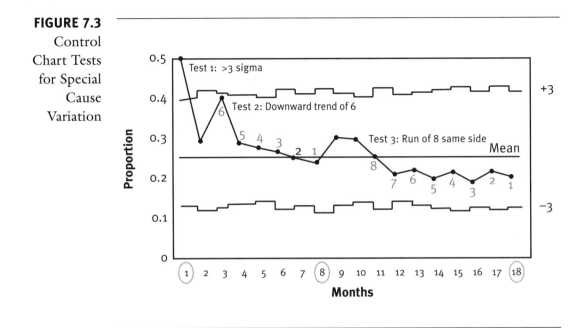

SOURCE: Data from Lee and McGreevey (2000).

Shewhart's disciples at Western Electric developed other tests, such as observation of eight consecutive points either above or below the mean, four of five consecutive points beyond one sigma, or two of three consecutive points beyond two sigmas.

A *trend* is defined as six consecutive data points incrementally increasing or decreasing. Those unfamiliar with control charts tend to see "trends" of fewer than six points, which often results in identifying common cause patterns as special causes. See Figure 7.3.

Number of Data Points

Shewhart recommended that 20 to 25 data points be used to evaluate the stability of a given process. If a process with 25 points has only common cause variation, one can be reasonably certain that a process is "in control." One then can estimate the capability of the process—that is, how it is likely to perform in the near future. Even with fewer than 25 points, examination of a process for the presence of special causes is useful. However, with fewer than 25 points, the upper and lower control limits should be referred to as *trial limits*. If one observes a special cause with, for example, only 12 points, one should take the time to investigate it. However, with only 12 data points, there is a higher probability of missing a special cause when it is present (Type II error), and one cannot estimate process capability confidently.

Choosing the Correct Control Chart

There are many different control charts. However, in its initial efforts, the average facility can manage well with only four:

- p-chart
- u-chart
- Individual values and moving range chart (XmR chart)
- X-bar and S chart

The first two analyze attributes data. The second two analyze variables data.

Attributes Data

Attributes data are discrete whole numbers, not continuous measurements. They are counts of an event of interest that can be considered desirable or undesirable. One can keep score of these counts in two ways:

- The number of times a unique event of interest occurs—for example, the patient had a pneumococcal vaccination during his or her stay (For any given patient, the event either did or did not occur and can be counted only one time per patient.)
- The total number of nonunique events—for example, the total number of patient falls (This event may occur multiple times for a patient.)

When counting unique events, one uses a p-chart. The number plotted on a chart would be either a proportion or a percentage. When counting total events (e.g., the number of falls per patient day each month), one plots a ratio on a u-chart.

Examples of attributes data plotted as percentages on p-charts include figures such as:

- percentage of patients who died;
- percentage of pneumonia patients receiving a pneumococcal vaccination;
- percentage of scripts that had one or more medication errors; and
- percentage of patients readmitted to the hospital within 30 days.

Examples of attributes data plotted as ratio data on u-charts include figures such as:

- total number of patient falls per patient day;
- total number of medication errors per total number of scripts; and

- total number of surgical complications divided by the total number of surgeries.

Variables Data

Variables data are measurements that can be plotted on a continuous scale. They can be either whole numbers or decimals. Variables data are plotted on either an X-bar and S chart or an XmR chart.

Examples of variables data include measurements such as:

- length of stay;
- length of intubation time; and
- average door-to-thrombolytic time for acute myocardial infarction patients.

An XmR chart is used when there is only one measurement for each period.

The X-bar and S charts are paired charts. In other words, the X-bar chart reveals whether there is a special cause across months, whereas the S chart reveals whether there are special causes within each month.

To interpret the X-bar chart successfully, the S chart must be free of data points beyond the upper control limit (the only test used on the S chart). If the S chart has a data point beyond three standard deviations from the mean, that data point or points should be investigated for a special cause. A special cause on the S chart must be identified and eliminated before the X-bar chart can be interpreted accurately (Lee and McGreevey 2000).

Comparison Chart Analysis

The objective of comparison analysis is to evaluate whether a healthcare organization's performance is different from the expected level derived from other organizations' data. This analysis is interorganizational because analysis is performed on the basis of data from multiple organizations. This analysis also is cross-sectional because comparisons are made at a specific point in time (e.g., month). When an organization's performance level is significantly different from the expected level, it is called an *outlier performance*. An outlier performance may be either favorable or unfavorable depending on the measure's "direction of improvement."

The use of comparison analysis in addition to the control chart can be a powerful approach. The two analyses are alike in that an organization's actual (or observed) performance level is evaluated against a comparative norm, but they are fundamentally different in how such a norm is established. In control chart analysis, the norm is determined from an organization's own historic data (i.e., process mean) to assess the organization's internal process stability. On the other hand, in comparison analysis, the norm is determined on the basis of several organizations' performance data to evaluate an organization's relative performance level. Therefore, the two analyses evaluate organizational performance from two distinct perspectives and, as a result, provide a more comprehensive framework to assess overall performance level.

Because of the analyses' different focuses, the control and comparison analyses may portray different pictures about an organization's performance. For example, an organization's control chart may show a favorable pattern (i.e., in control) at the same time the comparison chart shows unfavorable performance (i.e., a bad outlier). This apparent discrepancy may appear when an organization's performance is consistently lower than that of other organizations and suggests that a new process may need to be implemented to achieve a performance improvement. On the other hand, an organization without an outlier performance in the comparison analysis may show an out-of-control pattern in the control chart. In this case, the organization needs to investigate any presence of special cause variation in the process before making conclusions about its performance level. In general, the control chart analysis should be done before the comparison analysis to ensure process stability so that the observed performance data truly represent the organization's performance capability.

Statistical Assumptions About Data

Statistical analyses differ depending on assumptions made about data. For instance, if a normal distribution is assumed for a data set, comparison analysis is performed using a z-test. Different assumptions are made depending on the type of measure (i.e., proportion, ratio, or continuous variable) described below:

- Proportion measures: Proportion measures are assumed to follow a binomial distribution, which is the probability distribution of the number of "successes" (i.e., numerator) in a series of independent trials (i.e., denominator), each of which can result in either a "success" or a "failure" with a constant probability. For example, for a pneumococcal vaccination rate proportion measure, each individual is assumed to have an equal probability of receiving a pneumococcal vaccination under the binomial assumption. Under certain circumstances (e.g., large sample size), a binomial distribution can be approximated using a normal distribution to simplify statistical analysis.
- Ratio measures: The ratio measures are similar to the proportion measures in that both are based on count (or attributes) data but differ in that the numerator and the denominator address different attributes. An example is the number of adverse drug reactions (ADRs) per 1,000 patient days. For this type of measure, the probability of a "success" (e.g., an ADR) is very small, whereas the area of opportunity (e.g., patient days) is usually large. Ratio measures are assumed to follow a Poisson distri-

bution. Like binomial distribution, Poisson distribution can be approximated by normal distribution.

- Continuous variable measures: Continuous variable measures deal with interval scale data and generally are not restricted to particular values. Examples include CABG length of stay and the number of minutes before administration of antibiotics. An appropriate distribution assumption for this type of measure is a normal distribution (or t distribution for a small sample size).

What Data Are Compared?

The comparative norm (e.g., expected rate) in the comparison analysis is the *predicted rate* if the measure is risk adjusted and the *comparison group mean* if the measure is not risk adjusted. Because performance measurement systems develop the comparative data and The Joint Commission receives only summary-level data, the accuracy of comparison analysis depends on the quality of data submitted by individual measurement systems. Whenever appropriate, as a comparative norm, risk-adjusted data are preferable to the summary data from comparison groups because a valid and reliable risk adjustment procedure can reduce organization- or patient-level variability (e.g., different levels of severity of illness). In this case, the comparison data are customized for individual organizations and thus more accurate, fairer performance comparisons can be made.

How Are Statistical Outliers Determined?

In comparison analysis, the underlying hypothesis (i.e., null hypothesis) about an organization's performance is that the observed performance is not different (that is, statistically) from the expected level. By applying a set of statistical procedures (i.e., hypothesis testing) to actual performance data, one determines whether the null hypothesis is likely to be true for individual organizations. If it is not true, the performance is called an *outlier*. In general, statistical outliers can be determined using two approaches. One approach is based on the p-value, and the other is based on the expected range. These two approaches always result in the same conclusion about the outlier status.

- Outlier decision based on p-value: A p-value is the probability of obtaining data that are the same as or more extreme than the observed data when the null hypothesis is true (i.e., when the organization's actual performance is not different from the expected performance). Therefore, a p-value that is very small (e.g., less than 0.01) indicates that the actual performance is likely to be different from the expected level. In this case, the null hypothesis is rejected and an outlier is determined. A p-value is calculated on the basis of an assumption about the probability distribution

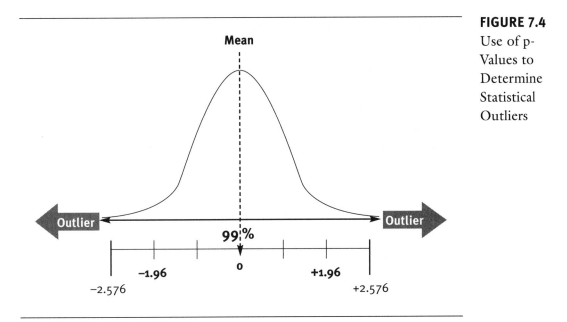

FIGURE 7.4

Use of p-Values to Determine Statistical Outliers

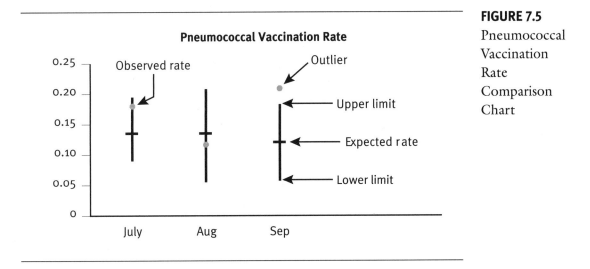

FIGURE 7.5

Pneumococcal Vaccination Rate Comparison Chart

of data. If a normal distribution is assumed, a p-value less than 0.01 is equivalent to a z-score greater than 2.576 or less than –2.576 (for a two-sided test). See Figure 7.4.

• Outlier decision based on expected range: An expected range (also called the *acceptance interval*) is an interval with upper and lower limits that represents the set of values for which the null hypothesis is accepted. Usually, the midpoint of the interval is the expected rate (or value) for the organization. When the observed data are outside the expected range, an outlier is determined. The expected range can be useful for displaying an organization's outlier status in a chart. See Figure 7.5.

Comparison Chart Construction

A comparison chart is a graphical summary of comparison analysis. It displays tabular information from the comparison analysis in a standardized graphical format so that a visually intuitive assessment may be made about an organization's performance.

A comparison chart consists of actual (or observed) rates, expected rates, and expected ranges (i.e., upper and lower limits) for a given time frame. Unlike control charts, which require at least 12 data points (i.e., months) for a meaningful interpretation, comparison charts can be created with just a single valid data point because of its cross-sectional nature.

To create a comparison chart, one must calculate the expected range. An expected range is determined using the two-step process described below.

- Step one: Calculate confidence limits for the observed rate (or value) using the formulas provided in Appendix 2. (Here, the observed rate is considered as a random variable, whereas the expected rate is assumed to be a constant value.) If the confidence interval includes values outside the allowable range, the interval must be truncated. For proportion measures, the values must be between 0 and 1. For ratio measures, the values must be zero or any positive numbers. Continuous variable measures may include any positive or negative numbers.
- Step two: Convert the confidence interval into the expected range.

Comparison Chart Interpretation

Depending on the direction of a measure's improvement, outlier interpretations can be positive, negative, or neutral.

- Positive measures: A rate increase signals improvement. In other words, a larger rate is better than a smaller rate. The pneumococcal vaccination measure is an example. For this measure, an observed rate above the expected range indicates a favorable outlier, whereas a rate below the range indicates an unfavorable outlier.
- Negative measures: A rate decrease signals improvement. In other words, a smaller rate is better than a larger rate. Mortality rate measures are an example. For these measures, an observed rate above the expected range indicates an unfavorable outlier, whereas a rate below the range indicates a favorable outlier.
- Neutral measures: Either an increase or a decrease in rate could be a signal of improvement. In other words, there is no clear direction of improvement for these measures. For example, whether a vaginal birth after Cesarean section (VBAC) rate of 5 percent is better (or worse) than a

VBAC rate of 95 percent is difficult to determine. In this case, an observed rate either above or below the expected range is an unfavorable outlier. For these measures, no favorable outliers can be identified.

The comparison analysis will result in one of the following scenarios, regardless of the type of measure.

- No outlier: Actual performance is within the expected range.
- Favorable outlier: Actual performance is better than the expected performance.
- Unfavorable outlier: Actual performance is worse than the expected performance.
- Incomplete data: Data cannot be analyzed because of a data error.
- Small sample size: Data cannot be analyzed because of a small sample size.

Data are "incomplete" if data elements used in the comparison analysis are missing or invalid. Small sample sizes are defined as fewer than 25 denominator cases for proportion measures, fewer than 4 numerator cases for ratio measures, and fewer than 10 cases for continuous variable measures. In addition, representation of fewer than 10 organizations in the comparison group data for non-risk-adjusted measures is considered as a small sample size (Lee and McGreevey 2000).

Using Data for Performance Improvement

Once collected, performance measurement data require interpretation and analysis if they are to be used to improve the processes and outcomes of healthcare. There are a number of ways to use data for improvement purposes, all of which involve comparison. Data can be used to compare (1) an organization's performance against itself over time, (2) the performance of one organization to the performance of a group of organizations collecting data on the same measures in the same way, and (3) an organization's performance against established benchmarks or guidelines.

As a first step, an organization must determine whether the process it is measuring is in control. To improve a process, it first must be understood. Processes characterized by special cause variation are unstable, unpredictable, and therefore difficult to understand. Control charts should be used to determine whether processes are stable and in statistical control or whether special cause variation exists. If special cause variation does exist, it must be investigated and eliminated. Once special cause variation has been eliminated, organizations can be confident that the data accurately reflect performance.

Consider a hypothetical situation in which a hospital measures its pneumococcal vaccination rates using a control chart. The control chart in Figure 7.6 indicates existence of special cause variation at time 8 as the

FIGURE 7.6

Control Chart
Reflecting a
Change in
Process

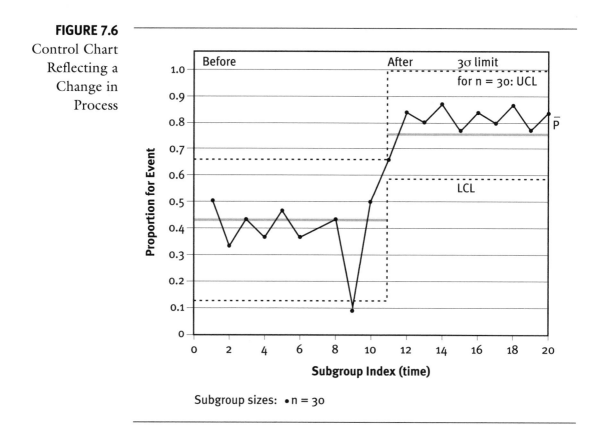

Subgroup sizes: •n = 30

observed rate deviates from the upper control limit. Suppose that the hospital conducted a root cause analysis after time 8 to identify the source of the special cause and found that there was a serious problem in the hospital's coding practice. The hospital then implemented an intervention plan at time 10, and the hospital's rates shifted to within the control limits (times 11 to 20). In addition, the process mean (i.e., centerline) shifted from 0.42 to 0.75 after the intervention. The hospital should continue to monitor its pneumococcal vaccination rates using the new process mean as part of a continuous quality improvement plan.

Control charts, however, tell us only about the stability of the process; they tell us nothing about quality of care. After determining that the process of interest is stable and in control, organizations need to use other SPC tools and data analysis techniques to determine whether they are performing as they want to perform. One way a healthcare organization can measure whether it is meeting its goals and targets is to compare its performance against itself over time. By consistently tracking the same measures on an ongoing basis, an organization can spot trends, cycles, and patterns, all of which will help determine whether it is meeting its preset targets and whether its performance is improving or declining. Importantly, it also can monitor the impact of quality improvement interventions it has implemented and track the sustainability of those improvements.

Another way to use data for improvement purposes is to compare the performance of one organization to the performance of a group of organizations collecting data on the same measures in the same way. In this way, the healthcare organization can track how it is performing as compared to other organizations providing the same services. These comparisons can be local, regional, national, or based on any number of other strata. Statistical analyses can pinpoint whether a healthcare entity is performing in a way that is comparable to other organizations or whether it is at a level that is, statistically speaking, significantly above or below others in the comparison group. An organization's discovery that it is performing at a level significantly below that of its peers is often a powerful incentive to improve.

A third method of comparing performance is through benchmarking. There are a variety of definitions of benchmarking but, generally speaking, it compares an organization's performance in relation to a specified service or function to that of industry leaders or exemplary organizations. Benchmarking is goal directed and promotes performance improvement by:

- providing an environment amenable to organizational change through continuous improvement and striving to match industry-leading practices and results;
- creating objective measures of performance that are driven by industry-leading targets instead of by past performance;
- providing a customer/external focus;
- substantiating the need for improvement; and
- establishing data-driven decision-making processes (Czarnecki 1994).

In healthcare, professional societies and expert panels routinely develop scientifically based guidelines of patient care practices for given treatments or procedures. The goal of these guideline-setting efforts is to provide healthcare organizations with tools that, if appropriately applied, can help raise their performance to the level of industry leaders. Organizations can use performance measure data to track how often, and how well, they comply with the guidelines.

Conclusion

This chapter provided a framework for performance measurement in the context of performance improvement and advice on the selection of performance measures. You are now familiar with two statistical tools, the control chart and the comparison chart, and their use in tracking performance measures data.

Study Questions

1. What are common data quality problems in healthcare performance measurement? How should the sufficiency of data quality be evaluated? What consequences are associated with the use of poor quality data?
2. When an organization uses sample data in performance measurement, how can it determine appropriate sample sizes and how can it ensure that the sample data represent the entire population? How should it handle small sample sizes in the analysis and use of control and comparison charts?
3. How does the rigorous use of control and comparison charts for performance management and improvement contradict, if at all, the art-of-medicine philosophy that each patient is unique?

Appendix 1: Control Chart Formulas[2]

Attributes Data: Proportion Measures (p-Chart)

Proportion measures are analyzed using a p-chart. The following data elements (organization level) are used to construct a p-chart.

Data Element	Notation[*]
Number of denominator cases for a month	n_i
Number of numerator cases for a month	x_i
Observed rate for a month	p_i

[*]The subscript i represents individual months.

Statistical formulas for calculating the centerline and control limits are given below. Note that the control limits are calculated for individual months and that the limits vary by month unless the number of denominator cases for each month is the same for all months.

Centerline of the Chart

$$\bar{p} = \frac{\sum x_i}{\sum n_i} = \frac{x_1 + x_2 + \ldots + x_m}{n_1 + n_2 + \ldots + n_m},$$

where m is the number of months (or data points).

Upper and Lower Control Limits for Each Month

$$\bar{p} \pm 3 \times \sqrt{\frac{\bar{p} \times (1 - \bar{p})}{n_i}}$$

Small Sample Size Adjustments

When the sample sizes are very small, a standard p-chart cannot be used because the statistical assumption needed to create a p-chart (i.e., normal approximation to the binomial distribution) is not valid. Specifically, the small sample sizes are defined as follows:

$$\bar{n} \times \bar{p} < 4 \text{ or } \bar{n} \times (1 - \bar{p}) < 4,$$

where n-bar is the average number of denominator cases and p-bar is the centerline (i.e., weighted average of individual months' observed rates).

In this situation, an adjusted p-chart using an exact binomial probability (i.e., probability limit method) is used. To calculate the upper and lower control limits using the probability limit method, the smallest x_U and the largest x_L satisfying the following two binomial probability distribution functions should be calculated first.

$$\sum_{x=x_u}^{n} \left[\frac{n}{x} \right] p^x (1 - p)^{n-x} \le 0.00135 \text{ and } \sum_{x=0}^{x_L} \left[\frac{n}{x} \right] p^x (1 - p)^{n-x} \le 0.00135$$

Next, the upper and the lower control limits for the observed rate are obtained by dividing x_U and x_L by the number of denominator cases n for the month. Alternatively, instead of the binomial probability distribution, an incomplete beta distribution may be used to calculate the probability limits (SAS Institute 1995).

Attributes Data: Ratio Measures (u-Chart)

Ratio measures are analyzed using the u-chart. A u-chart is created using the following data elements (organization level).

Data Element	Notation*
Number of denominator cases for a month	n_i
Number of numerator cases for a month	x_i
Observed rate for a month	u_i

*The subscript i represents individual months.

Centerline of a u-Chart

$$\bar{u} = \frac{\sum x_i}{\sum n_i} = \frac{x_1 + x_2 + \ldots + x_m}{n_1 + n_2 + \ldots + n_m},$$

where m is the number of months (or data points).

Control Limits for Each Month

$$\bar{u} \pm 3 \times \sqrt{\frac{\bar{u}}{n_i}}$$

If the ratio is to be calculated on a prespecified denominator basis (or on a scaling factor basis), the control chart must be scaled appropriately using that information. For example, the denominator basis for the ratio measure "number of falls per 100 resident days" is 100. In this case, all values in the control chart, including the centerline and control limits, and observed ratio must be multiplied by 100.

Small Sample Size Adjustments

Like p-charts, a standard u-chart should not be used when the sample size is very small because the statistical assumption for a u-chart (normal approximation to the Poisson distribution) fails if the sample size is very small. Small sample size for ratio measures is defined as:

$$\bar{n} \times \bar{u} < 4,$$

where n-bar is the average number of denominator cases and u-bar is the centerline of the u-chart.

In this situation, an adjusted u-chart based on Poisson probability is used. The upper and lower control limits are obtained by first calculating x_U and x_L and then dividing each value by the number of denominator cases n for the month. To obtain x_U and x_L, the following two Poisson probability distribution functions should be solved in such a way that the smallest x_U and the largest x_L satisfying these conditions are obtained.

$$\sum_{x=x_u}^{\infty} \frac{e^{-u}u^x}{x!} \leq 0.00135 \text{ and } \sum_{x=0}^{x_L} \frac{e^{-u}u^x}{x!} \leq 0.00135$$

Alternatively, a chi-square distribution may be used instead of the Poisson probability distribution to calculate the probability limits (SAS Institute 1995).

Variables Data (X-Bar and S Chart)

Variables data, or *continuous variable measures*, are analyzed using the X-bar and S chart. To construct an X-bar and S chart, the following data elements (organization level) are needed.

Data Element	Notation[*]
Number of cases for a month	n_i
Mean of observed values for a month	x_i
Standard deviation of observed values for a month	s_i

[*]The subscript *i* represents individual months.

The centerline and control limits for an X-bar and S chart are calculated using the following formulas. Note that the control limits vary by months depending on the denominator cases for individual months.

Centerline

1. X-bar chart

$$\bar{x} = \frac{\sum n_i \times x_i}{\sum n_i}$$

2. S-chart

a. Minimum variance linear unbiased estimate (SAS Institute 1995)

$$\bar{s}_i = c_4 \times \frac{\sum h_i \times \dfrac{s_i}{c_4}}{\sum h_i}, \text{ where } h_i = \frac{c_4^2}{1 - c_4^2}$$

b. Pooled standard deviation (Montgomery 1996)

$$\bar{s} = \sqrt{\frac{\sum (n_i - 1) \times s_i^2}{\sum n_i - m}}$$

These two methods result in slightly different values, but the differences generally are negligible.

c_4 is a constant that depends on the sample size. As the sample size increases, c_4 approaches 1. The exact formula for c_4 is:

$$c_4 = \sqrt{\frac{2}{n_i - 1}} \times \frac{\Gamma\left(\dfrac{n_i}{2}\right)}{\Gamma\left(\dfrac{n_i - 1}{2}\right)}$$

Control Limits

1. X-bar chart

$$\bar{x} \pm 3 \times \frac{\bar{s}}{c_4 \sqrt{n_i}}$$

2. S chart

$$\bar{s} \times \left(1 \pm \frac{3}{c_4} \times \sqrt{1 - c_4^2}\right)$$

Small Sample Size Adjustments

If the sample size is 1 for all data points, an XmR chart is used instead of an X-bar and S chart, assuming the observed mean value as a single observation for the month (Lee and McGreevey 2000).

Appendix 2: Comparison Chart Formulas[2]

Comparison Analysis: Proportion Measures

Three data elements (listed below) are used in the comparison chart analysis for proportion measures. The expected rate is either the risk-adjusted rate (if risk adjusted) or the overall observed rate for the comparison group (if not risk adjusted or if risk-adjusted data are not available).

Data Element Name	Notation
Number of denominator cases for a month	n
Observed rate for a month	p_0
Expected rate for a month A) Risk-adjusted rate; or B) Overall observed rate	p_e p_e

Analysis is based on the score test (Agresti and Coull 1998). This test is based on the difference between the observed and the expected rates, divided by the standard error of the expected rate as shown below.

$$Z = \frac{p_o - p_e}{\sqrt{\dfrac{p_e \times (1 - p_e)}{n}}}$$

This value (or Z-statistic) follows a normal distribution when the sample size is not very small. A value less than –2.576 or greater than 2.576 signals a statistically significant difference between the two rates at a 1 percent significance level.

The confidence interval for the observed rate is determined by expanding the above formula with respect to the expected rate (Agresti and Coull 1998; Bickel and Doksum 1977). Its upper limit (U_0) and lower limit (L_0) for a month are calculated as follows.

$$U_o = \frac{\left(p_o + \dfrac{Z^2_{1-\frac{\alpha}{2}}}{2 \times n} \right) + Z_{1-\frac{\alpha}{2}} \times \sqrt{\dfrac{Z^2_{1-\frac{\alpha}{2}}}{4 \times n^2} + \dfrac{p_o \times (1 - p_o)}{n}}}{1 + \dfrac{Z^2_{1-\frac{\alpha}{2}}}{n}}, \text{ where } Z_{1-\frac{\alpha}{2}} = 2.576$$

$$L_o = \frac{\left(p_o + \dfrac{Z^2_{1-\frac{\alpha}{2}}}{2 \times n} \right) - Z_{1-\frac{\alpha}{2}} \times \sqrt{\dfrac{Z^2_{1-\frac{\alpha}{2}}}{4 \times n^2} + \dfrac{p_o \times (1 - p_o)}{n}}}{1 + \dfrac{Z^2_{1-\frac{\alpha}{2}}}{n}}, \text{ where } Z_{1-\frac{\alpha}{2}} = 2.576$$

Statistical significance also can be determined by comparing the expected rate (p_e) with the confidence interval (L_0, U_0). If p_e is within the interval, the observed rate is not different from the expected rates; therefore, it is not an outlier. If p_e is outside the interval, it is an outlier.

This information is depicted on the comparison chart by converting the confidence interval around the observed rate into the expected range (or acceptance interval) around the expected rate (Holubkov et al. 1998). The upper limit (U_e) and lower limit (L_e) of the expected range are calculated as follows.

$$U_e = p_e + (p_o - L_o). \text{ [If } U_e > 1, \text{ then } U_e = 1.]$$

$$L_e = p_e + (p_o - U_o). \text{ [If } L_e < 0, \text{ then } L_e = 0.]$$

The interpretation of the comparison chart now involves the relative location of the observed rate with respect to the expected range. If the observed rate (p_0) is within the expected range (L_e, U_e), it is not a statistical outlier (i.e., not a statistically significant difference) at a 1 percent significance level. If the observed rate is outside the expected range, the observed rate is a statistical outlier.

Comparison Analysis: Ratio Measures

Three data elements are used in the comparison chart analysis for ratio measures. The expected rate is either the risk-adjusted rate (if risk adjusted) or the overall observed rate for the comparison group (if not risk adjusted or if risk-adjusted data are not available).

Data Element Name	Notation
Number of denominator cases for a month	n
Observed rate (ratio) for a month	u_0
Expected rate (ratio) for a month A) Risk-adjusted rate; or B) Overall observed rate	u_e u_e

Similarly to proportion measures, analysis for ratio measures is based on the score test (The Joint Commission 2000). This test is based on the difference between the observed and expected number of numerator cases divided by the standard error of the expected number of events.

This value (or Z-statistic) is assumed to follow a normal distribution when the sample size is not very small. A value less than –2.576 or greater than 2.576 signals a statistically significant difference between the two rates at a 1 percent significance level.

$$Z = \frac{n \times u_o - n \times u_e}{\sqrt{n \times u_e}}$$

The confidence interval is derived from the above test statistic (Agresti and Coull 1998; Bickel and Doksum 1977). The upper and lower limits of the confidence interval are calculated as follows.

$$U_o = \frac{(n \times u_o + \frac{Z^2_{1-\frac{\alpha}{2}}}{2}) + \frac{Z_{1-\frac{\alpha}{2}}}{2} \times \sqrt{Z^2_{1-\frac{\alpha}{2}} + 4 \times n \times u_o}}{n}, \text{ where } Z_{1-\frac{\alpha}{2}} = 2.576$$

$$L_o = \frac{(n \times u_o + \frac{Z^2_{1-\frac{\alpha}{2}}}{2}) - \frac{Z_{1-\frac{\alpha}{2}}}{2} \times \sqrt{Z^2_{1-\frac{\alpha}{2}} + 4 \times n \times u_o}}{n}, \text{ where } Z_{1-\frac{\alpha}{2}} = 2.576$$

The upper limit (U_e) and lower limit (L_e) of the expected range are calculated as follows (Holubkov et al. 1998).

$$U_e = u_e + (u_o - L_o).$$

$$L_e = u_e + (u_o - U_o). \text{ [If } L_e < 0, \text{ then } L_e = 0.]$$

Using the comparison chart, one can determine statistical significance by comparing the observed rate (u_o) to the expected range (L_e, U_e). If the observed ratio (u_o) is within the expected range (L_e, U_e), it is not a statistical outlier at a 1 percent significance level. If the observed ratio is outside the expected range, the observed rate is a statistical outlier.

Continuous Variable Measures

Four data elements (listed below) are used in the comparison chart analysis for continuous variable measures. The expected value is either the risk-adjusted value (if risk adjusted) or the overall mean observed value for the comparison group (if not risk adjusted or if risk-adjusted data are not available).

Data Element Name	Notation
Number of cases for a month	n
Mean of observed values for a month	x_0
Standard deviation of observed values	s_0
Mean of expected values for a month A) Mean risk-adjusted value; or B) Overall mean observed value	x_e x_e

1. The statistical test is based on normal distribution. Specifically, the following formulas are used depending on the sample size.

a. $n \geq 25$.

$$Z = \frac{X_o - X_e}{S_o / \sqrt{n}}$$

This value (or Z-statistic) is assumed to follow a normal distribution when the sample size is not very small. A value less than -2.576 or greater than 2.576 signals a statistically significant difference between the two rates at a 1 percent significance level.

b. $n < 25$.

$$t = \frac{X_o - X_e}{S_o / \sqrt{n}}$$

This value (or t-statistic) is assumed to follow a t distribution. Unlike a normal distribution, the t distribution depends on the sample size. For example, if the sample size is 15, a value less than -2.977 or greater than 2.977 signals a statistically significant difference between the two rates at a 1 percent significance level.

2. Based on the test statistic, the expected range is calculated using the following formula.

Expected upper limit: $U_e = x_e + (x_0 - L_0)$, and
expected lower limit: $L_e = x_e + (x_0 - U_0)$, where

$$U_o = x_o + Z_{1-\frac{\alpha}{2}} \times \frac{S_o}{\sqrt{n}} \text{ and } L_o = x_o - Z_{1-\frac{\alpha}{2}} \times \frac{S_o}{\sqrt{n}} \text{ if } n \geq 25$$

or

$$U_o = x_o + t_{1-\frac{\alpha}{2}, n-1} \times \frac{S_o}{\sqrt{n}} \text{ and } L_o = x_o - t_{1-\frac{\alpha}{2}, n-1} \times \frac{S_o}{\sqrt{n}} \text{ if } n < 25$$

If the observed value (x_0) is within the expected range (L_e, U_e), it is not a statistical outlier (i.e., not a statistically significant difference) at a 1 percent significance level. If the observed value is outside the expected range, the observed rate is a statistical outlier (Lee and McGreevey 2000).

Appendix 3: Case Studies[2]

Case 1: Pneumococcal Vaccination Rate—Proportion Measure

A healthcare organization started to collect data for the proportion measure "pneumococcal vaccination rate" on July 1, 1998. As of November 1,

1999, this organization collected 12 months of observed pneumococcal vaccination rates (p_0). The organization's calculated observed rates (p_0) for individual months are given below.

	7/98	8/98	9/98	10/98	11/98	12/98
n	81	75	88	89	66	67
x	13	14	18	8	9	7
p_0	0.1605	0.1867	0.2045	0.0899	0.1364	0.1045

	1/99	2/99	3/99	4/99	5/99	6/99
n	68	79	84	81	75	85
x	11	10	11	13	14	11
p_0	0.1618	0.1266	0.1310	0.1605	0.1867	0.1294

Control Chart (p-Chart)

A standard p-chart can be created for this organization because (1) at least 12 months passed since the data collection begin date, (2) more than two non-missing data points are available, and (3) the sample sizes are not small.

Centerline

$$\bar{p} = \frac{13+14+18+8+9+7+11+10+11+13+14+11}{81+75+88+89+66+67+68+79+84+81+75+85} = 0.1482$$

Control Limits

1. Upper control limit (UCL) for July 1998

$$UCL = 0.1482 + 3 \times \sqrt{\frac{0.1482 \times (1-0.1482)}{81}} = 0.2666$$

2. Lower control limit (LCL) for July 1998

$$LCL = 0.1482 - 3 \times \sqrt{\frac{0.1482 \times (1-0.1482)}{81}} = 0.0298$$

3. UCL for June 1999

$$UCL = 0.1482 + 3 \times \sqrt{\frac{0.1482 \times (1-0.1482)}{85}} = 0.2638$$

4. LCL for June 1999

$$LCL = 0.1482 - 3 \times \sqrt{\frac{0.1482 \times (1-0.1482)}{85}} = 0.0326$$

The calculations above were rounded to four decimal points for illustration. A p-chart using the above data is shown below. (The centerline is rounded to two decimal points.)

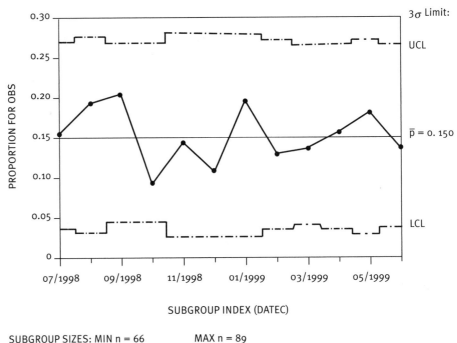

PMS ID = 1   HCO ID = 1   MEAS ID = 1

SUBGROUP SIZES: MIN n = 66   MAX n = 89

Comparison Chart

For July 1998:

$$U_o = \frac{0.1605 + \dfrac{2.576^2}{2 \times 81} + 2.576 \times \sqrt{\dfrac{2.576^2}{4 \times 81^2} + \dfrac{0.1605 \times (1 - 0.1605)}{81}}}{1 + \dfrac{2.576^2}{81}} = 0.2904$$

$$L_o = \frac{0.1605 + \dfrac{2.576^2}{2 \times 81} - 2.576 \times \sqrt{\dfrac{2.576^2}{4 \times 81^2} + \dfrac{0.1605 \times (1 - 0.1605)}{81}}}{1 + \dfrac{2.576^2}{81}} = 0.0820$$

The expected range is:

$U_e = 0.1605 + 0.1546 - 0.0820 = 0.2331$, and

$L_e = 0.1605 + 0.1546 - 0.2904 = 0.0247$.

Because $|Z| = 0.147 < 2.576$, the pneumococcal vaccination rate for July 1998 is not a statistical outlier at a 1 percent significance level. The same conclusion can be drawn about the July 1998 performance using the expected range approach because the observed rate 0.1605 is within the expected range (0.0247, 0.2331).

PMS ID = 1   HCO ID = 1   MEAS ID = 1

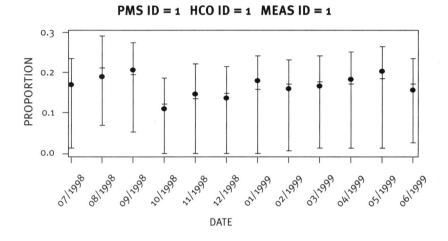

Case 2: Number of Adverse Drug Reactions per 100 Patient Days— Ratio Measure

Suppose a healthcare organization collected data for the ratio measure "number of adverse drug reactions per 100 patient days" for the period from July 1, 1998, to June 30, 1999. U_0 and U_e represent actual rate and comparison group rate, respectively.

	7/98	8/98	9/98	10/98	11/98	12/98
n	164	170	145	179	185	155
x	8	11	4	5	7	6
u_0	0.0488	0.0647	0.0276	0.0279	0.0378	0.0387
u_e	0.0315	0.0415	0.0415	0.0315	0.0425	0.0435

	1/99	2/99	3/99	4/99	5/99	6/99
n	165	189	175	166	156	176
x	9	4	7	5	6	9
u_0	0.0545	0.0212	0.0400	0.0301	0.0385	0.0511
u_e	0.0415	0.0315	0.0435	0.0415	0.0465	0.0485

Control Chart (u-Chart)

A standard u-chart can be created for this organization because (1) at least 12 months passed since the data collection begin date; (2) more than 2 non-missing data points are available; and (3) the sample sizes are not small.

Centerline

$$\bar{u} = \frac{8 + 4 + \ldots + 9}{164 + 189 + \ldots + 176} = 0.04 \ (4 \text{ ADRs per 100 patient days})$$

Control Limits for Each Month

1. UCL for July 1998

$$UCL = 0.04 + 3 \times \sqrt{\frac{0.04}{164}} = 0.0869 \ (8.69 \text{ ADRs per 100 patient days})$$

2. LCL for July 1998

$$LCL = 0.04 - 3 \times \sqrt{\frac{0.04}{164}} = -0.0069 \ (0)$$

3. UCL for June 1999

$$UCL = 0.04 + 3 \times \sqrt{\frac{0.04}{176}} = 0.0852 \ (8.52 \text{ ADRs per 100 patient days})$$

4. LCL for June 1999

$$UCL = 0.04 - 3 \times \sqrt{\frac{0.04}{176}} = -0.0052 \ (0)$$

Note that the LCL calculations for July 1998 and June 1999 resulted in negative values and were replaced by zero because a u-chart must include only nonnegative values. Below is a u-chart created using these data.

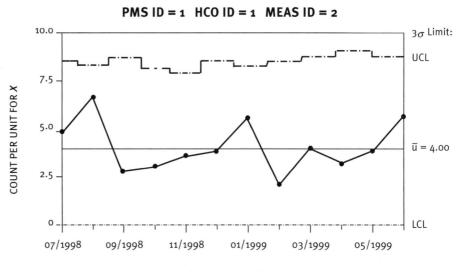

PMS ID = 1   HCO ID = 1   MEAS ID = 2

Comparison Analysis

For July 1998:

$$Z = \frac{164 \times 0.0488 - 164 \times 0.0315}{\sqrt{164 \times 0.0315}} = 1.248,$$

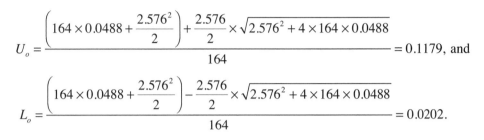

$$U_o = \frac{\left(164 \times 0.0488 + \dfrac{2.576^2}{2}\right) + \dfrac{2.576}{2} \times \sqrt{2.576^2 + 4 \times 164 \times 0.0488}}{164} = 0.1179, \text{ and}$$

$$L_o = \frac{\left(164 \times 0.0488 + \dfrac{2.576^2}{2}\right) - \dfrac{2.576}{2} \times \sqrt{2.576^2 + 4 \times 164 \times 0.0488}}{164} = 0.0202.$$

The expected range is:

U_e = 0.0488 + 0.0315 − 0.0202 = 0.0601 (6.01 ADRs per 100 patient days), and

L_e = 0.0488 + 0.0315 − 0.1179 = −0.0376 (0).

Because |Z| = 1.248 < 2.576, the observed ratio for July 1998 is not a statistical outlier at a 1 percent significance level. The same conclusion for July 1998 performance can be drawn using the expected range approach because the observed ratio 0.0488 (4.88 ADRs per 100 patient days) is within the expected range (0, 0.0601). The comparison chart using these data is shown below.

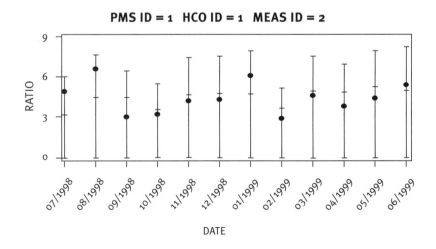

Case 3: CABG Length of Stay—Continuous Variable Measure

Suppose a healthcare organization has collected the following data for the continuous variable measure "CABG length of stay" during the 12-month period from July 1, 1998, to June 30, 1999.

	7/98	8/98	9/98	10/98	11/98	12/98
n	35	36	45	32	36	45
x_0	6.53	8.61	7.93	6.53	7.61	7.93
s_0	3.11	4.04	3.77	4.11	3.04	4.35
x_e	6.76	7.16	7.06	7.00	7.76	7.76

	1/99	2/99	3/99	4/99	5/99	6/99
n	32	36	45	32	36	45
x_0	6.53	8.61	7.93	6.53	7.61	7.93
s_0	3.11	3.04	3.71	3.11	3.04	3.57
x_e	7.16	7.96	7.56	7.46	7.76	7.76

Control Chart (X-Bar and S Chart)

An X-bar and S chart can be created for this organization because (1) at least 12 months passed since the data collection begin date, (2) more than two non-missing data points are available, and (3) the sample sizes are not small.

Centerline

X-bar chart

$$\bar{x} = \frac{35 \times 6.53 + 36 \times 8.61 + \ldots + 45 \times 7.93}{35 + 36 + \ldots + 45} = 7.58$$

S chart (June 1999)

$$\bar{s}_{12} = 0.9943 \times \left[\frac{\dfrac{0.9927^2}{1 - 0.9927^2} \times \dfrac{3.11}{0.9927} + \ldots + \dfrac{0.9943^2}{1 - 0.9943^2} \times \dfrac{3.57}{0.9943}}{\dfrac{0.9927^2}{1 - 0.9927^2} + \ldots + \dfrac{0.9943^2}{1 - 0.9943^2}} \right] = 3.53$$

c_4 is 0.9927 for $n = 35$ and 0.9943 for $n = 45$.

Control Limits

X-bar chart

$$UCL(\bar{x}) = 7.58 + 3 \times \frac{3.53}{0.9943 \sqrt{45}} = 9.17$$

$$LCL(\bar{x}) = 7.58 - 3 \times \frac{3.53}{0.9943 \sqrt{45}} = 5.99$$

S chart

$$UCL(\bar{s}) = 3.53 \times \left(1 + \frac{3}{0.9943}\sqrt{1 - 0.9943^2}\right) = 4.67$$

$$LCL(\bar{s}) = 3.53 \times \left(1 - \frac{3}{0.9943}\sqrt{1 - 0.9943^2}\right) = 2.39$$

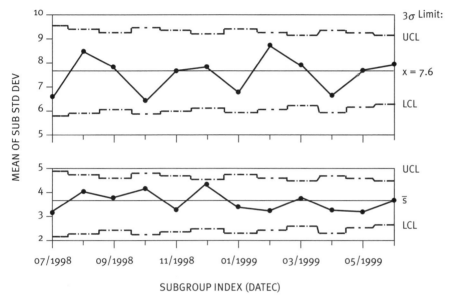

PMS ID = 1   HCO ID = 1   MEAS ID = 3

SUBGROUP INDEX (DATEC)

Subgroup Sizes: Min n=32   Max n=45

Comparison Analysis

For June 1999:

$$Z = \frac{7.93 - 7.76}{3.57 / \sqrt{45}} = 0.319$$

$$U_o = 7.93 + 2.576 \times \frac{3.57}{\sqrt{45}} = 9.30$$

$$L_o = 7.93 - 2.576 \times \frac{3.57}{\sqrt{45}} = 6.56$$

Then, the expected range is:

$$U_e = 7.76 + 7.93 - 6.56 = 9.13$$

$$L_e = 7.76 + 7.93 - 9.30 = 6.39$$

Because $|Z| = 0.319 < 2.576$, the observed value for June 1999 is not a statistical outlier at a 1 percent significance level. The same conclusion for June 1999 performance can be drawn using the expected range approach because the observed value 7.93 is within the expected rage (6.39, 9.13) (Lee and McGreevey 2000).

The comparison chart using these data is shown below.

PMS ID = 1   HCO ID = 1   MEAS ID = 4

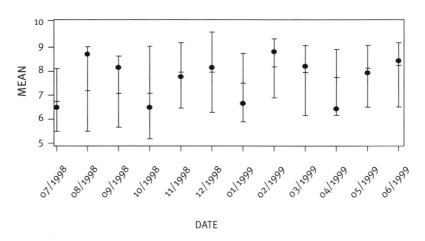

DATE

Notes

1. Kwan Y. Lee, formerly of The Joint Commission, contributed as the first author in the first edition of this chapter.
2. The content of Appendices 1, 2, and 3 is largely based on a Joint Commission specification manual titled *Mining ORYX Data 2000—A Guide for Performance Measurement Systems* (Lee and McGreevey 2000).

References

Agresti, A., and B. A. Coull. 1998. "Approximate Is Better than 'Exact' for Interval Estimation of Binomial Proportions." *The American Statistician* 52 (2): 119–25.

Bickel, P. J., and K. A. Doksum. 1977. *Mathematical Statistics.* San Francisco: Holden-Day.

Czarnecki. M. T. 1994. *Benchmarking Strategies for Health Care Management.* Gaithersburg, MD: Aspen.

Donabedian, A. 1980. *Explorations in Quality Assessment and Monitoring. Volume 1: The Definition of Quality and Approaches to Its Assessment.* Chicago: Health Administration Press.

Holubkov, R., V. L. Holt, F. A. Connell, and J. P. LoGerfo. 1998. "Analysis, Assessment, and Presentation of Risk-Adjusted Statewide Obstetrical Care Data: The StORQS II Study in Washington State." *Health Services Research* 33 (3, Pt. I): 531–48.

The Joint Commission. 1998. *Attributes of Core Performance Measures and Associated Evaluation Criteria.* Oakbrook Terrace, IL: The Joint Commission.

———. 2000. *A Guide to Performance Measurement for Hospitals.* Oakbrook Terrace, IL: The Joint Commission.

Lee, K. Y., and C. McGreevey. 2000. *Mining ORYX Data 2000—A Guide for Performance Measurement Systems.* Oakbrook Terrace, IL: The Joint Commission.

McNeese W. C., and R. A. Klein. 1991. *Statistical Methods for the Process Industries.* Boca Raton, FL: CRC Press.

Montgomery, D. C. 1996. *Introduction to Statistical Quality Control.* New York: Wiley & Sons.

SAS Institute. 1995. *SAS/QC Software: Usage and Reference, Version 6,* 1st ed., vol. 2. Cary, NC: SAS Institute.

PHYSICIAN AND PROVIDER PROFILING

David B. Nash, Adam Evans, and Richard Jacoby

Physician profiles can improve physician performance, especially in the context of continuous quality management and value-based purchasing of healthcare. Profile development is not without problems, however, and profiles are not always fully implemented in healthcare organizations.

Background and Terminology

Centers for Medicare & Medicaid Services (CMS 2007) has forecasted annual healthcare spending to increase from 16 percent of the gross domestic product in 2006 to 19.6 percent of the gross domestic product in 2016. With this increased spending on healthcare, many Americans are beginning to question whether they are receiving increased quality and value for their healthcare dollars. The Institute of Medicine (IOM 2000) detailed that anywhere from 44,000 to 98,000 people die each year from preventable medical errors. Because of increased reports like this one, which detail problems with medical errors and adverse events, the government, employers, and the public are demanding more affordable healthcare and improved quality.

The Physician's Role in Improving Quality

Physicians' actions have been noted to be a major contributor to unexplained clinical variation in healthcare (Dartmouth Institute 2007). Unexplained clinical variation leads to increased healthcare costs, medical errors, patient frustration, and poor clinical outcomes.

   The increase in information being collected on physician practice patterns has begun to expose widespread variations in practice. In healthcare, variation exists among providers by specialty, geographical region, and practice setting. Unexplained clinical variation is present among treatment options for patients with various conditions. Although variation can lead to similar outcomes, it often can lead to problems with care. Uniform medical treatments do not always exist, so unexplained clinical variation continues. If significant improvements are to be made in the healthcare system, physician behavior must be modified to reduce practice variation.

In response to the public's demand for greater physician accountability, initial attempts to change physician behavior resulted in the development of physician report cards (Ransom 1999). However, the medical community has found fault with these report cards. Complaints center largely on the gauges of quality used to measure physician performance and the inconsistencies in risk-adjustment methods comparing outcomes among physicians (University Health System Consortium 2003). As an alternative to report cards, the creation of physician profiles to measure performance can help to minimize variations in healthcare.

Physician Profiling

Physician profiling is the collection of data used to analyze physician practice patterns, utilization of services, and outcomes of care. The goal of physician profiling is to improve physician performance through accountability and feedback and to decrease practice variation through adherence to evidence-based standards of care.

The purpose of establishing consistent treatment methods for physicians is to achieve high-quality, low-cost healthcare. Through profiling, physicians' performance can be measured against their colleagues' performance on a local, state, and national level. The idea is that physicians, who are often highly driven, goal-oriented individuals, will be motivated to increase their performance in areas in which they do not currently rank the highest. Examples of categories in which physicians would be evaluated include patient satisfaction and amount of resources used (Gevirtz and Nash 2000).

Numerous studies have highlighted differences between what physicians think they do and what they actually do in practice (Gevirtz and Nash 2000). Many physicians overrate their performance. Profile development enables a physician's treatment pattern to be recorded. Profiling compares providers' actions to the current evidence-based best practices in medicine and helps to reduce practice variation. With this information, physicians can make changes to improve wasteful or unproductive practice patterns and to better satisfy their patients. Profile development also provides a framework for physician evaluation and quality improvement.

The establishment of measures to assess physician performance will lead to greater accountability and performance by physicians. Since the dissemination of IOM's 2001 publication *Crossing the Quality Chasm*, which detailed the problems with processes of care and unexplained clinical variation in the U.S. healthcare system, more employers, consumers, and patients have been seeking information on which to base healthcare and provider choices. Published information on the strengths and weaknesses of physicians will help healthcare purchasers make decisions based on quality. As physicians continue to decrease variation and improve outcomes in response to increased feedback and measurement of performance, the question of whether purchasers of healthcare are willing to pay for improved performance arises.

Scope and Use of Profiling in Healthcare

Value-Based Purchasing

The government, large employers, and the public are concerned about whether healthcare providers are offering high-quality, affordable care. Because many employees receive health insurance through their employers, employers have a vested interest in purchasing high-quality care. Employers recognize that workers who are satisfied with their health benefits will have a greater desire to remain with a company and will be more productive.

Evidence is growing that healthcare buyers are beginning to use value-based purchasing to make healthcare decisions. In addition to cost, employers are interested in incorporating outcomes and value into their decisions when selecting provider contracts.

Efforts to determine quality measures for hospitals and health plans are now being expanded to include physicians (*Consumer Driven Healthcare* 2003). Common strategies employers use to compare quality among physicians include collecting data on physicians, selective contracting with high-quality providers, partnering with providers to improve quality, and rewarding or penalizing providers to encourage quality (Maio et al. 2003).

These strategies have a significant effect on physician practice patterns and decision making. Information regarding higher-quality providers enables employers to make objective decisions regarding higher-quality care in the best interest of their employees. In addition, collection of reliable and accurate data on physician performance gives purchasers an advantage in contract negotiations with physicians.

In some situations, such data could facilitate a working relationship between healthcare purchasers and providers to improve the quality of care individuals are receiving. Physician performance measurement could lead to the development of continuous quality management programs that could improve various aspects of patient care and clinical outcomes. Financial rewards for physicians who meet the highest standards of performance also would encourage greater physician participation.

Profiling as Part of Continuous Quality Improvement (CQI)

Physicians realize that a problem with quality exists in the United States. Many physicians resent quality improvement efforts centered on them, but equally as many are willing to engage the issue. However, most physicians are suspicious of quality measures as an accurate reflection of the quality of care they provide and are skeptical that data sources other than medical records can provide accurate information about what really happens to patients (Teleki et al. 2006; Nash 2000). As a result, many physicians have dismissed conclusions on their performance as interpretations of inaccurate data.

Many healthcare organizations have developed a CQI strategy that encourages a systems solution to improving healthcare. CQI integrates structure, process, and outcomes of care into a management system that allows processes to be analyzed and outcomes to be improved (see Chapter 5). *Structure* relates to the array of organizational resources in place to provide healthcare to patients. *Process* measures interactions between individuals in the healthcare system. *Outcomes* include both patient response to treatment and how it affects their quality of life (Gevirtz and Nash 2000). This approach involves everyone in an organization and focuses on process failures, not individual failures. An understanding of process problems can help identify and improve factors that contribute to poor quality.

As part of their continuous total quality management strategies, healthcare organizations use several tools to maintain the most competent physician staffs. These tools, described briefly below, include credentialing, outcome management, physician report cards, benchmarking, and clinical pathways (Nash 2000).

Credentialing

Credentialing refers to the process of hiring a well-qualified medical staff that is able to deliver the highest-quality care. Physicians are offered positions on the basis of criteria such as peer review, board certification, and hours spent in continuing medical education. By developing standards for competency, the hospital is able to maintain the highest level of quality among the physicians in its system.

Outcomes Management

Outcomes management is the relationship between clinical outcomes and patient satisfaction. Besides measuring morbidity and mortality, outcomes management takes into account the quality of healthcare received from the patient's perspective (Nash 2000).

Physician Report Cards

Physician report cards (which may be a component of a physician profile) compare physicians on outcomes related to measures such as quality, patient satisfaction, and cost utilization patterns. This information can encourage changes in physician behavior because physicians typically are competitive people. Physicians who do not perform well in rankings against their peers likely will take steps to improve their performance.

However, providers have disapproved of report cards (Casalino et al. 2007). They claim that too much variation exists in the methodologies report cards use to evaluate provider outcomes (Landon et al. 2003). Report cards also do not explain variation among providers' outcomes and therefore make process of care improvement difficult. Another criticism is that they do not provide physicians with feedback alerting them to performance areas that need improvement.

Benchmarking

Benchmarking uses quantitative measures of best practices to evaluate physician performance. When physicians' performance is compared to the best practices of their peers, underperforming physicians may be more willing to change their practice patterns. For example, in ambulatory care, achieving and maintaining an optimal blood level of HbA1c has been identified as an important measurement in controlling the incidence of complications in diabetic patients. If a physician's rate of achieving this level for his or her diabetic population lags that of his or her peer group, the physician can identify and rectify the causes so that subsequent measurements more closely resemble the best practices of the peer group.

Clinical Pathways

Clinical pathways are treatment plans designed to reduce variation in clinical guidelines and protocols and facilitate their implementation. By combining physician input with evidence-based medicine, organizations create new treatment pathways to increase quality, improve outcomes, and decrease costs.

Use in Healthcare Organizations

Physician profiling is one of the many tools used in CQI. It is valuable to healthcare purchasers and in educating physicians. Because unexplained clinical variation can lead to poorer outcomes for patients, measuring the difference between what physicians think they do and what they actually do in practice is an essential part of improving physicians' performance and an organization's overall processes of care. Although physicians typically do not like to examine their own performance, numerous studies have documented that, when presented with information on their performance relative to that of their colleagues, physicians will change their behavior to meet a specified outcome (National Health Information 2003a).

The most effective profiles document variations in provider performance on an individual, local, and national basis. If shown how they perform versus a group of peers, physicians will be more likely to improve in areas in which they rank low. Profiles should be easy to understand and provide specific suggestions. If profiles outline physicians' strengths and weaknesses in a way that is easy to understand, physicians may be more likely to make changes in their behavior.

Healthcare organizations can use physician profiles as a valuable educational tool. Doing things correctly the first time will yield the lowest costs, but doing things correctly the first time is not always possible in medicine. Physician profiles provide physicians with the information to determine which conditions they are treating appropriately, how they compare to their peers, and areas in which they need improvement. Profile comparison displays current trends among specialists and can teach these physicians the most cost-effective practices. On the basis of these trends, an organization can develop quality improvement plans to educate physicians on how to improve their performance.

The creation of an information technology infrastructure to analyze the performance of all physicians in a healthcare system can be useful in identifying the diseases the hospital, physician, or physician group treats most. Organizations then can develop clinical pathways to treat these conditions and improve processes of care.

Patients also can benefit from the creation of physician profiles. Physician profiles would be valuable to a healthcare organization interested in increasing patient satisfaction. Through a survey, patients could evaluate things such as physician bedside manner, the amount of time they spent in the waiting room, and the amount of time they spent with the physician. These data could be analyzed and conveyed to physicians with suggestions for improvement. This commitment to improving physicians' customer service would increase the quality of patient care and patients' confidence in the healthcare they receive. Patient enrollment with physicians in the healthcare organization would increase, increasing system profits.

Clinical and Operational Issues

Best-practice standards in healthcare continue to evolve in response to new medicines and treatment options. Organizations can use physician profiles to compare various processes and determine the most efficient, cost-effective way to practice medicine. In addition, the development of ongoing measurements to evaluate physicians will encourage physicians to stay current on the latest trends in medicine.

Before encouraging the use of profiles, the organization and its physicians must adopt a commitment to CQI. This commitment entails improving patient satisfaction, drafting an agreement to work with the physicians on staff at the hospital or the group in question, and developing mutual quality indicators.

The following list details a number of concerns in the creation of physician profiles (Gevirtz and Nash 2000).

- What do you want to measure, and why is this important?
- Are these the most appropriate measures of quality improvement?
- How will you measure performance? (What is the gold standard?)
- How and when will you collect the measures?
- How reliable are the profiles you are creating?
- What are the most appropriate measures of physician performance?
- Can you measure these variables? (How will you collect the data?)
- What is the appropriate design (e.g., measuring percentages, means)?
- How will you interpret the results (e.g., risk adjustment, acceptable results)?
- How will these findings influence change?

The implementation and use of profiles should be part of a CQI process. A step-by-step approach is the most effective approach to profiling. An approach that moves slowly and involves a diverse group of members of the healthcare organization will be more likely to gain support and produce change within the system.

Choosing Which Measures to Profile

Within a healthcare organization, many areas lend themselves to quality improvement, such as appropriate prescription of antibiotics, surgical outcomes, patient safety, patient satisfaction, and decreased costs. The committee should identify the areas most appropriate for profiling and the areas in which it wants to improve quality. It must understand that not all medical conditions are appropriate for profiling. It should profile only diseases for which evidence-based guidelines exist. This information could come from nationally recognized practice guidelines or other practice parameters.

Guidelines serve as a checklist of objectives against which the team can compare its actions. Without guidelines, the team cannot be sure it is including all components of the care process. This emphasis on rational decision making will foster greater support from physicians in the organization and is more likely to bring about performance improvement.

Collecting the Data

The committee then should identify the techniques it will use to gather and disseminate the data. It should gather the information without interfering with the daily operations of patient care. Traditional methods of data collection have relied on medical records and claims data. In situations where these methods are not available or the most appropriate, direct observation or surveys can be used. Data collection by either method can be difficult, and the committee must assess which data are most applicable for measuring performance. The committee also should identify how much data it will need to gather to produce statistically valid results.

Interpreting the Results

Once the committee gathers the data, it must develop an objective and an appropriate way to interpret the results. It should assess physician performance in relation to the accepted national goals for the disease or whatever target the quality committee decides is appropriate. The committee should gather profiles only on physicians who have a large volume of patients with the disease (or other target). A physician who sees 200 patients with a condition is more likely to value the data on his or her performance than will a physician who sees 20 patients with the same condition. Physicians themselves can help the committee construct profiles by including diseases for which there is potential for improved treatment processes and outcomes, agreeing on benchmarks and gauges of quality, and encouraging other physicians to participate in the quality improvement process. From this information, the committee can determine outcomes that are both statistically and clinically significant.

The data also must be risk adjusted to compensate for the diverse populations of patients that physicians encounter. Risk adjusting will validate the physicians' results and prevent them from arguing that their patients are sicker.

Communicating the Results

Once the committee has developed the profile, it must decide which format will be most valuable to the physician. Graphical representations of data are the easiest to understand and will allow physicians to see their progress over a specific period. The information conveyed to the physician must be kept simple. Physicians are busy individuals; if given too much information, they may become overwhelmed and their efforts to improve quality may decrease. Figure 8.1 is an example of a physician profile that illustrates prescribing behaviors (National Health Information 2003a).

In addition, the committee must decide whether the information distributed in the profiles will be blinded or nonblinded. Some physicians may resent having their performance publicly available for other physicians to see, especially if they rank lower in certain areas. Ideally, physicians will use nonblinded information to find physicians who have better outcomes and to learn ways to improve. Also, physicians who rank lower will want to improve because they do not want to be seen as performing at a lower level than that of their peers. For this part of the process, physician buy-in is crucial.

Prescribed Medication Use
Prescriber: Jane Doe MD
Peer Group: Internal Medicine

FIGURE 8.1
Example of a
Physician
Profile

Report Period: April–June, 2003

of Your Regence patients who filled your prescription: 175   All Oregon prescription card claims

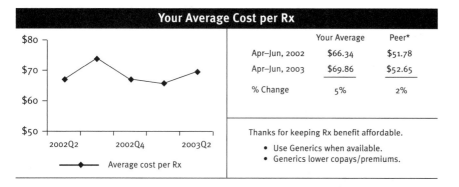

Your Average Cost per Rx

	Your Average	Peer*
Apr–Jun, 2002	$66.34	$51.78
Apr–Jun, 2003	$69.86	$52.65
% Change	5%	2%

Thanks for keeping Rx benefit affordable.
- Use Generics when available.
- Generics lower copays/premiums.

━━◆━━ Average cost per Rx

Prescribed Medication Opportunities

Use more generics in these drug classes:

Drug Class	Your Generic %	Peer* %	Consider these alternatives
Antidepressants	11%	38%	Use *fluoxetine*
Hypotensives–ACE Inhibitors/ARBs	13%	59%	Use *cuptopril, enalapril, listinopril, moexipril*
Lipid Lowering Agents	0%	17%	Use *lovastatin*

Use preferred drugs in place of these non-preferred drugs:

Non-preferred Drug	Rxs	Avg$/Rx	Consider these alternatives:
Non-preferred: ZOCOR	34	$159	Use *lavastatin (Mevacor), Lescol/XL, Lipitor*
Non-preferred: DIOVAN HCT	23	$79	Use *lisinopril + HCTZ, enalapril + HCTZ*
Non-preferred: AMBIEN	25	$70	Use *generic sedative-hypnotics*
Non-preferred: ADVIR DISKUS	12	$144	Use *Azmacort/Flovent/Pulmlcort + Serevent/ Foradil*
Non-preferred LEXAPRO	12	$97	Use *fluaxetine (Prozac)*

Class Overview: Lipid Lowering Agents

Drug Name		Rxs		Drug Cost	Avg$/Rx
LIPITOR		57	54%	$5,975	$105
ZOCOR	NP	34	32%	$5,402	$159
PRAVACHOL	NP	3	3%	$709	$236
LESCOL XL		9	9%	$634	$70
OTHER		2	2%	$182	$92
Total: This Class		**105**	**100%**	**$12,901**	**$123**

NP = non-preferred

Generic
lovastatin (Mevacor®)
has similar LDL reduction
to Pravachol® at less cost.

Lipitor® has highest LDL
reduction per cost.

% Preferred Rxs in Class

	Q2 '02	Q3 '02	Q4 '02	Q1 '03	Q2 '03
Your Rate	64%	57%	62%	61%	63%
Peer Rate*	95%	94%	94%	93%	92%

* The peer comparator is statistically derived at the 70th percentile of Oregon Internal Medicine prescribers.

SOURCE: David Clark, The Regence Group, Blue Cross Blue Shield of Oregon. Reprinted with permission.

Meetings should be scheduled on a weekly, monthly, or quarterly basis so that physicians have the opportunity to provide input on how the profiling system is working. These meetings also will provide time for physicians to obtain feedback on their performance and discuss ways to improve.

Keys to Successful Implementation and Lessons Learned

Implementation

Administrators or quality improvement teams that wish to develop profiles should work closely with physicians. At the start of the project, teams should approach physician leaders who express interest in quality improvement. Involvement of physicians who are open to change, respected by their peers, and knowledgeable about quality will increase the chance that other physicians in the organization will participate.

Specialists require different levels of information and different methodologies to analyze outcomes. In their use of physician profiles, individuals at Providence Medical Center in Seattle found that surgeons were more prone to focus on conclusions, whereas cardiologists were more interested in statistical significance (Bennett, McKee, and Kilberg 1996). Involvement of many different specialists in the quality process will result in greater data validity and increased physician participation.

After the committee develops a profile, it should determine a time frame for all physicians to review the information and submit complaints before the profile becomes an official tool of the organization. Remember, if the committee allows physicians to participate in profile development, they may be more likely to approve of profiling. Once the physicians have submitted their reviews, the committee should meet to finalize the profiles and set a time frame to begin using them.

After the profile has been in use for a defined period, the committee should organize multiple educational sessions. Organization of follow-up activity communicates to physicians that profiling is a program designed for quality improvement. Modification of physician behavior is a process that will happen over time, and organizations need to reassure physicians on a regular basis that they are following the best treatment protocols for their patients. Providing physicians with incentives to improve their performance, such as bonuses or award recognition, also will boost quality improvement.

The profiling system should not be threatening to physicians. If profiles are to be successful in improving healthcare processes and outcomes, physicians must see them as nonpunitive and primarily for educational purposes. Physicians have to believe that profiling is designed to help them improve their performance and target patients who may need more closely monitored care.

Lessons Learned

The use of profiling has many critics. No consensus exists as to what constitutes a profile, what it should measure, and the groups to which the information should be targeted. Employers and consumers want different levels of information with which to make healthcare decisions. Employers are interested in differences in quality and outcomes across providers. Consumers want to know how providers perform with respect to their specific conditions (*Consumer Driven Healthcare* 2003).

Many physicians are skeptical of profiling. They feel that they know what is best for their patients because they see them on a regular basis. Adherence to generally accepted guidelines may not be appropriate for the population of patients they serve.

Individuals with chronic conditions who see several doctors for their condition pose another problem. Examination of the practice pattern of a physician and related outcomes in this case may cause physicians to draw inaccurate conclusions. Also, because many patients constantly switch providers, developing profiles over a period long enough to be meaningful may be difficult (Gevirtz and Nash 2000).

Physicians also may be skeptical of employers' calculations of their results. Physicians who treat a small volume of patients with a specific condition may resent being compared to physicians who treat a larger volume of patients with the same condition.

Agreeing on the best treatment for a particular medical condition is a difficult task. The emergence of new technologies, drugs, and payment schemes on a yearly basis significantly affects a physician's practice and makes reaching consensus on a specific treatment challenging. For these reasons, some physicians may be reluctant to accept national treatment guidelines.

Finally, successful patient outcomes rely partly on patient compliance. The profile has to recognize a level where the physician's efforts to improve quality are at their maximum; beyond this mark, actions of the patient largely determine outcomes.

Case Study

This section highlights a theoretical scenario involving physician profiles in an ambulatory care setting. Two different payers developed the profiles, as part of pay-for-performance programs, for a group of primary care physicians practicing in a large academic group practice and for primary care physicians practicing both individually and in small groups in a private practice setting.

The first payer was a large Blue Cross/Blue Shield (BC/BS) health plan that dominated the local market. It developed its profiles using administrative claim data. The second payer was Medicare, which developed pro-

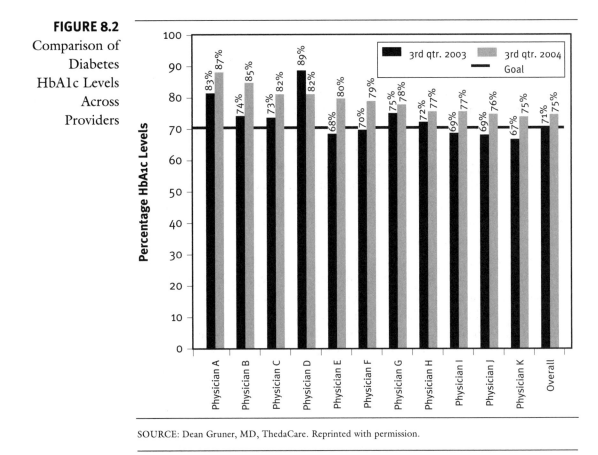

SOURCE: Dean Gruner, MD, ThedaCare. Reprinted with permission.

files from data submitted by physicians on HCFA 1500 billing forms as part of the CMS Physicians Quality Reporting Initiative (PQRI).

The BC/BS profiles involved a variety of measures from the Healthcare Effectiveness Data and Information Set (HEDIS). The measures and goals were chosen in conjunction with representatives from the academic group (for logistical reasons) and applied to all the academic and private practice physicians. BC/BS calculated performance on each measure for each physician. It displayed the information in graphical, nonblinded formats that compared the performance of individual physicians to that of their colleagues (National Health Information 2003b). A sample of the type of data physicians received is shown in Figure 8.2. The physicians received this report quarterly.

A second report, also sent quarterly, not only provided their numerical score for each measure but also benchmarked their performance (scores) against local scores for other physicians in their specialty as well as against national benchmarks. This report also contained information on their pay-for-performance bonuses. For purposes of determining the bonus amounts, each of the measure scores was given a "weight." A weighted average of a physician's scores was then developed, displayed in a profile, and compared to the appropriate aggregated benchmarks (Figure 8.3). Bonuses were paid on a sliding scale based on their performance relative to the benchmarks at the conclusion of the measurement cycle. The maximum achievable bonus represented 5 percent of the total fees the BC/BS plan paid the physician for that cycle. A small percentage of their bonus calculation was allocated to their performance on episode treatment groups, a form of relative cost of care index (Forthman, Dove, and Wooster 2000). Physicians whose performance did not qualify them for a bonus were not penalized.

In graphics like those shown in Figures 8.2 and 8.3, physicians could see whether they were performing up to the best standards and how they compared to the rest of their peers. Some physicians did not like being compared to their peers and having their results shown publicly, but BC/BS emphasized that this report was meant to be nonpunitive and aimed at CQI.

A quality improvement team trained in CQI supported the physicians in the academic group practice. When the initial results were received, the team instituted a CQI education and implementation program. As a result, over the next several years, the practice incrementally improved its performance on the quality measures and eventually received the maximum bonus from the pay-for-performance program. The physicians took pride in their accomplishments.

The physicians in the private practice settings had a slightly different experience. Although their performance on quality measures in the first year paralleled that of their colleagues practicing in the academic setting, they did not perform as well in subsequent years. Lack of an infrastructure supporting CQI caused their performance on the measures to stagnate. They did not qualify for bonus payments and their profiles reflected subpar performance when compared to national and local benchmarks.

Both the academic and private practice groups had more difficulty implementing the Medicare PQRI program (more accurately described as a pay-for-reporting program than a pay-for-performance program when initiated) because the program required more active engagement on the part of physicians and their staffs. This lack of engagement resulted because the physicians' offices had to gather and submit the data on HCFA 1500 billing forms, whereas the BC/BS plan simply aggregated administrative data. Neither the academic nor private practice physicians used electronic medical records, which made data collection labor intensive.

Initially, the participation in the PQRI program was voluntary and required physicians and staff to be educated in quality and quality measures. Physicians primarily used the CMS website to acquire this education. CMS reported the results once per year.

In the academic practice group, the quality improvement team provided supplemental educational materials to physicians, as well as chart tools that facilitated identification and capture of the data required to report the measures.

Quality Measures	Weights	Target Local Peer Group Performance	Target HEDIS 90th Percentile Benchmark Performance	Dr. C Results
Persistence of beta-blocker treatment after a heart attack	11.2%	51.5%	81.0%	57.1%
Comprehensive diabetes care: LDL-C screening performed	11.2%	95.4%	96.0%	83.3%
Colorectal cancer screening	11.2%	56.8%	63.5%	57.9%
Use of appropriate medications for people with asthma	11.2%	91.8%	94.1%	89.5%
Breast cancer screening	11.2%	70.6%	80.1%	73.0%
Comprehensive diabetes care: HbA1c control (<9.0%)	6.0%	70.0%	86.1%	82.0%
Comprehensive diabetes care: eye exam (retinal) performed	6.0%	62.7%	69.3%	43.6%
Osteoporosis management in women who had a fracture	6.0%	29.0%	30.4%	30.0%
Cholesterol management for patients with cardiovascular conditions	6.0%	54.4%	56.5%	46.5%
Resource Management Measures				
Pharmacy management	10.0%	53.18%	55.20%	52.8%
Relative cost of care index (ETGs)	10.0%			Calculated at year-end

FIGURE 8.3
Physician C Profile: Pay-for-Performance Results Through Third Quarter—2006

Initially, the physicians used the tools inconsistently. As a result, relatively few physicians reported on enough measures to earn bonuses in the program. Physician profiles developed by Medicare were incomplete.

In an attempt to monitor the performance in an ongoing manner, the quality improvement team developed a database by using reports from the billing system. It programmed a sophisticated analytic tool to capture the data and report it in a format that could be monitored quarterly so that CQI could be implemented. With this feedback and support, physicians in the academic group practice began to consistently report on measures. Through monitoring, feedback, and interaction between the quality improvement team and the physicians, physicians were able to improve their performance where indicated and receive bonus payments. In addition, their Medicare profiles identified them as physicians practicing high-quality medicine.

The primary care physicians practicing both individually and in small groups in private practice participated minimally in the PQRI program. Many were not aware of the program. Many who were aware of the program found it difficult to comprehend. Of the few who took the time to understand it, most concluded that the 1.5 percent bonus being offered did not cover the costs of gathering the data required to be reported. Occasional physicians and physician groups reported on the required measures, figuring that this type of reporting and profiling would be mandatory at some time in the near future. They appreciated that these quality performance measures would benefit their patients and decided that learning the program was worth the effort, sooner rather than later. In general, the lack of a supporting educational infrastructure had a negative impact on adoption of PQRI in the private practice group.

The success of the academic group practice in both the BC/BS and PQRI profiling programs is a good example of how fostering and supporting a culture of quality in an organization can enhance the delivery of healthcare. Development of incentives to improve physician performance and investment in information systems are valuable initiatives that will help to improve outcomes and make processes of care more efficient.

Study Questions

1. What challenges may an administrator who attempts to measure physician performance encounter?
2. Describe the relationship between continuous quality management and physician profiling.
3. Describe the strengths and weaknesses of the profiles discussed in this chapter.

References

Bennett, G., W. McKee, and L. Kilberg. 1996. "Physician Profiling in Seattle: A Case Study." In *Physician Profiling and Risk Adjustment*, edited by N. Goldfield and P. Boland, 317–31. Gaithersburg, MD: Aspen.

Casalino, L. P., G. C. Alexander, L. Jin, and R. T. Konetzka. 2007. "General Internists' Views on Pay-for-Performance and Public Reporting of Quality Scores: A National Survey." *Health Affairs* 26 (2): 492–99.

Centers for Medicare & Medicaid Services. 2007. "National Health Expenditure Data: Projected." [Online information; retrieved 12/07.] www.cms.hhs.gov/NationalHealthExpendData/03_NationalHealthAcco untsProjected.asp#TopOfPage.

Consumer Driven Healthcare. 2003. Editorial. *Consumer Driven Healthcare* 2 (7): 99–100.

Dartmouth Institute for Health Policy & Clinical Practice. 2007. *Dartmouth Atlas of Health Care.* [Online information; retrieved 12/07.] www.dartmouthatlas.org.

Forthman, T., H. Dove, and D. Wooster. 2000. "Episode Treatment Groups (ETGs): A Patient Classification System for Measuring Outcomes Performance by Episode of Illness." *Topics in Health Information Management* 21 (2): 51–61.

Gevirtz, F., and D. B. Nash. 2000. "Enhancing Physician Performance Through Practice Profiling." In *Enhancing Physician Performance: Advanced Principles of Medical Management*, edited by S. Ransom, W. Pinsky, and J. Tropman, 91–116. Tampa, FL: American College of Physician Executives.

Institute of Medicine. 2000. *To Err Is Human: Building a Safer Health System.* Washington, DC: National Academies Press.

———. 2001. *Crossing the Quality Chasm: A New Health System for the 21st Century.* Washington, DC: National Academies Press.

Landon, B. E., T. Normand, D. Blumenthal, and J. Daley. 2003. "Physician Clinical Performance Assessment Prospects and Barriers." *Journal of the American Medical Association* 290: 1183–89.

Maio, V., N. I. Goldfarb, C. T. Carter, and D. B. Nash. 2003. "Value-Based Purchasing: A Review of the Literature." *Commonwealth Fund Report* 636 (May). [Online information; retrieved 03/08.] www.commonwealth fund.org/publications/publications_show.htm? doc_id=221339.

Nash, D. B. 2000. "The Elements of Medical Quality Management." In *Fundamentals of Medical Quality Management*, edited by J. Hammons, 259–69. Tampa, FL: American College of Physician Executives.

National Health Information. 2003a. "Wrestle Down Drug Costs with Profiling, Education." In *Physician Profiling and Performance:*

Changing Practice Patterns Under Managed Care, vol. II, 29–32. Atlanta, GA: National Health Information.

———. 2003b. "Touchpoint Docs Respond to Feedback Data." In *Physician Profiling and Performance: Changing Practice Patterns Under Managed Care*, vol. II, 4–7. Atlanta, GA: National Health Information.

Ransom, S. 1999. "Enhancing Physician Performance." In *Clinical Resource and Quality Management*, edited by S. Ransom and W. Pinsky, 139–69. Tampa, FL: American College of Physician Executives.

Teleki, S. S., C. L. Damberg, C. Pham, and S. H. Berry. 2006. "Will Financial Incentives Stimulate Quality Improvement? Reactions from Frontline Physicians." *American Journal of Medical Quality* 21: 367–74.

University Health System Consortium. 2003. "Health Care Report Cards: Too Soon for a Passing Grade." White paper, July. Oak Brook, IL: University Health System Consortium.

MEASURING AND IMPROVING PATIENT EXPERIENCES OF CARE

Susan Edgman-Levitan

Quality in health care has two dimensions. Technical excellence: the skill and competence of health professionals and the ability of diagnostic or therapeutic equipment, procedures, and systems to accomplish what they are meant to accomplish, reliably and effectively. The other dimension relates to the subjective experience, and in health care, it is quality in this subjective dimension that patients experience most directly—in their perception of illness or well-being and in their encounters with health care professionals and institutions, i.e., the experience of illness and healthcare *through the patient's eyes.* Health care professionals and managers are often uneasy about addressing this "soft" subject, given the hard, intractable, and unyielding problems of financing, access, and clinical effectiveness in health care. But the experiential dimension of quality is not trivial. It is the heart of what patients want from health care—enhancement of their sense of well-being, relief from their suffering. *Any* health care system, however it may be financed or structured, must address both aspects of quality to achieve legitimacy in the eyes of those it serves. (Gerteis et al. 1993)

Patient satisfaction or patient experience-of-care surveys are the most common method used to evaluate quality from the patient's perspective. Since the 1980s, there has been a strong push to develop surveys that measure the processes of care that matter most to patients and their families in place of older instruments that tended to focus on processes of care or departments that healthcare managers had some control over or decided on their own were important (e.g., food services, housekeeping, admitting). These departments and services all contribute to a positive experience, but they may or may not be what matters most to patients and their families.

In 1987, the Picker/Commonwealth Program for Patient-Centered Care set out to explore patients' needs and concerns, as patients themselves define them, to inform the development of new surveys that could be linked to quality improvement efforts to enhance the patient's experience of care. Through extensive interviews and focus groups with a diverse group of patients and their families, the research program defined eight dimensions of measurable patient-centered care:

1. Access to care
2. Respect for patients' values, preferences, and expressed needs
3. Coordination of care and integration of services
4. Information, communication, and education
5. Physical comfort
6. Emotional support and alleviation of fear and anxiety
7. Involvement of family and friends
8. Transition and continuity

The Picker Institute further explored and enhanced these dimensions of care, and the Institute of Medicine used them as the basis of its definition of patient centeredness in its 2001 publication *Crossing the Quality Chasm*.

An important design feature of these survey instruments is the use of a combination of *reports* and *ratings* to assess patients' experiences within important dimensions of care, their overall satisfaction with services, and the relative importance of each dimension in relation to satisfaction. In focus groups of healthcare managers, physicians, and nurses organized to facilitate the design of "actionable" responses, complaints about the difficulty of interpreting *ratings of satisfaction* came up repeatedly. Clinicians and managers expressed well-founded concern about the inherent bias in ratings of satisfaction and asked for more objective measures describing what did and did not happen from the patient's perspective. The end result has been the development of questions that enable patients to *report* their experiences with care. For example, a report-style question asks, "Did you doctor explain your diagnosis to you in a way you could understand?" instead of, "Rate your satisfaction with the quality of information you received from your doctor."

Regulatory and Federal Patient Survey Initiatives

Most healthcare organizations and settings in the United States routinely measure patient experiences of care in some fashion. Nationally, much of the standardization of survey instruments and processes has occurred as a result of the Consumer Assessment of Healthcare Providers and Systems (CAHPS) initiative, funded by the Agency for Healthcare Research and Quality. The CAHPS program is a multiyear public-private initiative to develop standardized surveys of patients' experiences with ambulatory and facility-level care. Healthcare organizations, public and private purchasers, consumers, and researchers use CAHPS results to:

- assess the patient-centeredness of care;
- compare and report on performance; and
- improve quality of care.

Additional information can be found at www.cahps.ahrq.gov.

As explained above, by providing consumers with standardized data and presenting them in a way that is easy to understand and use, CAHPS can help people make decisions that support better healthcare and better health. This emphasis on the consumer's point of view differentiates CAHPS reports from other sources of information about clinical measures of quality. The CAHPS program is also working to integrate CAHPS results into the quality improvement programs of sponsors and healthcare providers. Centers for Medicare & Medicaid Services (CMS) and the CAHPS team also published *The CAHPS Improvement Guide* (Edgman-Levitan et al. 2003) to help health plans and group practices improve their performance on the surveys. All CAHPS products are in the public domain, free, and available for use by anyone.[1]

CAHPS has been tested more completely than any previously used consumer survey (Hays et al. 1999). Surveys and consumer reports are now completed to measure and report customers' experience of care with health plans for the commercially insured, Medicare and Medicaid populations, and behavioral health services. Over a dozen CAHPS surveys have been developed or are in development for different healthcare settings. Common CAHPS surveys currently used include a hospital survey, a nursing home survey, a health plan survey, and a clinician and group survey. These instruments are being developed as part of a national plan to publicly report results to consumers to foster quality improvement and help consumers improve their decision making about choice of plan, hospital, or provider.

The value of national efforts such as CAHPS lies in the development of standardized surveys and data collection protocols that enable rigorous comparisons among organizations and the creation of trustworthy, accurate benchmark data. Standardized surveys also allow healthcare organizations to share strategies that are known to improve scores and enable consumers to make better choices of plans and clinicians when the data are publicly reported. Publicly reported quality measures enable consumers to make better plan and clinician choices. They also have proven to be a powerful stimulant to internal quality improvement efforts and frequently result in increased budgets for quality improvement work.

The National Committee for Quality Assurance requires that all health plans submit CAHPS data as part of their Healthcare Effectiveness Data and Information Set (HEDIS) submission for accreditation. CMS uses CAHPS to collect data from all Medicare beneficiaries in both managed care plans and fee-for-service settings, and approximately half of state Medicaid programs collect CAHPS data from Medicaid recipients. The CAHPS Hospital Survey, also known as HCAHPS, is a standardized survey instrument and data collection methodology for measuring and publicly reporting patients' perspectives of hospital care. Although many hospitals collect information on patient satisfaction, until the HCAHPS initiative, there had been no national standard for collecting or publicly reporting information that would allow valid comparisons to be made among hospitals.

The HCAHPS survey is composed of 27 questions: 18 substantive items that encompass critical aspects of the hospital experience (communication with doctors, communication with nurses, responsiveness of hospital staff, cleanliness and quietness of hospital environment, pain management, communication about medicines, discharge information, overall rating of hospital, and recommendation of hospital), 4 items that skip patients to appropriate questions, 3 items that adjust for the mix of patients across hospitals, and 2 items that support congressionally mandated reports. There are four approved modes of administration of HCAHPS: (1) mail only; (2) telephone only; (3) mixed (mail followed by telephone); and (4) active interactive voice response (IVR). Hospitals will be reporting HCAHPS data publicly in 2008 to allow consumers to make "apples to apples" comparisons on patients' perspectives of hospital care. Additional information can be found at www.hcahpsonline.org.

Collecting patient experience-of-care data also is becoming a standard evaluation measure in the education and certification of medical, nursing, and allied health students. The American College of Graduate Medical Education has incorporated extensive standards into its requirements for residency training that focus on the doctor-patient relationship, and the American Board of Internal Medicine is piloting patient experience-of-care surveys for incorporation into the recertification process for Board-certified physicians.

Using Patient Feedback for Quality Improvement

Although nationally standardized instruments and comparative databases are essential for public accountability and benchmarking, measurement for the purposes of monitoring quality improvement interventions does not necessarily require the same sort of standardized data collection and sampling. Many institutions prefer more frequent feedback of results (e.g., quarterly, monthly, weekly), with more precise, in-depth sampling (e.g., at the unit or clinic level) to target areas that need improvement. Staff usually is eager to obtain data frequently, but the cost of administration and the burden of response on patients must be weighed against the knowledge that substantial changes in scores usually take at least a quarter, if not longer, to appear in the data.

Survey Terminology

Familiarity with terms describing the psychometric properties of survey instruments and methods for data collection can help an organization choose a survey that will provide it with credible information for quality improvement. There are two different and complementary approaches to assessing the reliability and validity of a questionnaire: (1) cognitive testing, which bases its assessments on feedback from interviews with people who are asked to react to the survey questions; and (2) psychometric testing, which bases its assessments on the analysis of data collected by the questionnaire. Although many existing consumer questionnaires about healthcare have been tested primarily or exclusively using a psychometric approach, many survey researchers view the combination of cognitive and psychometric approaches as essential to producing the best possible survey instruments. Consequently, both methods have been included in the development of CAHPS and other instruments (Fowler 1995, 2001).

The cognitive testing method provides useful information on respondents' perceptions of the response task, how respondents recall and report events, and how they interpret specified reference periods. It also helps identify words that can be used to describe healthcare providers accurately and consistently across a range of consumers (e.g., commercially insured, Medicaid, fee for service, managed care; lower socioeconomic status, middle socioeconomic status; low literacy, high literacy) and helps determine whether key words and concepts included in the core questions work equally well in English and Spanish. For example, in the cognitive interviews to test CAHPS, researchers learned that parents did not think pediatricians were primary care providers. They evaluated the care they were receiving from pediatricians in the questions about specialists, not primary care doctors. Survey language was amended to ask about "your personal doctor," not "your primary care provider," as a result of this discovery (Fowler 1992).

Validity

In conventional use, the term *validity* refers to the extent to which an empirical measure accurately reflects the meaning of the concept under consideration (Babbie 1995). In other words, validity refers to the degree to which the measurement made by a survey corresponds to some true or real value. For example, a bathroom scale that always reads 185 pounds is reliable. Although the scale may be reliable and consistent, it is not valid if the person does not weigh 185 pounds.

The different types of validity are described below.

- *Face validity* is the agreement between empirical measurers and mental images associated with a particular concept. Does the measure look valid to the people who will be using it? A survey has face validity if it appears on the surface to measure what it has been designed to measure.
- *Construct validity* is based on the logical relationships among variables (or questions) and refers to the extent to which a scale measures the construct, or theoretical framework, it is designed to measure (e.g., satisfaction). Valid

questions should have answers that correspond to what they are intended to measure. Researchers measure construct validity by testing the correlations between different items and other established constructs. Because there is no objective way of validating answers to the majority of survey questions, researchers can assess *answer validity* only through their correlations with other answers a person gives. We would expect high *convergent validity*, or strong correlation, between survey items such as waiting times and overall ratings of access. We would expect *discriminant validity*, or little correlation, between patient reports about coordination of care in the emergency room and the adequacy of pain control on an inpatient unit.

- *Content validity* refers to the degree to which a measure covers the range of meanings included within the concept. A survey with high content validity would represent topics related to satisfaction in appropriate proportions. For example, we would expect an inpatient survey to have a number of questions about nursing care, but we would not expect a majority of the questions to ask about telephone service in the patient's room.

- *Criterion validity* refers to whether a newly developed scale is strongly correlated with another measure that already has been demonstrated to be highly reliable and valid. Criterion validity can be viewed as how well a question measures up to a gold standard. For example, if you wanted to ask patients about the interns and residents who cared for them, you would want to be sure that patients could distinguish between staff and trainee physicians. You could measure the criterion validity of questions that ask about the identity of physicians by comparing patients' answers to hospital records.

- *Discriminant validity* is the degree of difference between survey results when the scales are applied in different settings. Survey scores should reflect differences among different institutions, where care is presumably different. Discriminant validity is the extent to which groups of respondents who are expected to differ on a certain measure do in fact differ in their answers (Fowler 1995).

Reliability

Reliability is a matter of whether a particular technique applied repeatedly to the same object yields the same results each time. The reliability of a survey instrument is initially addressed within the questionnaire development phase. Use of ambiguous questions, words with many different meanings, or words that are not universally understood will yield unreliable results. Use of simple, short words that are widely understood is a sound approach to questionnaire design, even with well-educated sample populations (Fowler 1992). An instrument is reliable if consistency across respondents exists (i.e., the questions mean the same thing to every respondent). This consistency will ensure that differences in answers can be attributed to differences in respondents or their experiences.

Instrument reliability, or the reliability of a measure, refers to the stability and equivalence of repeated measures of the same concept. In other words, instrument reliability is the reliability of the answers people give to the same question when they are asked it at different points in time, assuming no real changes have occurred that should cause them to answer the questions differently. Reliable survey questions always produce the same answers from the same respondents when answered under similar circumstances. Thus, reliability is also the degree to which respondents answer survey questions consistently in similar situations. Inadequate wording of questions and poorly defined terms can compromise reliability. The goal is to ensure (through pilot testing) that questions mean the same thing to all respondents.

The *test-retest reliability coefficient* is a method to measure instrument reliability. This method measures the degree of correspondence between answers to the same questions asked of the same respondents at different points in time. If there is no reason to expect the information to change (and the methodology for obtaining the information is correct), the same responses should result at all points in time. If answers vary, the measurement is unstable and thus unreliable.

Internal consistency is the intercorrelation among a number of different questions intended to measure (or reflect) the same concept. The internal consistency of a measurement tool may be assessed using *Cronbach's alpha reliability coefficient*. Cronbach's alpha tests the internal consistency of a model or survey. Sometimes called a *scale reliability coefficient*, Cronbach's alpha assesses the reliability of a rating summarizing a group of test or survey answers that measure some underlying factor (e.g., some attribute of the test taker) (Cortina 1993; Cronbach 1951).

Readability of Survey Instruments

The readability of survey questions has a direct effect on the reliability of the instrument. Unreliable survey questions use words that are ambiguous and not universally understood. No simple measure of literacy exists. The Microsoft Word program comes with a spelling and grammar checker that will produce a statistical analysis of a document. The spelling/grammar checker can calculate the Flesch-Kincaid index for any document, including questionnaires. The Flesch-Kincaid index (Flesch 1948) is a formula that uses sentence length (words per sentence) and complexity, along with the number of syllables per word, to derive a number corresponding to grade level. Documents containing shorter sentences with shorter words have lower Flesch-Kincaid scores.

Weighting Survey Results

Weighting of scores is frequently recommended if members of a (patient) population have unequal probabilities of being selected for the sample. If necessary, weights are assigned to the different observations to provide a representative picture of the total population. The weight assigned to a particular sample member should be the inverse of its probability of selection.

Weighting should be considered when an unequal distribution of patients exists by discharge service, nursing unit, or clinic. When computing an overall score for a hospital or a group of clinics with an unequal distribution of patients, weighting by probability of selection is appropriate. The probability of selection is estimated by dividing the number of patients sampled by the total number of patients. When the probability of selection of patients from different services or units is equal, patients from different services or units will be represented in the sample in the same proportion they occur in the population. If the probability of selection of patients from different hospitals or medical groups is the same, the sample size for different hospitals or medical groups will vary according to the number of total discharges from each.

Similarity—presenting results stratified by service, unit, or clinic—provides an accurate and representative picture of the total population. For example, the most straightforward method for comparing units to an overall score is to compare medical units to all medical patients, surgical units to all surgical patients, and childbirth units to all childbirth patients.

The weighting issue also arises when comparing hospitals or clinics within a system. If the service case mix is similar, we can compare by hospital without accounting for case-mix difference. If service case mix is not similar across institutions, scores should be weighted before comparisons are made among hospitals. Alternatively, comparisons could be made at the service level.

Response Rates

The response rate for mailed surveys is calculated by dividing the number of useable returned questionnaires by the number of patients who were mailed questionnaires. Adjustments are made to the denominator to exclude ineligible cases—questionnaires that were not delivered and patients who should not have been sent a questionnaire, such as deceased patients.

The calculation is different for telephone surveys. The following cases are often removed before calculating rates: nonworking numbers, numbers that were never answered or were answered by a machine, patients who were too ill or confused to be interviewed, and patients the interviewer determined were ineligible for some other reason.

Low response rates compromise the internal validity of the sample. Survey results based on response rates of 30 percent or less may not be representative of patient satisfaction (at that institution). Although a representative sample is chosen, certain population groups are more likely to self-select out of the survey process. An expected (and typical) response bias is seen in all mailed surveys. For example, young people and Medicaid patients are less likely to respond to mailed surveys.

An optimal response rate is necessary to have a representative sample; therefore, boosting response rates should be a priority. Methods to improve response rates include:

- making telephone reminder calls for certain types of surveys;
- using the Dillman (1978) method, a three-wave mailing protocol designed to boost response rates;
- ensuring that telephone numbers or addresses are drawn from as accurate a source as possible; and
- offering incentives appropriate for the survey population (e.g., drugstore coupons, free parking coupons).

Survey Bias

Bias refers to the extent to which survey results do not accurately represent a population. A perfectly unbiased survey is impossible to conduct. Considering potential sources of bias during the survey design phase can minimize its effect. The potential biases in survey results should be considered as well.

Sampling Bias

All patients who have been selected to provide feedback should have an equal opportunity to respond. Any situation that makes certain patients less likely to be included in a sample leads to bias. For example, patients whose addresses are outdated or whose phone numbers are obsolete or incomplete in the database are less likely to be reached. Up-to-date patient lists are essential. Survey vendors also can minimize sampling bias through probability sampling—that is, giving all patients who meet the study criteria an opportunity to be included in the sample.

Nonresponse Bias

In every survey, some people agree to be respondents but do not answer every question. Although nonresponse to individual questions is usually low, occasionally it can be high and can affect estimates. Three categories of patients selected to be in the sample do not actually provide data:

- Patients the data collection procedures do not reach, thereby not giving them a chance to answer questions
- Patients asked to provide data who refuse to do so (do not respond to the survey)

- Patients asked to provide data who are unable to perform the task required of them (e.g., people who are too ill to respond to a survey or whose reading and writing skills preclude them from filling out self-administered questionnaires)

Regardless of how representative the sampling frame is, bias usually is introduced by selected patients' choice not to respond to the survey. Demographic information on all patients in the sample pool can help estimate the size and type of nonresponse bias. You should consider the profile of respondents and nonrespondents in relation to demographic variables that are important to you (e.g., age, gender, payer, or discharge service).

Administration Method Bias or Mode Effects

The way a survey is administered inevitably introduces bias of one sort or another. Comparison of data that have been collected using different modes of administration (e.g., mail and telephone) will reveal differences that are either real or the result of different modes of administration. An instrument that produces comparable data regardless of mode effect introduces no bias. For example, patients who are not literate or do not have a mailing address are excluded from mail surveys. People who do not have phones introduce bias in telephone surveys. In face-to-face interviews, interviewers can influence respondents by their body language and facial expressions. In surveys conducted at the clinic or hospital, respondents may be reluctant to answer questions candidly. A combination of methods, such as phone follow-up to mailed surveys or phone interviews for low-literacy patients, can reduce some of these biases.

A major concern about comparability is that telephone interviews often collect more favorable responses (or answers that reflect more positively on respondents) than do mail surveys. CAHPS testing showed that the majority of the differences could be linked to the way question skips were handled. The telephone interview used explicit screening questions, whereas the mail version asked respondents to check a box labeled "inapplicable" when the question did not apply. The explicit screening question identified many more people to whom questions did not apply than were reflected in the mail data.

Proxy-Response Bias

Studies comparing self-reports with proxy reports do not consistently support the hypothesis that self-reports are more accurate than proxy reports. However, conclusions drawn from studies in which responses were verified using hospital and physician records show that, on average, (1) self-reports tend to be more accurate than proxy reports and (2) health events are underreported in both populations. In terms of reporting problems with care, most studies comparing proxy responses to patients' responses show that proxies tend to report more problems with care than patients do (Vom Eigen et al. 1999). Therefore, the percentage of response by proxy needs to be taken into consideration in the interpretation of survey results.

Recall Bias

Typically, patients receive questionnaires from two weeks to four months after discharge from the hospital. This delay raises concern about the reliability of the patient's memory. Memory studies have shown that the greater the effect of the hospitalization and the nature of the condition are, the greater the patient's ability is to recall health events. Studies also suggest that most people find it difficult to remember precise details, such as minor symptoms or the number of times a specific event occurred. For ambulatory surveys, patients should be surveyed as soon after the visit or event as possible.

Case-Mix Adjustment

Case-mix adjustment accounts for the different types of patients in institutions. Adjustments should be considered when hospital survey results are being released to the public. The characteristics commonly associated with patient reports on quality of care are (1) patient age (i.e., older patients tend to report fewer problems with care) and (2) discharge service (e.g., childbirth patients evaluate their experience more favorably than do medical or surgical patients; medical patients report the most problems with care) (Hargraves et al. 2001).

Scope and Use of Patient Experiences in Healthcare

Customer Service and Patient Satisfaction

Healthcare organizations' ability to deliver high-quality, patient-centered care to their members and patients depends in part on their understanding of basic customer service principles and their ability to integrate these principles into clinical settings.

Healthcare organizations should pay attention to customer service for several reasons. First, better service translates into higher satisfaction for the patient and, subsequently, for the employer who pays most of the bills. Second, as in any other service industry, a satisfied (and loyal) member or patient creates value over the course of a lifetime. In the context of healthcare, this value may manifest itself in the form of repeat visits, trusting relationships, and positive word of mouth. A dissatisfied member or patient, on the other hand, generates potential new costs. Many health plans, for example, have found that the cost of replacing members lost to disenrollment can be high. Patients who are not involved in decision making

FIGURE 9.1

Relationship Between Patient/ Member Satisfaction and Retention

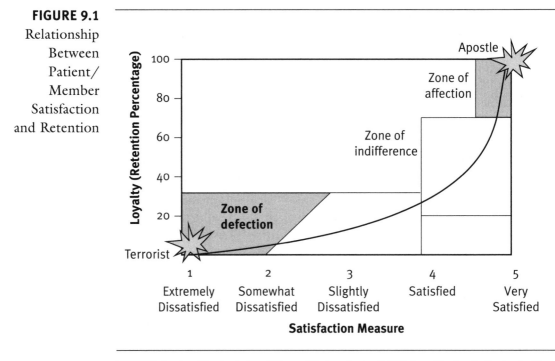

the way they want to be; who cannot get an appointment with their clinician when they are sick; or who are not treated with respect and dignity by their hospital, plan, or clinician may not follow clinical advice, can develop worse outcomes, and frequently share their negative stories with friends and family members. Third, existing patients and members are an invaluable source of information healthcare organizations can use to learn how to improve what they do and reduce waste by eliminating services that are unnecessary or not valued (Heskett et al. 1994).

Figure 9.1 depicts the relationship between satisfaction and loyalty. Individuals who are the most satisfied have the highest correlation to loyalty to a product, service, or provider (the zone of affection). Accordingly, individuals who are the most dissatisfied have the highest correlation to abandonment of their current service, product, or provider (the zone of defection). The zone of indifference reflects the greatest percentage of people who are neither highly satisfied (loyal) nor highly dissatisfied (disloyal).

Finally, poor customer service raises the risk of a negative "grapevine effect." More than 50 percent of people who have bad experiences will not complain openly to the plan or the medical group. However, research shows that nearly all (96 percent) are likely to tell at least ten other people about them. Several years of experience in collecting CAHPS data have revealed that even patient surveys do not adequately capture the full story about problems because, contrary to what many staff and clinicians think, the angriest patients are often the least likely to respond to patient surveys.

Word-of-mouth reputation is important because studies continue to find that the most trusted sources of information for people choosing a health plan, medical group, doctor, or hospital are close family, friends, and work colleagues. When a survey asked people whom they would go to for this kind of information, more than two-thirds of respondents said they would rely on the opinions of family members and friends (Kaiser Family Foundation and Agency for Healthcare Research and Quality 2000). General Electric concluded from one of its studies that "The impact of word-of-mouth on a customer's purchase decision was twice as important as corporate advertising" (Goodman 1987).

Healthcare organizations also need to pay attention to customer service because service quality and employee satisfaction go hand in hand. When employee satisfaction is low, an organization with satisfied patients is almost impossible to find. Employees often are frustrated and angry about the same issues that bother patients and members: chaotic work environments, poor systems, and ineffective training. No amount of money, signing bonuses, or other tools currently used to recruit hard-to-find staff will offset the negative effect of these problems on employees. The real cost of high turnover may not be the replacement costs of finding new staff but the expenses associated with lost organizational knowledge, lower productivity, and decreased customer satisfaction.

Achieving Better Customer Service

The most successful service organizations pay attention to the factors that ensure their success: investing in people with an aptitude for service, technology that supports frontline staff, training practices that incorporate well-designed experiences for the patient or member, and compensation linked to performance. In particular, they recognize that their staffs value achievement of good results, and they equip them to meet the needs of members and patients. For health plans, better customer service could mean developing information systems that allow staff to answer members' questions and settle claims quickly and easily; for provider organizations, better customer service could mean providing the resources and materials that clinicians need to provide high-quality care in a compassionate, safe environment.

Experts on delivering superior customer service suggest that healthcare organizations adopt the following set of principles (Leebov, Scott, and Olson 1998).

1. Hire service-savvy people. Aptitude is everything; people can be taught technical skills.
2. Establish high standards of customer service.

3. Help staff hear the voice of the customer.
4. Remove barriers so staff can serve customers.
5. Design processes of care to reduce patient and family anxiety and thus increase satisfaction.
6. Help staff cope better in a stressful atmosphere.
7. Maintain a focus on service.

Many customer service programs have been developed for companies outside healthcare. Although the strategies are similar, Leebov, Scott, and Olson (1998) have adapted this work for healthcare settings in ways that increase its credibility and buy-in, especially from clinical staff. Their books and articles include practical, step-by-step instructions about how to identify and solve customer service problems in the healthcare delivery system (Leebov 1998).

"Listening Posts" Used to Incorporate Patient and Family Perspective into Quality Improvement Work

Patient satisfaction and patient experience-of-care surveys are the most common *quantitative* measures healthcare organizations use, but they can use other important *qualitative* methods, or *listening posts*, to obtain important information from patients and their families to guide improvement work. Although patient satisfaction surveys provide useful data, they are not the best source of information for innovative ideas about improving the delivery of care. Also, even healthcare organizations with high satisfaction scores have opportunities to improve services, which survey data may not reveal.

Quality improvement activities that focus on the needs and experiences of customers (i.e., members and patients) are effective only in environments that emphasize the concepts and responsibilities of customer service. One critical element of effective customer service is the capacity to elicit detailed, constructive feedback in a way that assures people that someone is listening to them. Members and patients are more likely to report a positive experience to customer service teams that have this skill.

However, this hands-on approach can be a major challenge for healthcare organizations that are not accustomed to communicating with their members or patients in this way. Many assume they understand how to fix the problem and do not probe beneath the surface of complaints and survey responses. Organizations should not be surprised by negative reports. Complaints about unhelpful office staff could stem from many sources.

- Employees did not provide clear directions to patients on how to get to the practice.
- Patients were not able to get an appointment when they needed one.
- Employees put patients on hold in the middle of medical emergencies.
- An employee was rude or disrespectful during a visit or on the phone.

The solutions to these problems vary. Without consulting with patients or members further to understand the true problem, healthcare organizations or quality improvement teams could waste a lot of money on the wrong fixes.

The term *listening posts* refers to a variety of ways to learn about the experiences of patients and staff and involve them in the improvement process. Listening posts already exist in some form in most health plans or clinical practices. The most difficult issue with listening posts is building a system to routinely synthesize the feedback received from them into a coherent picture of what they reveal about the delivery of care. Once this system is in place, root-cause analyses can be performed to identify particular problems, such as a staff member or medical group that contributes to problems, or problems that are systemic to the delivery of care, such as an antiquated manual appointment system. Listening post strategies include:

- surveys;
- focus groups;
- walk-throughs;
- complaint/compliment letters; and
- patient and family advisory councils.

Surveys

Analyzing data from the CAHPS and other patient satisfaction or patient experience-of-care surveys can be beneficial, as can more frequent, small-scale use of individual questions to monitor a specific intervention.

Focus Groups

Staff or patients can be brought together in a moderator-led discussion group to collect more precise information about a specific problem and new ideas for improvement strategies. A focus group allows for more in-depth exploration of the causes of dissatisfaction and can provide excellent ideas for reengineering services. In addition, videotapes of focus groups can be effective at changing the attitudes and beliefs of staff members because the stories participants tell animate the emotional effect of excellent service as well as service failures (Bader and Rossi 2001; Krueger and Casey 2000).

Walk-Throughs

A walk-through may be the fastest way to identify system, flow, and attitude problems, many of which can be fixed almost overnight. Performing a walk-through is an effective way of recreating for staff the emotional and physical experiences of being a patient or family member. Walk-throughs provide a different perspective and uncover rules and procedures that may have outlived their usefulness. This method of observation was developed by David Gustafson, PhD, at the University of Wisconsin in Madison (Ford et al. 2007) and adapted here to incorporate the staff perspective.

During a walk-through, one staff member plays the role of the patient and another accompanies him or her as the family member. They go through a clinic, service, or procedure exactly as a patient and family do, and they follow the same rules. They do this openly, not as a mystery patient and family, and ask staff questions throughout the process to encourage reflection on the systems of care and identify improvement opportunities.

The staff members conducting the walk-through take notes to document what they see and how they feel during the process. They then share these notes with the leadership of the organization and quality improvement teams to help develop improvement plans. For many conducting walk-throughs, they will enter their clinics, procedure rooms, or labs for the first time as a patient and family member. Clinicians are routinely surprised at how clearly they can hear staff comments about patients from public areas and waiting rooms. Walk-throughs usually reveal problems with flow and signage and wasteful procedures and policies that can be fixed promptly.

An alternative to a walk-through is a similar technique called *patient shadowing*. A staff member asks permission to accompany a patient through the visit and take notes on the patient's experience. Because this approach does not take a slot away from a real patient, it can be useful in settings where visits are at a premium.

Complaint/Compliment Letters

Systematic review of letters can provide a better picture of where more background research is needed with staff and patient focus groups or a walk-through versus when a manager should be involved to address a personnel problem.

Patient and Family Advisory Councils

Some patients and health plan members are not concerned with being heard. Rather, their dissatisfaction with their healthcare experience reflects frustration with a system that does not involve them in decisions that will affect the design and delivery of care. From their perspective, the system is superficially responsive; it acknowledges that a problem with service or care exists but does not bother to investigate whether a proposed solution will really address the problem from the patient's or member's point of view.

A patient and family advisory council is one of the most effective strategies for involving families and patients in the design of care (Webster and Johnson 2000). First designed and advanced by the Institute for Family-Centered Care, these councils are composed of patients and families who represent the constituencies served by the plan or medical group. Families and patients both should be involved because they see different things, and each have an important perspective to consider.

The goal of the councils is to integrate patients and families into the healthcare organization's evaluation and redesign processes to improve the experience of care and customer service. In addition to meeting regularly with senior leadership, council members serve as listening posts for the staff and provide a structure and process for ongoing dialogue and creative problem solving between the organization and its patients and families. The councils can play many roles, but they do not function as boards, nor do they have fiduciary responsibility for the organization.

Council responsibilities may include input on or involvement in:

- program development, implementation, and evaluation;
- planning for major renovation or the design of a new building or service;
- staff selection and training;
- marketing plan or practice services;
- participation in staff orientation and in-service training programs; and
- design of new materials or tools that support the doctor-patient relationship.[2]

These councils help organizations overcome a common problem that they face when they begin to develop patient- and family-centered processes—they do not have direct experience of illness or the healthcare system. Consequently, healthcare professionals often approach the design process from their own perspective, not those of patients or families. Improvement committees with the best of intentions may disagree about who understands the needs of the family and patient best. Family members and patients rarely understand professional boundaries. Their suggestions are usually inexpensive, straightforward, and easy to implement because they are not bound by the usual rules and sensitivities.

Usually, employees recommend potential members of the family advisory council, and then those family members form the group. Depending on the size of the organization, most councils have between 12 and 30 patient or family members and 3 or 4 members from the staff of the organization. The council members are usually asked to commit to one two- to three-hour meeting per month, usually over dinner, and participation on one committee. Most councils start with one-year terms for all members to allow for departures in case a member is not well suited for the council.

People who can listen and respect different opinions should be sought. They should offer constructive input and be supportive of the institution's mission. Staff members frequently describe good council members as people who know how to provide constructive critiques. Council members also need to be comfortable speaking to groups and in front of professionals.

Keys to Successful Implementation

Avoid Failure by Establishing Clear Goals

Feedback from patients and their families will provide rich information for quality improvement work. For these efforts to be successful, you should consider the following questions.

- What is your aim for improvement?
- What types of information from patients, families, and staff will help you achieve your aim?
- How frequently do you need to measure your performance to achieve your aim?
- Who will review the data?
- What is your budget?

Once you know the answers to these questions, you can plan your data collection strategy.

What Is Your Aim for Improvement?

If you are trying to improve overall satisfaction with care, or your patients' willingness to recommend your organization to their family members and friends, or both, you must focus your measurement efforts on all dimensions of care that matter to patients and choose a survey that accurately measures these dimensions. If you are trying to improve a specific dimension of the patient's experience of care or the performance of a specific unit (e.g., emergency room, surgical unit, outpatient clinic), you must think carefully about what type of survey you need.

Be sure to determine the strongest drivers of overall satisfaction from the results of the survey you are using and focus on them. In general, many studies document the importance of access to care, doctor-patient communication, and respect for patient preferences; however, you may decide that preparing patients for discharge from the hospital is so important to clinical outcomes that it will take precedence over the other dimensions.

What Type of Information Will Help You Achieve Your Aim?

Match the type of feedback you are collecting to your aim. If you are trying to improve overall satisfaction with care, you may need a combination of survey data, focus group information, and information from compliment/complaint letters. If you are trying to improve a specific unit, you may need a combination of survey data, focus group information, walk-through results, and information from a targeted patient and family advisory council.

Choose a survey instrument that measures the processes of care that matter most to your patients. Make sure it is a validated instrument and that the comparative data are truly comparable. Determine how many organizations like yours are in the database and whether the data can be broken down to give you customized benchmarks. For example, a community hospital near a ski resort measuring patient experiences of emergency room care is probably more interested in benchmarks from other emergency rooms that see lots of orthopedic problems than benchmarks from large urban emergency rooms with many trauma victims.

Pick a survey that has a mode of administration that suits your patient population, and make sure you have tested the questions for administration in that mode. For example, if you have a patient population with low literacy, you may want to choose a telephone survey or a survey that is administered through IVR.

How Frequently Do You Need to Measure Your Performance?

Plan your data collection carefully. Avoid asking patients to answer too many surveys or appearing uncoordinated in your efforts to improve care. If you are trying to improve overall satisfaction with care, quarterly surveys are appropriate; you are unlikely to see changes in the data with more frequent data collection. One the other hand, you may determine that continuous sampling is more appropriate than a onetime snapshot in a quarter, or that you need to survey or interview five patients every Monday, ten patients a week, or all of the patients seen in a specific clinic. If you are testing a specific intervention, try various small tests. Develop a sampling strategy by service, unit, or condition, depending on your aim.

Never underestimate the potential for response bias when surveying patients about their experiences. Many people are concerned that negative responses will jeopardize the quality of care they receive in the future. Make sure that the surveys are administered in a way that provides anonymity and confidentiality. Also, ensure that the measures are taken at a time when the person can evaluate his or her experiences clearly. For example, many vendors try to send surveys to recently discharged patients as quickly as possible. However, patients may not have recovered enough to know whether they have received all the information they need to manage their condition or to know when they may resume activities of daily living or return to work.

Who Will Review the Data?

Make sure you understand the needs and perspectives of the audience who will receive the data. Include open-ended comments, stories, and anecdotes wherever possible in reports; they are powerful motivators for behavior change, and most staff members enjoy reading them. In his studies, Richard Nisbett at the University of Michigan found that data alone were the least persuasive motivator of cultural or behavioral change; stories combined with data were moderately persuasive; and stories alone were the most persuasive (Nisbett and Borgida 1975). Consider how you can combine stories from your walk-throughs, focus groups, and patient-family advisory councils to enrich your staff's understanding of the experiences of care, both positive and negative. If you are trying to attract the attention of senior leaders or clinicians, the scientific rigor of the data collection is important, and comparative data are usually essential to clarify whether the myths about the organization's performance measure up to reality.

You also should consider how the reports are formatted and presented to different audiences. Web-based reports support widespread and rapid dissemination of data. Some audiences need sophisticated graphical presentations; others are most interested in open-ended comments.

What Is Your Budget?

Do everything you can to create a budget that supports the type of data collection necessary to achieve your goals. If you are reporting patient experience-of-care data to the public, you need to maximize the rigor of the data collection to ensure excellent response rates and sampling, and you may need to spend more money to accomplish that goal. If you are collecting the data primarily for quality improvement purposes, you need to consider vendors that can supply the data via the Internet using reporting formats that facilitate quality improvement, such as putting the results into control charts. All these features have different budget implications that need to be considered before putting together a request for proposal.

Be careful not to include any in-house data collection activities (postage, printing the surveys, and mailing them) or analyses as "free." Sometimes organizations actually spend more money by choosing a lower-cost vendor that requires a lot of in-house support and in-kind contributions that are not factored into the overall cost of the data collection. Most healthcare organizations are not sophisticated about these issues, and their internal staff often takes far longer to accomplish the same tasks a good survey vendor could complete much more economically. For example, vendors sometimes drop the cost of postage and mailing the surveys out of their overall budget for a project, expecting the healthcare organization to pick up these costs. These tactics can lower a project bid falsely and need to be screened carefully.

Lessons Learned, or "The Roads Not to Take"

Honest criticism is hard to take, particularly from a relative, a friend, an acquaintance, or a stranger.

—Franklin P. Jones

Resistance to lower-than-expected results is common and reasonable. It is not necessarily a sign of complacency or lack of commitment to high-quality, patient-centered care. Most healthcare clinicians and staff are working harder than they ever have, and the systems they are using to deliver care are not necessarily designed to give patients or staff a positive experience. The expectations of patients and families also have increased over the last decade in response to greater access to clinical information and excellent service experiences in other industries such as banking, financial services, retail stores, and web-based retailers.

Feedback from patients stating that their clinical care falls short of expectations is frustrating and demoralizing for healthcare clinicians and employees to receive. With this in mind, both positive and negative results from patient surveys or listening posts should be presented and, whenever possible, strategies and systematic supports that make it easier for staff to perform at the levels they desire should be included. Executives, senior clinicians, and managers need to be prepared to respond effectively to the common arguments clinical and administrative staff use to deny the validity of patients' feedback. Most of this resistance comes in two forms: *people resistance*, arguments about patients' ability to accurately judge their interactions with healthcare clinicians and staff or the importance of such perceptions, and *data resistance*, arguments that attempt to undermine the scientific credibility of the data.

How to Address People Resistance

- "No one comes here for a good time." One certainly does not, and patients and family members will be the first to agree. Most people want to have as little contact with the healthcare system as possible, but when they need care, they want patient- and family-centered care designed to meet their needs, and they want it delivered in a compassionate, considerate manner.
- "But I was very nice." *Nice* is not the only aspect of quality care. Patients and their families have clearly articulated needs with respect to the care they receive. If the staff members they encounter are nice but do not meet their needs, these staff members have delivered care ineffectively. Usually, staff members emphasize this point when "being nice" was their only recourse to redress other important service failures (e.g., delays, absence of equipment the patient needed, missing lab work or X-rays). To solve this problem, staff must have the resources, systems, and training it requires to meet the needs of patients.
- "This patient/family is very difficult or dysfunctional." Asking staff members to describe patients or families they like and do not like can be helpful. They usually like patients and families who are grateful, patients from the same culture, or patients who speak the same language, but beyond those characteristics, the attributes of popular patients and families become pretty grim. The most popular patients never ring their call lights, never

ask for help, never ask questions or challenge their nurses and doctors, never read medical books, and never use the Internet for help. Their families are not present, and they do not have friends. In fact, they are as close to dead as possible.

- Many people who work in healthcare forget how anxiety-provoking an encounter with the healthcare system is, from finding a parking spot to receiving bad news. For most patients and families, a visit to the doctor or hospital is more like visiting a foreign country or going to jail than a positive, healing experience. They do not speak the same language, and few helpful guidebooks exist to show patients the way.

- We also do everything we can to force people to comply with our rules and regulations, no matter how outdated or meaningless they are, and then we are surprised when they react in anger or dismay. Why should a heart patient have to use a wheelchair to enter the hospital when he or she has been walking around the community for months and then be required to walk out the door only a few days after surgery? Why are we surprised when families fight over chairs or sofas in an ICU waiting room when we provide only a fraction of the chairs or couches necessary for at least two family members per patient? Why do we characterize patients as difficult when they express anger at being forced to go to the emergency room for a simple acute problem after office hours?

- Pointing out the effect of these unspoken beliefs and rules is helpful, as well as reminding everyone that the patients who are least likely to get better are the ones we like. Passive patients rarely do as well in the long run as active, assertive patients who want to learn as much as possible about how to improve their health or be more autonomous.

- "How can patients rate the skill of their doctors/nurses?" Patient and family surveys and the other listening posts described in this chapter are not designed to evaluate the technical skills of clinicians, and patients are the first to acknowledge that they do not know how to do so. Surveys ask patients to evaluate the processes of care and their communication with doctors and nurses (as well as the communication between doctors and nurses)—aspects of care that only they can evaluate. Chart documentation about patient education is worthless if the patient did not understand what was being taught.

How to Address Resistance to Data

- "The sample size is too small—you can't learn anything from it." Interestingly, doctors and other clinical staff trained in statistical methods are often the first to say they will not believe survey data until every patient has been interviewed. Sampling methodology in the social sciences and for survey research is no different from the sampling used in the diagnostic and laboratory tests clinicians trust every day. No one draws all of someone's blood to check hematocrit; a teaspoon or two is plenty.

- "Only angry people respond to surveys." Actually, the opposite is often true. Patients sometimes are afraid that negative responses to surveys will affect the quality of care they receive—a sad indicator of the trust they have in their healthcare providers—and we never hear from patients who likely had problems, such as patients who were discharged to nursing homes, people who speak foreign languages, and patients who died. In fact, the data most people see represent the happiest patients. This inherent bias is another important reason to draw samples that are as representative as possible of the patient population.

- "You really can't determine where something went wrong." Well-designed survey tools that measure things patients care about can provide a good picture of where to start looking. Also, remember to use the other listening posts to determine the sources of the problems, as well as ways to fix them, from the perspective of staff and patients.

- "It's not statistically significant." Again, if you pay attention to the reliability and validity of your survey tools, the sampling strategy, and the quality of your vendor's comparative database, and do everything you can to increase response rates, you will have an excellent idea about the statistical significance of trends and comparative benchmarks.

- "These patients aren't mine; my patients are different." Most people think their patients are different and that all survey data come from someone else's service or patient panel. Stratified results and comparative data can quiet some of these protests. A synthesis of data sources also can be helpful. Staff is more likely to believe that the problems are real if survey data reveal problems in the same areas addressed by complaint letters.

Other Reasons for Failure

- "We survey only because we have to." Organizations that survey only because an outside entity requires them to will never be successful in their efforts to become truly patient centered. Surveying is a waste of time and money until leadership takes the importance of patient- and family-centered care seriously.

- "Our bonuses are based on the results. We have to look good whether we are or not." When the incentives are aligned to reward people for appearing to be excellent instead of for collecting honest feedback and working to improve it, improvement efforts will never be successful. As with efforts to improve patient safety, rewarding people for continuing the status quo or hiding problems will never work.

- "The report sits on the shelf." Reports must be user friendly and easily accessible. Fortunately, most survey results are now available on the Internet, facilitating dissemination across an organization and customization of results to meet the needs of different audiences. The chief of primary care probably does not care about the results of the orthopedic clinic; doctors want to see results about the dimensions of care important to them, not dimensions that evaluate other disciplines or things over which they have no control (e.g., the claims processing service in a health plan).

- "Patient experience-of-care data do not appear credible to clinicians and senior leaders." If data and stories collected from patients and their families meet rigorous scientific standards and focus on issues that have relevance to clinicians, clinicians and senior leaders are more likely to take them seriously. The more they perceive the information to have relevance to clinical outcomes (help to reduce pain and suffering and improve patients' ability to manage their ongoing health problems), the more the organization will value it. If feedback is only collected about "safe" issues (e.g., food and parking), staff will be less willing to use it for improvement. Involve all of the end users of the data in the process of selecting survey instruments and vendors. Have them participate in other listening post activities. Videotape focus groups, and have clinical staff do walk-throughs or attend patient and family advisory council meetings.

- "Patient satisfaction is valued more than employee and clinical satisfaction." Again, patient satisfaction will never be high unless staff and clinicians feel nurtured and supported by the organization as well. Patient and staff satisfaction go hand in hand, and acknowledgment of this relationship will reinforce and motivate improvement efforts in both areas.

Case Study

A walk-through is an excellent method to use at the start of a quality improvement project because it is a simple and inexpensive but powerful way to provide clinicians and other staff with insights about the experience of care. Walk-throughs always yield ideas for improvement, many of which can be implemented quickly. Walk-throughs also build support and enthusiasm for redesigning care through the eyes of the patient much more rapidly than do data or directives from managers to "be nice to patients."

As you do the walk-through, ask questions of staff you encounter. The following questions incorporate the staff's perspective about its own work improvement opportunities into the process.

- What made you mad today?
- What took too long?
- What caused complaints today?
- What was misunderstood today?
- What cost too much?
- What was wasted?
- What was too complicated?

- What was just plain silly?
- What job involved too many people?
- What job involved too many actions?

Keep careful notes, and you will have a long list of things you can fix the next day.

Several years ago, the medical director and head nurse of a public community hospital emergency room joined an Institute for Healthcare Improvement Service Excellence Collaborative to improve the care in their emergency room. At the start of the collaborative, they did a walk-through in which the doctor played a patient with asthma and the nurse was his family member. They encountered several surprises along the way, and their experience ultimately guided a redesign of the emergency room's physical environment and processes of care. They came to one realization right at the beginning of the walk-through—the "patient" and the "family member," both clinical leaders of the emergency room, never had entered the emergency room through the patient entrance.

When the patient called the hospital number (from his office) and told the operator he was having an acute asthma attack, the operator put him on hold without explanation for several minutes. The operator did transfer his call to the emergency room, but his anxiety increased because he did not understand what was happening.

When he was finally connected to the emergency room, his family member took the phone to get directions to the entrance from an address in the neighborhood. The person was incapable of helping her and finally found someone else to give her directions. After this delay, as they followed the directions, they discovered they were incorrect. Also, as they drove up to the hospital, they realized that all of the signage to the emergency room entrance was covered with shrubs and plants. They had no idea where to park or what to do.

The emergency room entrance and waiting area were filthy and chaotic. The signage was menacing and told them what not to do rather than where they could find help. They felt like they had arrived at the county jail.

As the patient was gasping for air, they were told to wait and not to ask for how long. At this point in the walk-through, the doctor described his anxiety as so intense he thought he actually might need care.

The family member went to the restroom, but it was so dirty she had to leave; she realized that this simple but important condition made her lose all confidence in the clinical care at the emergency room. If staff could not keep the bathroom clean, how could it do a good job with more complicated clinical problems?

The most painful part of the walk-through occurred when the nurse told the patient to take his clothes off. He realized there was no hook, hanger, or place for them; he had to put them on the floor. For years he had judged his patients negatively because of the way they threw their clothes on the floor, only to discover that this behavior was, in essence, his fault.

The story could continue indefinitely. Many of the problems the medical director and head nurse experienced were relatively easy to fix quickly: standardized, written directions to the emergency department in different languages for staff to read, different signage in the waiting areas and outside the hospital, and better housekeeping and other comfort issues such as clothes hooks in the exam areas. Other problems took longer to redress, but one simple walk-through helped refocus the hospital's improvement aims and its perspective on the importance of the patient's experience of care.

Conclusion

Apart from the obvious humane desire to be compassionate toward people who are sick, improving the patient experience of care results in better clinical outcomes, reduced medical errors, and increased market share. The leadership, focus, and human resource strategies required to build a patient-centered culture also result in improved employee satisfaction because we cannot begin to meet the needs of our patients until we provide excellent training and support for our clinical staff and all employees. Improving the patient's experience of care could be the key to transforming our current healthcare systems into the healthcare systems we all seek.

Study Questions

1. What is the difference between patient reports about experiences with care and patient ratings of satisfaction?
2. What criteria should you use when selecting a patient survey?
3. List four methods other than surveys to acquire feedback from patients and families to help improve care.
4. What are four arguments for the importance of collecting feedback from patients and families about their experiences with care?

Notes

1. The CAHPS Survey and Reporting Kit 2002 contains everything necessary to conduct a CAHPS survey, including the CAHPS 3.0 questionnaires in English and Spanish. To learn more about CAHPS, access a bibliography of publications about the CAHPS products, or order a free copy of the kit, go to www.cahps.ahrq.gov.
2. The Peace Health Shared Care Plan is an example of such material and is available at www.peoplepowered.org.

References

Babbie, E. R. 1995. *Survey Research Methods*, 2nd ed. Belmont, CA: Wadsworth.

Bader, G. E., and C. A. Rossi. 2001. *Focus Groups: A Step-by-Step Guide*, 3rd ed. San Diego: Bader Group.

Cortina, J. M. 1993. "What Is Co-Efficient Alpha? An Examination of Theory and Applications." *Journal of Applied Psychology* 78: 98–104.

Cronbach, L. J. 1951. "Coefficient Alpha and the Internal Structure of Tests." *Psychometrika* 16: 297–334.

Dillman, D. A. 1978. *Mail and Telephone Surveys: The Total Design Method*. New York: John Wiley & Sons.

Edgman-Levitan, S., D. Shaller, K. McInnes, R. Joyce, K. Coltin, and P. D. Cleary. 2003. *The CAHPS Improvement Guide: Practical Strategies for Improving the Patient Care Experience*. Baltimore, MD: Centers for Medicare & Medicaid Services.

Flesch, R. F. 1948. "A New Readability Yardstick." *Journal of Applied Psychology* 32: 221–33.

Ford J. H., C. Green, K. Hoffman, J. Wisdom, K. Riley, L. Bergmann, and T. Molfenter. 2007. "Process Improvement Needs in Substance Abuse Treatment: Admissions Walk-Through Results." *Journal of Substance Abuse Treatment* 33 (4): 379–89.

Fowler, F. J., Jr. 1992. "How Unclear Terms Affect Survey Data." *Public Opinion Quarterly* 56 (2): 218–31.

———. 1995. *Improving Survey Questions: Design and Evaluation*. Thousand Oaks, CA: Sage.

———. 2001. *Survey Research Methods*. Thousand Oaks, CA: Sage.

Gerteis, M., S. Edgman-Levitan, J. Daley, and T. Delbanco. 1993. *Through the Patient's Eyes: Understanding and Promoting Patient-Centered Care*. San Francisco: Jossey-Bass.

Goodman, J. 1987. "Setting Priorities for Satisfaction Improvement." *Quality Review* (Winter).

Hargraves, J. L., I. B. Wilson, A. Zaslavsky, C. James, J. D. Walker, G. Rogers, and P. D. Cleary. 2001. "Adjusting for Patient Characteristics when Analyzing Reports from Patients About Hospital Care." *Medical Care* 39 (6): 635–41.

Hays, R. D., J. A. Shaul, V. S. Williams, J. S. Lubalin, L. D. Harris-Kojetin, S. F. Sweeny, and P. D. Cleary. 1999. "Psychometric Properties of the CAHPS 1.0 Survey Measures. Consumer Assessment of Health Plans Study." *Medical Care* 37 (3, Suppl.): MS22–MS31.

Heskett, J. L., T. O. Jones, G. Loveman, E. Sasser, Jr., and J. A. Schlesinger. 1994. "Putting the Service-Profit Chain to Work." *Harvard Business Review* 167 (Mar./Apr.).

Institute of Medicine. 2001. *Crossing the Quality Chasm: A New Health System for the 21st Century.* Washington, DC: National Academies Press.

Kaiser Family Foundation and Agency for Healthcare Research and Quality. 2000. *Americans as Health Care Consumers: An Update on the Role of Quality Information, 2000.* Rockville, MD: Agency for Healthcare Research and Quality.

Krueger, R. A., and M. A. Casey. 2000. *Focus Groups: A Practical Guide for Applied Research.* Thousand Oaks, CA: Sage.

Leebov, W. 1998. *Service Savvy Health Care: One Goal at a Time.* San Francisco: Jossey-Bass/AHA Press.

Leebov, W., G. Scott, and L. Olson. 1998. *Achieving Impressive Customer Service: 7 Strategies for the Health Care Manager.* San Francisco: Jossey-Bass.

Nisbett, R., and E. Borgida. 1975. "Attribution and the Psychology of Prediction." *Journal of Personality and Social Psychology* 32: 932–43.

Vom Eigen, K. A., J. D. Walker, S. Edgman-Levitan, P. D. Cleary, and T. L. Delbanco. 1999. "Carepartner Experiences with Hospital Care." *Medical Care* 37 (1): 33–38.

Webster, P. D., and B. Johnson. 2000. *Developing and Sustaining a Patient and Family Advisory Council.* Bethesda, MD: Institute for Family-Centered Care.

Other Useful Resources

Charles, C., M. Gauld, L. Chambers, B. O'Brien, R. B. Haynes, and R. Labelle. 1994. "How Was Your Hospital Stay? Patients' Reports About Their Care in Canadian Hospitals." *Canadian Medical Association Journal* 150 (11): 1813–22.

Cleary, P. D. 2003. "A Hospitalization from Hell: A Patient's Perspective on Quality." *Annals of Internal Medicine* 138 (1): 33–39.

Cleary, P. D., and S. Edgman-Levitan. 1997. "Health Care Quality. Incorporating Consumer Perspectives." *Journal of the American Medical Association* 278 (19): 1608–12.

Cleary, P. D., S. Edgman-Levitan, J. D. Walker, M. Gerteis, and T. L. Delbanco. 1993. "Using Patient Reports to Improve Medical Care: A Preliminary Report from 10 Hospitals." *Quality Management in Health Care* 2 (1): 31–38.

Coulter, A., and P. D. Cleary. 2001. "Patients' Experiences with Hospital Care in Five Countries." *Health Affairs (Millwood)* 20 (3): 244–52.

Delbanco, T. L., D. M. Stokes, P. D. Cleary, S. Edgman-Levitan, J. D. Walker, M. Gerteis, and J. Daley. 1995. "Medical Patients' Assessments of Their Care During Hospitalization: Insights for Internists." *Journal of General Internal Medicine* 10 (12): 679–85.

Edgman-Levitan, S. 1996. "What Information Do Consumers Want and Need?" *Health Affairs (Millwood)* 15 (4): 42–56.

Frampton, S., L. Gilpin, and P. Charmel. 2003. *Putting Patients First: Designing and Practicing Patient-Centered Care.* San Francisco: Jossey-Bass.

Fremont, A. M., P. D. Cleary, J. L. Hargraves, R. M. Rowe, N. B. Jacobson, and J. Z. Ayanian. 2001. "Patient-Centered Processes of Care and Long-Term Outcomes of Myocardial Infarction." *Journal of General Internal Medicine* 16 (12): 800–808.

Fremont, A. M., P. D. Cleary, J. L. Hargraves, R. M. Rowe, N. B. Jacobson, J. Z. Ayanian, J. H. Gilmore, and B. J. Pine II. 1997. "The Four Faces of Mass Customization." *Harvard Business Review* 75 (1): 91–101.

Goodman, J. 1999. "Basic Facts on Customer Complaint Behavior and the Impact of Service on the Bottom Line." *Competitive Advantage: ASQ Newsletter* 8: 1.

Homer, C. J., B. Marino, P. D. Cleary, H. R. Alpert, B. Smith, C. M. Crowley Ganser, R. M. Brustowicz, and D. A. Goldmann. 1999. "Quality of Care at a Children's Hospital: The Parent's Perspective." *Archives of Pediatric and Adolescent Medicine* 153 (11): 1123–29.

Larson, C. O., E. C. Nelson, D. Gustafson, and P. B. Batalden. 1996. "The Relationship Between Meeting Patients' Information Needs and Their Satisfaction with Hospital Care and General Health Status Outcomes." *International Journal of Quality in Health Care* 8 (5): 447–56.

Leebov, W., and G. Scott. 1993. *Service Quality Improvement: The Customer Satisfaction Strategy for Health Care.* San Francisco: Jossey-Bass/AHA Press.

Roth, M. S., and W. P. Amoroso. 1993. "Linking Core Competencies to Customer Needs: Strategic Marketing of Health Care Services." *Journal of Health Care Marketing* 13 (2): 49–54.

Seelos, L., and C. Adamson. 1994. "Redefining NHS Complaint Handling— The Real Challenge." *International Journal of Health Care Quality Assurance* 7 (6): 26–31.

Seybold, P. B. 2001. "Get Inside the Lives of Your Customers." *Harvard Business Review* 79 (5): 80–89, 164.

Veroff, D. R., P. M. Gallagher, V. Wilson, M. Uyeda, J. Merselis, E. Guadagnoli, S. Edgman-Levitan, A. Zaslavsky, S. Kleimann, and P. D. Cleary. 1998. "Effective Reports for Health Care Quality Data: Lessons from a CAHPS Demonstration in Washington State." *International Journal of Quality in Health Care* 10 (6): 555–60.

Wasson, J. H., M. M. Godfrey, E. C. Nelson, J. J. Mohr, and P. B. Batalden. 2003. "Microsystems in Health Care: Part 4. Planning Patient-Centered Care." *Joint Commission Journal of Quality and Safety* 29 (5): 227–37.

10

DASHBOARDS AND SCORECARDS: TOOLS FOR CREATING ALIGNMENT

Michael D. Pugh

Measurement is a critical leadership function. As a means of organizing and using measurement to drive change, dashboards and scorecards are useful tools. When used properly, they can contribute to accelerated rates of improvement and better alignment of effort.

Background and Terminology

Many healthcare organizations use some form of cross-functional or multidimensional measurement tool. Robert S. Kaplan and David P. Norton first used the term *Balanced Scorecard* in their January–February 1992 *Harvard Business Review* article, "The Balanced Scorecard—Measures That Drive Performance." Based on a multicompany study, the article examines approaches to organizational performance management beyond the use of standard financial and accounting measures. Kaplan and Norton's theory was that reliance on traditional financial measures alone to drive performance limits a company's ability to increase shareholder value. This investigational premise is consistent with quality guru Dr. W. Edwards Deming's idea that companies cannot be run by visible numbers alone (Aguayo 1991). To overcome this limitation, successful companies use a broader index of performance metrics to create a balance between financial and other important dimensions of organizational performance.

Kaplan and Norton's 1996 follow-up book, *The Balanced Scorecard—Translating Strategy into Action*, further examines the development of performance measures linked to organizational strategy. To achieve results, Kaplan and Norton observe that the Balanced Scorecard should be central to the leadership system rather than function simply as a balanced set of outcome measures for the organization. The above-referenced work is the original text on the deployment of strategy and development and use of balanced sets of measures at the organizational level to drive performance.

Kaplan and Norton (1996) observe that most organizations collect nonfinancial performance measures that reflect important dimensions such as customers, service, and product quality. However, these measures generally are reviewed independently from financial results and with decreased leadership emphasis. Kaplan and Norton also observe that leaders can increase organizational alignment by simultaneously reviewing and monitoring the critical measures across multiple dimensions of performance, not just financial dimensions. Kaplan and Norton see the Balanced Scorecard as central to deploying organizational strategy rather than simply as a monitor of a broader set of outcome or process measures.

Dashboards

Although the terms *dashboard* and *scorecard*[1] are used interchangeably in practice, the words have two different meanings. The term *dashboard* brings to mind the indicator panel on an automobile, which is most useful when the car is moving as a way for the driver to monitor key performance metrics such as speed, fuel level, engine temperature, and direction from digital display units. The driver also could monitor other metrics, such as tire pressure, manifold temperature, oil viscosity, or transmission efficiency. These measures may be useful to a NASCAR driver in a high-performance race car, but they are not critical to the average driver's journey from point A to point B. Instead, drivers rely on a core set of important high-level measures to inform the real-time process of driving the car.

The cockpit of an airplane is a more complex example of a collection of instruments that reports information critical to successful air travel. The driver of a car or the pilot of an airplane monitors multiple indicators of performance simultaneously to arrive at the intended destination successfully. At any given point in the journey, the driver or pilot may focus on one indicator, but overall success depends on the collective performance of the systems represented by the indicators. Dashboards are tools that report on the ongoing performance of the critical processes that lead to organizational success rather than on the success itself.

Scorecards

The term *scorecard* brings to mind a different image. Scorecards are used to record and report on prior periods or past performance rather than on real-time performance. Generally, they are outcome measures rather than process measures. School report cards, for example, report how an individual student performed against a specific grading standard and are issued at some point after all work is completed. Although there is a lag time in reporting, changes can be made to influence future outcomes, such as changes in study habits, class attendance, allocation of study time to a specific subject matter, outside tutoring, or homework preparation. However, these possible changes are the result of investigation of the current process rather than review of information available on the report card.

Golf scorecards are another example. They reflect the outcome of the previous holes played, compare the score for each hole to a target score (par), and compare performance against other players or an overall stroke target for the game. In a competitive match, a player can use this report of past performance to influence the level of aggressive play on future holes. Also, a player can monitor the cumulative score during play to judge the likelihood of achieving a desired overall score for the round. However, the scores from past holes generally do not tell a player much about the changes he or she needs to make to improve success on future holes. Instead, the focus is on results. For many of us, golf might be more fun if we did not keep score. If we never keep score, however, we will never know how our play compares to the target (par) or other players' performance, or how our play varies from round to round.

Although the above differences between scorecards as outcome or results measures and dashboards as process measures may be logical, in practical application within healthcare they are rarely distinct. Healthcare organizations are complex, and a metric often is a process measure and an outcome measure at the same time. As a result, many organizational scorecards contain a mix of outcome-, strategic-, and process-related measures. The key issue is how leadership uses the measures and measurement sets to align priorities and achieve desired organizational results.

Scope and Use of Dashboards and Scorecards in Healthcare

Common Uses of Dashboards and Scorecards

A typical hospital routinely collects and reports on hundreds of quality and performance measures for external reporting to regulatory agencies and for internal quality monitoring. Although most healthcare organizations use some form of a dashboard/scorecard at the senior leadership level, there often is a wide gap between the existence of a measurement set that an organization calls a scorecard/dashboard and the actual use of the tool to create alignment.

Commonly Used Measurement Sets

Hospitals routinely collect and review patient satisfaction and financial indicators and generally monitor a large, diverse set of quality indicators. As a condition of accreditation, The Joint Commission requires organizations to collect and monitor a specific set of quality indicators and provide them to survey teams. This required set of indicators aligns closely with quality indicators for specific clinical conditions (e.g., pneumonia and heart failure) promulgated by the Centers for Medicare & Medicaid Services (CMS) and collected on hospitals by CMS-contracted professional review organizations (PROs) in the late 1990s.

In 2003, the American Hospital Association organized an effort to report a set of common quality indicators publicly in response to growing concern that CMS would at some point require public disclosure of a broad set of quality indicators. Currently, CMS requires both hospitals and long-term care facilities to collect a core set of quality and clinical indicators that are made publicly available through the CMS website. Multiple states, as well as state hospital associations, hospital trade groups, commercial sites such as HealthGrades.com, and business coalitions such as the Leapfrog Group, are publishing sets of quality measures. Although transparency is intended to spur healthcare organizations to pay attention to important quality indicators, many view public reporting of performance data as a questionable regulatory process rather than a meaningful reflection of an organization's performance. There is a significant difference between compliance with regulatory reporting and creating an organizational focus around a set of key performance indicators that leadership uses to guide improvement efforts.

Other healthcare organizations collect a variety of measures to judge organizational performance and manage operations. Managed care organizations generally participate in a national data set known as the Healthcare Effectiveness Data and Information Set (HEDIS), which compares a variety of outpatient clinical performance indicators at the physician practice level, such as immunization rates and breast cancer screening rates in the covered population. Organized medical groups also may collect some form of patient satisfaction data as well as the HEDIS clinical data set. Other nonclinical indicators that health plans and physicians may use include waiting time to next appointment and medical cost per member, per month.

Quality Scorecards and Dashboards

Most commonly, healthcare organizations use some form of quality scorecard/dashboard at the senior leadership level to support the governance function. These scorecards tend to be reports of past achievement or quality control measures rather than drivers of future efforts, and they are not used routinely in the strategic manner contemplated by Kaplan and Norton. They often are populated with outcome and process-based measures. For example, inclusion of a quality control measure such as the nosocomial infection rate on a governance dashboard is not unusual, even absent an active improvement effort or link to organizational strategy. Healthcare organizations have monitored infection rates for years, but they generally react to them only when an outbreak occurs. Some organizations may include infection rates on their scorecards by default because of the absence of more important clinical outcome measures.

Organizing by Categories of Measures

Healthcare organizations traditionally sort the measures they collect into the categories of financial, volume, satisfaction, and clinical quality. Leadership often views these categories as independent sets, useful in day-to-day management. Some organizations have developed summary dashboards of key indicators, organized by category to facilitate review. For instance, leaders may receive and review a financial report routinely. At a different time, leadership may receive a customer/patient satisfaction or workforce report and then, through a committee review process, receive a report on clinical quality indicators. All these reports may be organized into scorecard or dashboard formats that highlight the key indicators. Quality scorecards and dashboards have become popular ways of reporting on clinical quality to medical staff committees and to the board. Although these approaches may be useful for these groups' review, format alone does not impart usefulness. Scorecards and dashboards should drive leadership behavior.

Financial and volume measures traditionally have driven management behavior in healthcare. One indicator of the emphasis on business in healthcare in the late 1970s and the 1980s was healthcare governing boards' tendency to spend considerably more time discussing financial reports and indicators than quality or satisfaction reports. Even though financial review still dominates, boards and senior leadership teams are now devoting more time to reviewing quality, workplace culture, and patient satisfaction data to balance their view of the important dimensions of performance. Although patient satisfaction measures are well developed and commonly used, widely accepted measures of clinical effectiveness remain underdeveloped. Despite the increased emphasis on patient safety and harm prevention, safety metrics are generally underrepresented on organizational performance scorecards.

Dashboards and scorecards may be organized in a variety of formats ranging from simple tables to web-based graphical reports embedded in computerized decision support systems. Data report formats include tables, radar charts, bar graphs, run or control charts, and color-coded indicators designed to highlight metrics that do not meet targets or expectations.[2] In some organizations, each operating unit has a scorecard of key indicators that mirrors the organizational or corporate scorecard.

Formatting available measures into a summary dashboard (either department/category specific or cross-dimensional) is a start. However, senior leaders can harness the real power of measures by organizing their leadership systems to achieve results. Figure 10.1 is one depiction of the leadership system in a healthcare organization. The leadership system drives both organizational culture and alignment in daily work to achieve a desired level of organizational performance. One of the key elements of the leadership system is the measurement process, which includes the tools of dashboards and scorecards.

FIGURE 10.1

Balanced
Scorecard
Central to
Strategic
Leadership
System

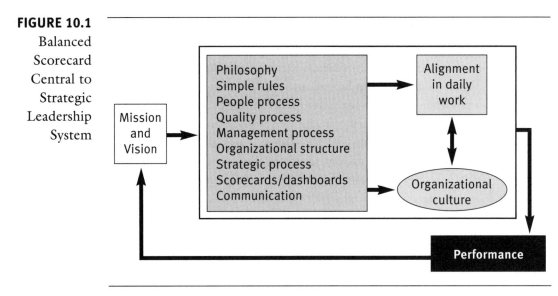

SOURCE: Pugh Ettinger McCarthy Associates, LLC. Used with permission.

The challenge for healthcare leaders is to make sense of the multitude of measures and metrics that exist and are routinely available in most organizations. Scorecards and dashboards are useful tools for organizing important metrics. However, healthcare leaders struggle with this question: What should we measure? The answer is tied to the answer to another question: For what purpose? Form should follow function.

Applications of Scorecards and Dashboards
Governance and Leadership Measures

Healthcare organizations should consider the use of three basic sets of measures in a scorecard or dashboard format. Figure 10.2 summarizes the three basic types of performance metrics and the relationships between the different types. At the governance level, a set of organizational performance measures should be defined and monitored. The organization should link these measures to how it defines performance within the context of its mission, vision, and values. A governance-level scorecard of performance measures should be a basic tool for all healthcare governing boards.

At the senior leadership level, a different set of measures should be used to align priorities, lead the organization, and embody the concept of a Balanced Scorecard. The organization should link these measures to its critical strategies, or *vital few* initiatives, and use them to drive desired results. As Kaplan and Norton (1992, 1996) suggest, strategic measures should be at the center of the organization's leadership system. Although

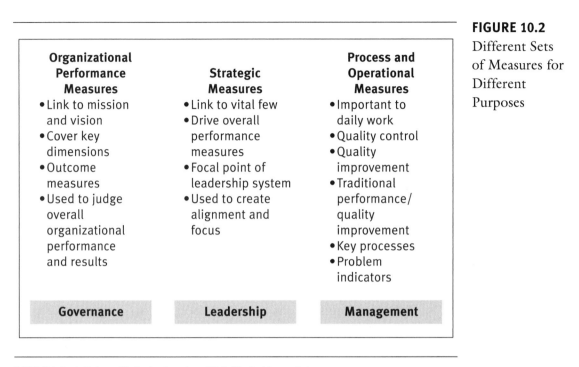

SOURCE: Pugh Ettinger McCarthy Associates, LLC. Used with permission.

leadership's role is to deploy strategy, monitoring deployment is also a governance responsibility. A dashboard of strategic measures is a tool leaders can use to set priorities and drive change.

The board also may use the same dashboard as a scorecard to monitor the deployment of strategy and assess leadership effectiveness. An important relationship exists between the overall organizational performance measures and the strategic measures. Strategy should focus on what drives desired organizational results. The test of good strategy and strategic measures is whether successful deployment of the strategies results in improved performance as measured by the scorecard.

Process and Management Measures

Typical metrics found on dashboards of critical process measures include quality control metrics, efficiency metrics, traditional quality/performance improvement measures, labor statistics, customer satisfaction indexes, and other routine statistics used in day-to-day operation. The monitored operational/process measures should be linked to the strategic measures. Organizational alignment is enhanced when, at the day-to-day work level, key processes that have a direct link to a specific organizational strategy are monitored and the successful deployment of strategy improves one or more organizational performance metrics.

FIGURE 10.3
Critical
Dimensions of
Healthcare
Organizational
Performance

- Patient and customer (satisfaction)
- Effectiveness (clinical outcomes)
- Appropriateness (evidence and process)
- Safety (patient and staff)
- Equity

- Employee and staff satisfaction (culture)
- Efficiency (cost)
- Financial
- Flow (wait times, cycle times, and throughput)
- Community/population health

SOURCE: Pugh Ettinger McCarthy Associates, LLC. Used with permission.

Dimensions of Performance in Healthcare

What is good performance in healthcare? How do we know whether we are doing a good job? How should we organize our important measures to have the greatest effect? What should be on our organizational scorecard?

These questions are critical for healthcare leaders. Figure 10.2 indicates that performance is an outcome of the leadership process and ultimately should be measured by the organization's ability to meet its mission and vision. Another way to think about performance is by important dimensions. Healthcare is about more than bottom line. Use of the word *performance* here instead of the term *quality* emphasizes that performance is a broader term that encompasses quality, although some advocates of quality improvement theory may disagree. The point is that performance and quality in healthcare should be considered broadly; therefore, organizations should identify the multiple dimensions of performance.

One method of defining performance is in terms of traditional financial, satisfaction, human resources, and clinical dimensions. However, many organizations have benefited from a broader consideration of what constitutes the important dimensions of performance in healthcare. Figure 10.3 lists some of the critical dimensions that healthcare organizations can use to define performance.

In *Crossing the Quality Chasm*, the Institute of Medicine (IOM) (2001) suggests a different approach to thinking about performance in healthcare. IOM recommends that patient care be reorganized and redesigned to achieve six specific aims:

- Safety
- Effectiveness
- Patient centeredness
- Timeliness
- Efficiency
- Equity

Some organizations have found these six aims useful in defining organizational performance and the type of metrics that should be included on their scorecards.

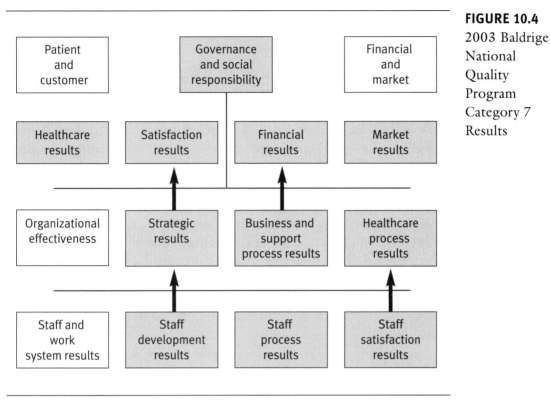

SOURCE: Pugh Ettinger McCarthy Associates, LLC. Used with permission.

FIGURE 10.4

2003 Baldrige National Quality Program Category 7 Results

A third approach to organizing performance results is the Baldrige National Quality Program (BNQP) framework. The criteria for Category 7, Organizational Performance, define specific classes of performance results that applicants are expected to track and report. Figure 10.4 shows the relationships between the various results required by BNQP.

Aside from the three examples discussed here, organizations can use other methods to develop and define the important dimensions of performance. Traditional financial, human resources, satisfaction, and clinical dimensions are the foundations of most methods. In addition, religiously affiliated healthcare organizations often include dimensions of performance related to the mission of the sponsoring organization.

Clinical and Operational Issues

Creating an Organizational Scorecard

The development of an organizational scorecard should involve more than simple organization of existing measures into a new format or framework. The first step is to decide on an appropriate framework for the scorecard. Next, senior leadership and the governing body should define the dimensions of performance relevant to the mission of the organization and the results they wish to achieve. Once they agree on these dimensions, leaders and governing boards should attempt to select appropriate outcome measures for each of the chosen dimensions.

At the organizational level, the ideal cycle time for performance measurement is quarterly. However, some metrics may be difficult or too expensive to obtain on a quarterly basis, and the organization may be forced to default to one or more annual measures. Sometimes the appropriate outcome measure for a dimension does not exist; the organization then must use a proxy measure or invest in the development of new metrics.

Healthcare leaders and trustees should include enough measures in an organizational scorecard to define the desired results in each of the important dimensions. Initially, in their enthusiasm for the process and desire to include great detail, most organizations nominate more measures than are practical and tend to include multiple process measures rather than outcome measures. Additional measures may be interesting, but the focus should remain on results. Organizations can maintain this focus in the measure selection process by concentrating on the results they want to achieve rather than on potential good measures. In the for-profit corporate world, the aim is fairly straightforward—increased shareholder value (defined as more than temporary stock price). In the not-for-profit healthcare provider world, the aims may be numerous, but they are just as measurable.

The governing body and senior leadership should use the organizational scorecard to monitor overall performance in a balanced manner. They also should use it to assess CEO and leadership performance. Although boards and senior leadership will continue to look at supporting reports of financial and clinical quality and other sources of additional performance detail, they should focus on the results they wish to achieve, as defined by the set of organizational performance measures.

When possible, organizations should compare their performance measures to the benchmarks of similar types of organizations and specific targets noted on the scorecard. Benchmarking does not mean comparing to the average. Instead, benchmarking should identify great or best levels of reported performance. Organizations then should deploy strategies to close the gap between current performance and the benchmark. Benchmarking in healthcare is a challenge, but it is becoming easier in some areas. Information on patient and employee satisfaction benchmark performance is available through the proprietary databases maintained by survey companies. Comparative financial and workforce information is also available through multiple sources, some free and some available by subscription. Comparative clinical outcome metrics are becoming more widely available as well.

However, for some clinical and safety issues, the target should be 100 percent. What level of medication error is acceptable to patients? How do you choose which qualified cardiac patient should not receive evidence-based clinical care? Setting best-in-class targets and high expectations on performance scorecards will help organizations achieve their desired results and thus increase healthcare reliability in these key areas.

One could begin to create an organizational scorecard by creating potential measures for each of the six IOM aims, such as:

- adverse drug events per 1,000 doses (safety);
- functional outcomes as defined by SF-12 health surveys, hospital mortality rates, compliance with best-practice guidelines, and disease-specific measures (effectiveness);
- patient satisfaction (patient centeredness);
- number of days until the third next available appointment (timeliness);
- hospital costs per discharge (efficiency); and
- effectiveness indicators by race/ethnicity and gender (equity).

Minimal agreement exists regarding the important outcome measures for an organization. An understanding of the critical dimensions of performance and the use of emerging national conventions (e.g., the IOM aims) can guide their development.

Creating Alignment

Creating alignment in organizations is a critical leadership function. Leadership has been a hot topic for many years, especially discussion of how to create and communicate a compelling vision. Innumerable works have been written about managing people and organizations and executing change. However, less literature exists on the leadership function of creating alignment between the compelling vision and the day-to-day work of organizations.

Figure 10.5 identifies the important leadership actions that create alignment. Scorecards and dashboards can be useful tools supporting the measurement, executive review, and strategy processes used to link overall direction to the day-to-day work of the organization. Different measurement sets organized into scorecards or dashboards support the three core leadership functions (see Figure 10.6).

One approach to creating alignment is to use the identified organizational performance dimensions as a framework for measurement throughout the organization. Metrics may be different in every department or division, but they are linked by consistent focus at every level of the organization.

For example, many healthcare organizations have identified patient satisfaction as a key dimension of performance. In a competitive market, the organization also may determine that one of its critical strategies is to improve patient satisfaction to build market share. The strategic dashboard could feature a set of metrics that confirm that improvement in satisfaction is taking place. To link this strategy to daily work, every operating unit could monitor some metric that relates to patient satisfaction with the services the

FIGURE 10.5

Leadership
Functions

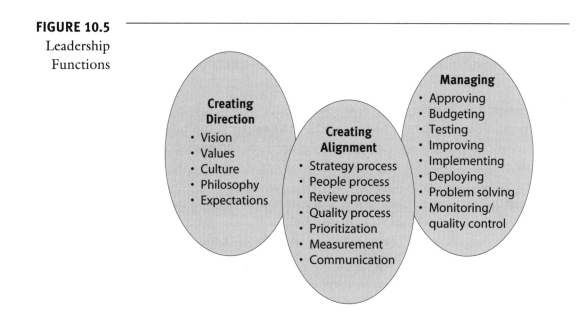

SOURCE: Pugh Ettinger McCarthy Associates, LLC. Used with permission.

FIGURE 10.6

Different
Measurement
Sets Support
Different
Leadership
Functions

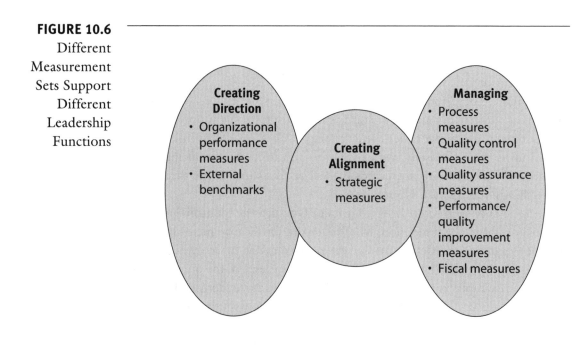

SOURCE: Pugh Ettinger McCarthy Associates, LLC. Used with permission.

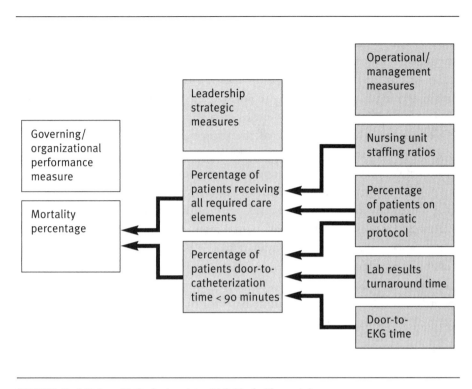

FIGURE 10.7
Creating Organizational Alignment Around a Critical Project: Cardiac Mortality

SOURCE: Pugh Ettinger McCarthy Associates, LLC. Used with permission.

department provides as well as monitor and improve processes known to affect satisfaction positively. An emergency room could monitor patient satisfaction information for its service, and the departmental operating dashboard could contain the appropriate metric. The emergency room also could be working on a project to improve flow, which in turn would reduce waiting time, a key process that affects the satisfaction of emergency patients. In this example, clear links exist among the organizational performance dimension of satisfaction, strategic measures, and the day-to-day improvement efforts and operation of the emergency room.

Figure 10.7 depicts a second method of creating organizational alignment in a critical strategy or project. This fictitious organization has determined that reducing mortality among heart attack patients is an important aim for the population it serves. At the governance level, overall cardiac mortality could be monitored as an organizational performance measure. In this example, the hospital has determined that the two key leverage points, or critical strategies, for reducing cardiac mortality in its organization are to (1) ensure that all cardiac care is delivered per evidence-based care plans and (2) reduce the time from presentation in the emergency room to initiation of interventional therapy.

Successful deployment of the two critical strategies is defined by the percentage of patients who received 100 percent of the required care elements and the percentage of patients with door-to-catheterization lab times of less than 90 minutes. These metrics are included on a strategic dashboard and regularly reviewed by senior management and the board. Through review and inclusion of these metrics on a strategic dashboard, senior leaders emphasize the importance of the project, have a method of monitoring the deployment progress, and have a method to link desired results (lower mortality) to specific actions (strategies and tactics).

The targets associated with the two strategies are important because they alert management to the significance of the change and desired results. Informed by these results, departmental management and clinical leadership then can organize efforts to understand the key processes and the levels of reliability at which these processes must operate. Once leadership identifies key process measures, it can add them to the appropriate management dashboards and use them on a real-time basis for further improvement or process control. For purposes of this example, the processes on the far right of Figure 10.7 are identified as the critical supporting processes. The theory is that improvement and control of these processes will bring about the desired results in the strategic measures, ultimately affecting overall cardiac mortality.

Keys to Successful Implementation and Lessons Learned

Successful development of performance scorecards and dashboards is dependent on many factors. This section describes some of the critical issues and problems organizations face in the development and use of performance measures.

Develop a Clear Understanding of the Intended Use

Healthcare management tends to be faddish. In some organizations, creation of the first scorecard is assigned to a member of the management team after a senior leader or board member has read or heard at a conference that healthcare organizations should have a performance scorecard. These efforts are doomed to failure. The CEO, senior leadership team, and board must have a clear understanding of why a scorecard is being created and how the board and senior leaders intend to use the scorecard. Many scorecards developed by organizations are sitting on shelves gathering dust, next to the strategic plans.

Engage the Governing Board Early in Development of Performance Measures

Organizations repeatedly make the mistake of having senior leadership present a performance scorecard to the board as an item of new business without adequate predevelopment discussion or involvement by the board. Ultimately, the governing body is responsible for the performance of the organization. This responsibility extends beyond simple fiduciary duties and includes clinical and service performance. Performance scorecards should reflect desired organizational results. Governing bodies must be involved in defining the important dimensions and choosing the relevant measures. Much of the work of development may be assigned to leadership and clinical teams, but final determination of the important dimensions and measures is the board's responsibility.

Use the Scorecard to Evaluate Organizational and Leadership Performance

Once developed, the organizational performance scorecard should be central to the organization's governance system. The scorecard should reflect the mission of the organization and be used by the board and leadership to evaluate progress toward achieving that mission. The governing board should review the scorecard at least quarterly. Because scorecards are about results, they can be useful in the CEO performance evaluation process and provide a balanced set of objective measures that can be tied to compensation plans and performance review criteria.

Be Prepared to Change the Measures

Developing a good organizational performance scorecard is a simple idea but difficult to do. An organization is unlikely to achieve a "perfect" set of measures the first time. Often measures that reflect the real results desired for a performance dimension do not exist and have to be developed. Other times, organizations realize after a couple of review cycles that they want better measures than those they currently use. Scorecard development is usually an iterative process rather than a single-shot approach. Organizations should continue to improve their scorecards as new understanding of the desired results linked to each dimension surfaces and as better metrics are developed. To quote the philosopher Voltaire, "Perfect is the enemy of good." Organizations should work toward creating a good scorecard, not a perfect one.

Make the Data Useful, Not Pretty

Formats should be useful and understandable. Many organizations struggle with fancy formats and attempts to create online versions. A good starting point is to construct simple run charts that display the measures over time and the desired target for each measure. Simple spreadsheet graphs can be dropped into a text document, four or six per page. The information conveyed, not the format, is important. Organizations have had mixed success with more sophisticated formats such as radar charts. Some boards find radar charts invaluable because they display all the metrics and targets on a single page. Other boards have difficulty interpreting this type of graph. The admonition to start simple does not imply that other approaches will not work. One innovative computer-based display (see the Case Study section) uses a radar chart backed by hot-linked run and control charts for each performance metric.

Integrate the Measures to Achieve a Balanced View

Although some organizations like to use scorecard and dashboard formats for financial and quality reports, the routine display of metrics in separate category-driven reports may reflect a lack of integration. If an organization has developed a broader set of high-level measures and the category-based reports support the key measures, this characterization is likely invalid. However, if an organization chooses to use separate detailed scorecards of financial, quality, and service metrics and reviews each independently, as tradition dictates, it probably will place more emphasis on financial results and pay less attention to clinical, satisfaction, and other dimensions, except when there is a crisis in a given area.

Develop Clear and Measurable Strategies

Kaplan and Norton (1992, 1996) contend that strategic measures should be central to the leadership system. Strategic dashboards and Balanced Scorecards are key tools that leaders can use to create alignment of effort. Unfortunately, in healthcare, strategy and strategic planning are generally underdeveloped. Many organizations engage in a superficial annual process that results in a set of vague objectives that are task oriented rather than strategic. Often, the strategic plan sits on a shelf until it is time to dust it off in preparation for the next board retreat. Organizations will have difficulty developing a Balanced Scorecard as envisioned by Kaplan and Norton if strategies are not clear, measurable, and truly strategic. In most organizations, a simple set of critical, or vital few, strategies exist; if successfully deployed, these strategies will accelerate an organization's progress toward achieving its mission and vision. Organizations should identify these critical strategies or strategic themes and develop a set of specific measures for each strategy.

Some organizations find tracking deployment progress on a specifically designed strategic dashboard useful. Choice of the measures is important because the measures help to define what the strategy is intended to accomplish. For most critical strategies, innumerable ideas and potential tactics exist. All proposed tactics, initiatives, or projects should affect one or more of the strategic measures directly. If not, leadership should look elsewhere to invest resources.

Use the Organizational Performance Dimensions to Create Alignment of Effort

One strategy for using scorecards and dashboards to create alignment is to build cascading sets of metrics consistent with the key dimensions of performance on the organizational scorecard. Each operating unit or department is required to develop a set of metrics for each of the key dimensions. For example, if patient safety is a key dimension, each nursing unit could track and seek to improve its fall rate or adverse drug event rate. If employee well-being is a key performance dimension, each department could track voluntary turnover rates. One important caveat is that measures should not be collected on departments; instead, each department or operating unit should develop and "own" a set of measures or dashboard consistent with the key performance dimensions. Executive review of departmental performance should include the entire set of measures rather than focus on the financial dimension this month and a service or clinical quality dimension next month.

Avoid Using Indicators Based on Averages

Averages mask variation, are misleading, and should be avoided when possible in developing scorecards and dashboards. For example, the average time from door to drug in the emergency room may be below a preset operating standard. However, examination of the data may reveal that a significant percentage of patients do not receive treatment within the prescribed standard. A better approach is to measure the percentage of patients who receive treatment within a specified standard. Average waiting times, average length of stay, average satisfaction scores, and average cost are all suspect indicators.

When Possible, Develop Composite Clinical Indicators for Processes and Outcome Indicators for Results

The whole issue of clinical indicators is difficult. Healthcare organizations are complex and generally provide care across a wide continuum of patient conditions and treatment regimens. They often have difficulty determining which clinical indicators are truly important and representative of the process of care provided. One approach is to develop composite indicators for high-volume, high-profile conditions. For example, the CMS/PRO review set contains six cardiac indicators. Most hospital organizations track their performance against each of the indicators, which is appropriate at the operational level.

However, at the senior leadership level, tracking the percentage of cardiac patients who received all six required elements may be more useful. This tracking accomplishes two things. First, it limits the number of metrics on a senior leadership or governing board scorecard. Second, it emphasizes that all patients should receive all required aspects of care, not just four out of six. Organizations can use the same approach to track performance for chronic diseases such as diabetes. They can establish the critical aspects of care that should always happen (e.g., timely hemoglobin testing, referral to the diabetes educator, eye and foot exams) and develop a composite measure that reflects the percentage of patients who receive complete care.

Another approach to developing clinical performance metrics is to consider the results rather than the process. Mortality and readmission rates are obvious results. Some organizations are beginning to look beyond these types of measures and are considering clinical results from the perspective of the patient. Development of experimental questionnaires and approaches to assessing patient function is underway and may include the following types of patient-centered questions.

- Was pain controlled to my expectations?
- Am I better today as a result of the treatment I received?
- Am I able to function today at the level I expected?
- Is my function restored to the level it was at before I became ill or was injured?
- Did I receive the help I need to manage my ongoing condition?
- Am I aware of anything that went wrong in the course of my treatment that delayed my recovery or compromised my condition?

When Possible, Use Comparative Data and External Benchmarks

When possible, use external benchmark data to establish standards and targets. Many organizations track mortality and readmission rates on their scorecards. Mortality is a much stronger performance measure when it is risk adjusted and compared to other organizations to establish a frame of reference. Without that frame of reference, mortality tracking provides little useful information except to note directional trends. However, beyond establishing a frame of reference, organizations should set targets based on best performance in class rather than peer-group averages. Comparison to a peer-group mean tends to reinforce mediocrity and deflects attention from the importance of the desired result monitored by the performance measure. One of the best examples is the peer averages and percentiles that most of the national patient satisfaction survey vendors provide. Being above average or in the top quartile does not necessarily equate to high patient satisfaction. A significant percentage of patients may be indifferent about the care they received or dissatisfied. Instead of percentile-based targets (targets based on ranking), average raw score or the percentage of patients who express dissatisfaction may be better indicators.

Change Your Leadership System

There is a saying that goes something like, "If you always do what you have always done, you will always get what you always got." One mistake some organizations have made is to roll out an elaborate set of cascading dashboards and scorecards and then fail to change the way the leadership system functions. Scorecards and dashboards quickly can become another compliance effort or something done for The Joint Commission outside the organization's "real work." Leadership must make the review of measurement sets an integral part of its function. When senior leaders review departments or operating units, the unit scorecard/dashboard should be their primary focus. If a strategic dashboard is developed, progress review should occur at least monthly or be coordinated with the measurement cycles of the indicators. Governing boards should review the organizational performance measures at least quarterly. Review should not be for the sake of review only but for the purposes of driving change and setting priorities.

Focus on Results, Not on Activities

A well-developed system of dashboards and scorecards allows leadership to focus on results instead of activities. Many results-oriented, high-performing organizations work from a leadership philosophy of tight-loose-tight. Senior leaders are very clear and "tight" about the results they wish to achieve and can measure them through the use of strategic and operational dashboards. At the same time, they are "loose" about the direct control of those doing the work, creating a sense of empowerment in those charged with achieving the results. In the absence of clear measures, leaders tend to control activities, micromanage, and disempower others in the organization. When desired results are clear, senior leaders can be "tight" about holding individuals and teams accountable for achieving them.

Cultivate Transparency

One characteristic of high-performing organizations such as BNQP winners is that every employee knows how his or her individual efforts fit into the bigger picture. Healthcare has a long tradition of secrecy about results, in part a reflection of the historical view that quality is about physician peer review and in part a reaction to the malpractice environment. Transparency is a big step for some organizations, but the results posted on the organizational scorecard should be discussed openly and shared with employees and clinical staff. Ideally, the results also should be shared with the community served. Employees and clinical staff need to know what dimensions of performance are important to the organization and the results, as well as the important process and management indicators and dashboards related to their daily work.

The same is true for strategic measures. Many organizations consider strategy confidentiality a ludicrous idea; successful deployment of strategy generally depends on what an organization does itself, not on what its competitors may do. Sometimes, a specific tactic such as building a new clinic in a competitive part of town may need to be closely held because of market issues, but the critical strategy relating to growth of the enterprise should not be a secret. Awareness and improvements of key processes that support a strategy are difficult to create if the strategy and strategic measures are secret.

Case Study: St. Joseph Hospital[3]

St. Joseph Hospital (SJH) in Orange, California, is the flagship hospital of the St. Joseph Health System (SJHS), sponsored by the sisters of St. Joseph of Orange. The system consists of 14 hospitals, all located in California, with the exception of Covenant Health, which is located in Texas. SJH and the Covenant Health operation are the two largest healthcare organizations in the system.

SJHS was an early adopter and developer of a systemwide approach to collecting and reporting a set of common performance indicators. Using the four dimensions of the quality compass framework (financial, human resources, clinical, and satisfaction), the corporate office collects a common set of performance indicators monthly from each hospital in the system. Known internally as "the web," individual hospital radar charts are developed. On a periodic basis, the information is shared with the corporate health system board. Hospital leadership and the local governing boards of each hospital use the charts to track progress, and the results are used in the individual CEO performance review process. A run or control chart backs each indicator on the radar chart. SJHS has been innovative in the development of its scorecard tool, using the system information to post monthly updates, which are accessible through the system intranet. The indicators are fairly traditional, but SJHS continues to modify and change indicators as the state of its art advances. Figure 10.8 is a representation of the monthly performance web for SJH.

Although both the corporate office and the governing boards of the hospitals considered the web useful for tracking performance across the system, they viewed it as a helpful but insufficient tool for driving change at SJH. Larry Ainsworth, CEO, realized early in 2002 that a different set of measures tied to organizational strategy were required to continue to progress and remain competitive in the Orange County marketplace. Traditionally, SJH used an annual planning process that yielded a business plan of more than 20 pages of objectives and proposed actions. Management spent an

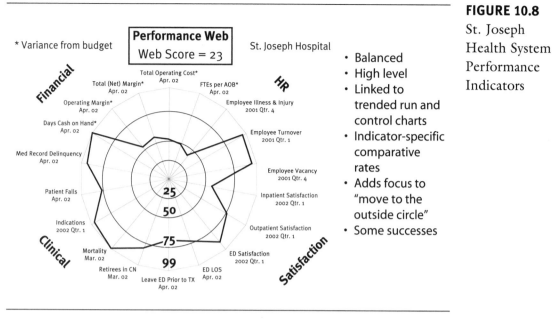

SOURCE: St. Joseph Health System. Used with permission.

FIGURE 10.8
St. Joseph
Health System
Performance
Indicators

enormous amount of time developing and tracking activities and objectives and reporting monthly to the board.

Instead of starting over, senior leadership examined the business plan and from it concluded that all of the proposed objectives could be sorted into five strategic themes. The five vital few strategies identified by the SJH leadership team are displayed in Figure 10.9.

For each strategy, a team of senior leaders and clinicians was formed to develop specific proposed strategic measures and identify the required tactics for deployment. Many of the tactics were modifications of previously identified objectives and actions, but the team developed many new ones in consideration of how they would affect the strategic measures directly. Development of visual strategy maps and associated measures for each tactic helped the hospital accomplish its aim of integrating previously separate quality, business, and strategic plans into a single approach. Hospital leadership viewed the strategy maps as critical to creating alignment and focus.

For each strategy, a dashboard of key measures was developed. The senior leadership team reviews this dashboard monthly and shares results with the governing board on a quarterly basis. Figure 10.10 is a sample of the strategic dashboard used to drive progress on SJH's oncology strategy. The strategies must be measurable, and each proposed tactic is required to have a set of associated measures to guide deployment.

Ainsworth and his leadership team made changes in the leadership system and began routine, scheduled, in-depth review of each strategy. The review started with the results of each of the strategic dashboard

FIGURE 10.9

St. Joseph
Hospital
Strategy Map:
Vital Few

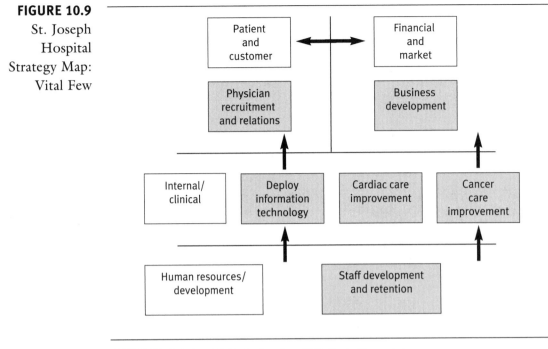

SOURCE: Pugh Ettinger McCarthy Associates, LLC. Used with permission.

measures and continued with discussions of specific tactics and review of associated tactical measures. Identification of the five critical strategies and development of the strategy maps also changed the process by which the hospital board monitors progress.

Clarifying the key organizational strategies, developing key strategic measures for each, using the strategic measures to prioritize proposed tactics, and implementing changes in the leadership system to focus on strategy resulted in increased organizational alignment in SJHS's improvement of important processes and increased organizational effectiveness. SJHS also noticed positive effects on the system-required web of performance indicators.

Conclusion

Healthcare organizations are complex service delivery organizations. Performance is measured across multiple dimensions, including financial, patient experience, clinical outcomes, employee engagement, and patient safety. Scorecards and dashboards are useful leadership and governance tools for creating focus and alignment within the organization on what needs to be improved and are critical to tracking progress on strategic objectives. There should be a direct link between an organization's strategy and quality improvement efforts so that resources are committed to improvements that move the organizational and governance performance measures in the desired direction.

FIGURE 10.10
Strategic
Dashboard
Used to Drive
Progress on
Oncology
Strategy at
St. Joseph
Hospital

What are we trying to accomplish:

To be recognized for clinical excellence with increased market share in the provision of coordinated cancer care (oncology) services for Orange County and surrounding communities

Promise:

You will receive timely, comprehensive, current knowledge-based, and compassionate care at St. Joseph Hospital

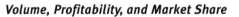

Volume, Profitability, and Market Share

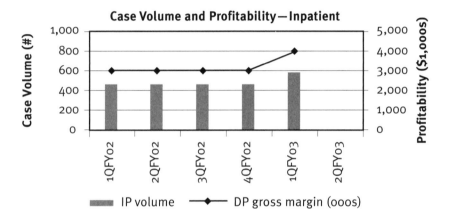

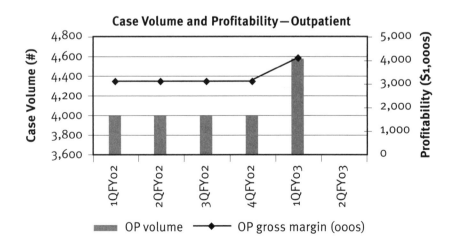

(continued)

FIGURE 10.10
(continued)

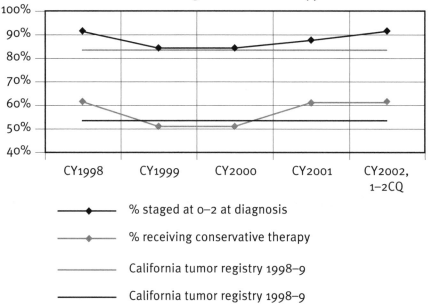

Outcomes and Safety

**Lung Cancer Survival—Comparative
(By Year After Diagnosis, by Stage)**

Y-axis: % Alive after "X" Years (0% to 80%)
X-axis: Year 1, Year 2, Year 3, Year 4, Year 5

Legend:
— SJH Stage 1
— SJH Stage 2
— National Stage 1
— National Stage 2

**Breast Care—Percentage Diagnosed at Stage 0–2 and Percentage
Receiving Conservative Therapy**

Y-axis: 40% to 100%
X-axis: CY1998, CY1999, CY2000, CY2001, CY2002, 1–2CQ

Legend:
— % staged at 0–2 at diagnosis
— % receiving conservative therapy
— California tumor registry 1998–9
— California tumor registry 1998–9

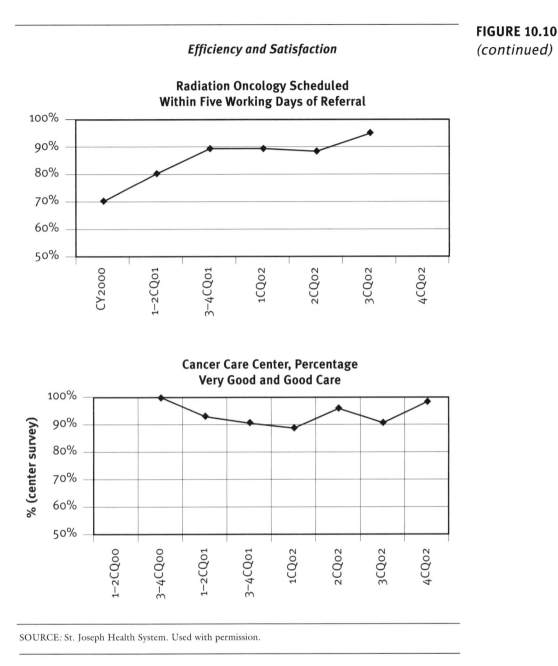

FIGURE 10.10
(*continued*)

Efficiency and Satisfaction

SOURCE: St. Joseph Health System. Used with permission.

Study Questions

1. In your experience with healthcare, what are the important dimensions of performance? How would you know whether an organization is performing well? What indicators do you think are important for a hospital to track? A physician practice? A home care agency? A long-term care facility? A managed care organization?

2. What could be good indicators reflecting patient centeredness as recommended by IOM?

3. What are some of the pitfalls of overmeasurement? How do you determine what is important to measure in an organization?

4. Why is creating alignment an important leadership function? What are other methods of creating alignment, and how can the use of measurement support their deployment?

Notes

1. In deference to the work of Kaplan and Norton (1992, 1996) and the specific concept of leaders using a Balanced Scorecard of strategic measures, this chapter does not use the term *Balanced Scorecard* except in direct reference to Kaplan and Norton's concept. Instead, it discusses the use of dashboards and scorecards in broader, generic terms in its exploration of a variety of applications that create focus and alignment in healthcare organizations.

2. A popular approach has been to use the stoplight color scheme of red, yellow, and green to highlight indicators where performance is judged against a predetermined standard. Indicators that reflect negative performance are highlighted in red, whereas indicators judged to be satisfactory or above expectations are highlighted in green. Yellow can mean caution or need for further review. Although useful for identifying problems or failure to meet a target, this format does not provide trended information useful for assessing progress or decline and, depending on the standard chosen, may reinforce poor actual results.

3. This case study was developed from the author's consulting work with St. Joseph Health System. Used with permission.

References

Aguayo, R. 1991. *Dr. Deming: The American Who Taught the Japanese About Quality.* New York: Simon & Schuster.

Institute of Medicine (IOM). 2001. *Crossing the Quality Chasm: A New Health System for the 21st Century.* Washington, DC: National Academies Press.

Kaplan, R. S., and D. P. Norton. 1992. "The Balanced Scorecard—Measures That Drive Performance." *Harvard Business Review* 70 (1): 71–79.

———. 1996. *The Balanced Scorecard—Translating Strategy into Action.* Boston: HBS Press.

11

PATIENT SAFETY AND MEDICAL ERRORS

Frances A. Griffin and Carol Haraden

Background and Terminology

Harm is never the intention in healthcare delivery, but unfortunately it is sometimes the outcome. In addition to fears of a terminal diagnosis and debilitating disease and pain, one of patients' greatest fears is that a mistake will occur and that the mistake will harm them. Horror stories of patients waking up in the middle of surgical procedures or having the wrong limb amputated, although rare, instill anxiety in individuals accessing the healthcare system. Fear of such events also plays on the minds of healthcare practitioners, who worry about malpractice claims, loss of licensure, and, worst of all, the guilt of having caused harm rather than having provided care and healing.

In 2000, a landmark study on patient safety titled *To Err Is Human* was published. Media attention to the report was swift and widespread, resulting in sudden public awareness that there was a problem. The public expressed shock at the estimate of up to 98,000 annual deaths in U.S. hospitals resulting from medical errors (Kohn, Corrigan, and Donaldson 2000). Reactions among healthcare providers ranged from those who argued, and continue to argue, that the numbers were grossly overestimated (Hayward and Hofer 2001) to those who were not surprised and even relieved that the information was now public, in hopes that action would be taken.

Published studies regarding medical errors, medication errors, and adverse events had been appearing in the literature for decades, providing the basis for the estimates in the report. In 1991, Dr. Lucian Leape, a leading expert on medical errors and author of many studies and articles, was one of the principal authors of the Harvard Medical Practice Study in which hospital records had been reviewed retrospectively for evidence of errors and adverse events (Brennan et al. 1991). Their findings indicated that medical errors and adverse events were occurring far more often than reported and contributing to unnecessary deaths. Further studies have demonstrated that errors and adverse events commonly occur in other healthcare settings besides hospitals. In 2003, a published study reported that 25 percent of patients in ambulatory care practices had experienced adverse drug events (Gandhi et al. 2003). Other studies, in both the United States and Australia, have reported how adverse drug

events result in additional visits to physician offices and emergency departments and increase hospital admissions (Kohn, Corrigan, and Donaldson
2000). The Commonwealth Fund found in 2002 that 25 percent of patients
across four countries reported that they had experienced some form of
medical error in the past two years (Blendon et al. 2003).

Patient Safety Defined

Patient safety is defined as "freedom from accidental injury" (Kohn, Corrigan,
and Donaldson 2000). At the core is the experience of the patient, with the
goal that no patient will experience unnecessary harm, pain, or other suffering. A patient's experience of harm or injury from a medical intervention
is an adverse event (i.e., not caused by an underlying medical condition)
(Kohn, Corrigan, and Donaldson 2000). Adverse events sometimes are the
result of an error, in which case they would be considered preventable.
However, not all adverse events are the result of error; some medical interventions can cause harm (Shojania et al. 2002), even when planned and executed correctly. Some argue that such events are not adverse and should not
be considered as harm; instead, they see such events are known complications or associated risks of certain procedures and interventions. However,
these consequences are still unintended, and the patient who experiences
the adverse event receives little comfort from this explanation.

Practitioners often link the determination of preventability of the
harm with the determination of culpability for the harm, though they are
not related. Acceptance that most harm is unpreventable can stop the
search for improved practices that create desired outcomes with no associated adverse events. For example, the early use of cancer chemotherapy,
particularly antimetabolitic agents, caused a good deal of harm in the form
of hyperemesis; patients were terribly ill and sometimes died from the
treatment. Hyperemesis was a known and associated risk of chemotherapy and, though unpreventable at times, was judged unacceptable. Years
of research have been conducted to develop classes of antiemetic agents
that prevent such harm.

Errors do not always reach patients, such as when the wrong dose of
a medication is dispensed but detected before administration and corrected.
Even when errors do reach the patient, they may not cause harm or injury;
for example, if the incorrect dose of a medication is administered, it may not
be enough of a difference from the intended dose to affect the patient adversely.

In the past few decades, much research has been conducted on human
factors and the cognitive processes associated with errors. James Reason
(1990), renowned expert in human factors and error, defines *error* as an
occasion in which a planned sequence of events fails to achieve its intended
outcome. According to Reason (1990), errors originate from two basic
types of failure: a planning failure or an execution failure. An example in

healthcare would be the use of antibiotics to treat an infection. When an antibiotic is prescribed, it should be one that is effective against the bacteria causing the patient's infection. However, sometimes an antibiotic must be selected on the basis of the physician's assessment of the most likely type of bacteria involved because results of laboratory cultures may not be available at the time of prescription. The selected antibiotic may be dispensed and administered in accordance with the physician's order but later turn out not to be the best choice. A planning error has occurred because the physician initiated the wrong plan, even though the plan was carried out as intended. An execution error occurs when the plan is correct but not carried out as intended. For example, if the physician selects the correct antibiotic, but the antibiotic is either not dispensed or not administered according to the order (e.g., wrong drug, wrong dose, wrong frequency), an error has occurred and the patient is at risk.

Etiology of Patient Errors

Addressing patient safety and medical error first requires an understanding of the underlying causes that contribute to errors and adverse events. Healthcare processes have become enormously complex over time, and the volume of information and knowledge currently available to practitioners is overwhelming, especially with the explosion of the Internet. New and rapidly advancing technologies have led to new treatments that offer many benefits but require training and expertise to be used effectively and safely. Thousands of new medications are introduced each year, far more than anyone could recall accurately from memory. Working conditions play an important role as well. Shortages of clinical personnel, high patient ratios, and long work hours all contribute to the risk that complex processes may not be executed as intended (i.e., an error may occur).

When an error occurs, whether in planning or execution, it is most often a systems problem (Leape, Berwick, and Bates 2002). Healthcare seldom has recognized this important correlation. Traditional response has been to blame an individual, usually the person at the end of a process that went wrong in many places, and often many times previously. When an error leads to an adverse event, or harm, emotions contribute to the situation: anger from patients and families, fear of lawsuits from risk managers and practitioners, and guilt from those involved. The common response has been to identify a person at fault and to take punitive action against that person, such as licensure removal, fines, suspension, or employment termination. Taking this sort of action prevents a deeper understanding of the real drivers of the event and mistakenly allows organizations and patients to feel safer until the same event occurs again but with different actors. Punishment for being involved in an error discourages people from reporting (Findlay 2000).

Punitive action is appropriate if an individual has knowingly and intentionally taken action to cause harm, which would be criminal or negligent behavior. An example is the case of a practitioner who injects a patient with a paralytic medication so that he or she can be the one to "save" the patient from the pulmonary arrest that occurs. Fortunately, such cases are the exception and do warrant disciplinary and legal action. However, most adverse events do not fit into this category but rather are the result of a process breakdown. Blaming and punishing an individual and failing to change the process do not reverse the harm that has occurred and do nothing to decrease the likelihood of the same adverse event occurring again elsewhere in the organization.

Reporting of errors and adverse events is essential to know where changes and improvements can be made. Unfortunately, reporting of healthcare errors and events has been and remains infrequent, within individual organizations as well as at state and national levels. This infrequency can be attributed to the structure and response of the existing reporting systems, the majority of which are voluntary.

Some state regulatory agencies, such as state departments of health, have mandatory reporting for certain types of adverse events. The Joint Commission has attempted to gain further information from accredited organizations through its Sentinel Event standards. Excessive jury awards and high settlements in malpractice cases have contributed to the lack of reporting. When an error occurs that causes no harm, there may be little incentive to report it, if it is even recognized. The result is that the process remains unchanged; the same error recurs and ultimately may cause harm. In addition, because only a minority of events actually is reported, these data cannot be used to track improvement robustly and to determine whether an institution is operating more safely today than it was at the same time last year.

In response to *To Err Is Human*, the Agency for Healthcare Research and Quality (AHRQ) released a report in 2001 that provided information on evidence-based safety practices (Shojania et al. 2002). In this report, AHRQ defined a patient safety practice as "a type of process or structure whose application reduces the probability of adverse events resulting from exposure to the health care system" (Shojania et al. 2002). Note that this definition does not reference error. Errors will continue to exist in healthcare. Processes will continue to have the potential to fail, and human factors always will contribute. However, adverse events and harm need not continue to occur (Nolan 2000). A system designed for patient safety is one in which errors are anticipated to occur, processes are designed and improved with human factors and safety in mind, and reporting is encouraged and rewarded. When safety is part of everyone's daily routine, errors exist but adverse events do not.

Scope and Use in Healthcare Organizations

Healthcare is not the only industry to have struggled with a poor safety record and public image problem. There was a period when aviation had nowhere near the safety record that it has today. During the mid-twentieth century, as commercial air travel increased in popularity, accidents and deaths occurred at significantly higher rates than those we see today. To survive, this industry had to make significant changes. It accomplished these changes by focusing on making systems safer and on developing a different culture. The results are obvious, considering the number of planes flown every day, the volume of passengers they transport, and the number of passengers who are injured or killed in airplane accidents. In the first half of the 1990s, the number of deaths was one-third what it had been in the mid-twentieth century (Kohn, Corrigan, and Donaldson 2000). We cannot say the same for healthcare and even wonder whether the opposite may be true.

Although the healthcare and aviation industries are different and the analogy is not perfect, much that the aviation industry learned is applicable. In fact, anesthesiology already has applied these lessons and is now considered the benchmark for safe delivery of medical care, which was not always the case. Fifty years ago, patients receiving general anesthesia were at a much greater risk of dying from the anesthesia than they are today. From the 1950s to the 1970s, changes were made that decreased the rate of anesthesia-related deaths from 1 in 3,500 to 1 in 10,000 (Findlay 2000), a significant improvement. Anesthesiologists themselves led the initiative, which was a major factor in its success. They developed standards of practice and guidelines that were not imposed on them by outside regulatory agencies. Protocol was adopted from the practices developed in aviation, such as use of standardized procedures and safety checklists. More recent data now show that anesthesia-related deaths have decreased to 1 in 300,000, a staggering difference from 40 years earlier (Findlay 2000). There is no single breakthrough technology or newly discovered drug that has been responsible for this improvement. Rather, this improvement results from the combination of a focus on a system of care that recognizes human frailties and accounts for them in the design of care and many small changes made over time that led to safer practices (Leape, Berwick, and Bates 2002).

Teamwork and Patient Safety

The interaction of a team, in any setting, affects the success of that team. When the members of a team do not function well together or are not perceived by each other as having equally important roles, they do not handle unexpected situations well. The aviation industry learned this lesson the hard way. Reviews of the events in a cockpit before a plane accident or crash revealed that copilots and engineers often were unable to communicate warnings effectively to the pilot, the senior member of the team, or received negative responses when they did. Warnings that could have prevented the death of hundreds of passengers, plus the crew itself, were frequently disregarded, poorly communicated, or not communicated. To change this environment, the industry initiated cockpit resource management, later renamed crew resource management (CRM). In CRM, crews learn how to interact as a team, and all members have equally important roles and responsibilities to ensure the safety of all on board. Appropriate assertion of concerns is more than encouraged; it is expected.

Healthcare has incorporated CRM and is using it in a variety of settings. Operating room teams can be compared to airline crews, and CRM training is improving how surgeons, anesthesiologists, nurses, and technicians work together to ensure the provision of safe care to the patient. Faculty at the University of Texas Center of Excellence in Patient Safety Research has studied airline crews and operating room teams to evaluate how they interact with each other and respond to errors and unexpected events. Team members' perceptions of teamwork, hierarchy, and culture were collected by survey and assessed, and then the teams were observed in their actual work environments to determine how many errors occurred, how many were serious, and how well the team resolved them. Teams that reported high levels of teamwork still had errors but had fewer serious ones compared to those that scored poorly on teamwork. In addition, teams scoring high on teamwork were able to resolve conflict more often and prevent small errors from becoming adverse events; however, this correlation appears to be true more often with airplane crews than operating room teams because they have been receiving CRM training for much longer (Sexton, Thomas, and Helmreich 2000).

People derive their attitudes about teamwork from the overall culture of an organization or unit. There can be enormous differences in culture from one unit or department to another, even within the same organization. Individuals are most affected by the culture of the department in which they spend most of their time. Culture in a unit may not be obvious. On the surface, it may be deemed good if disputes and arguments between staff, physicians, and managers are not frequent. Absence of such overt problems, however, does not necessarily indicate that there is a good underlying culture. Every department, unit, and organization should be developing and enhancing its culture constantly, regardless of how good it may appear or actually be, by focusing on and improving how all members of the healthcare team interact and communicate with each other. This focus on culture improves patient care, and it has many other benefits as well. When every member of the team feels valued and able to contribute, work satisfaction improves, thereby decreasing turnover, a costly issue in any organization. Improved communication between practitioners results in better coordination of care, early recognition of errors, and more rapid interventions, which contribute to operational benefits. At Johns Hopkins Hospital in Baltimore, Maryland, a comprehensive program to improve teamwork and culture in the intensive care unit resulted in a 50 percent decrease in length of stay, providing access for more than 650 additional admissions and $7 million in additional revenue (Pronovost et al. 2003). Other hospitals have used similar approaches to improve teamwork and communication among operating room teams. One technique is the adoption of pre-procedural safety briefings before every operation, during which the entire team meets to review the case and potential safety issues. Following implementation of this and other changes, staff members usually report that they had less difficulty speaking up if they perceived a problem. Even more interesting, though, was that staff's perception of high workload decreased, even though no changes to workload or staffing levels were made (Sexton 2002).

Leading Improved Patient Safety

Leadership of an organization is the driving force behind the culture that exists and the perceptions that it creates. For staff in any healthcare organization to believe that patient safety is a priority, that message must come from the CEO, medical staff leaders, and the board. Furthermore, that message must be visible and consistent. A visible approach to patient safety does not mean memos sent out by the CEO emphasizing its importance or a periodic column in a staff newsletter. The only way frontline staff will know and believe that safety is important to the organization's senior leaders is if the senior leaders visit the departments and units where the work occurs and talk directly with the staff about safety. Through unit rounds and by soliciting input from staff, senior leaders can gain tremendous knowledge about what is happening in their organizations and take steps to make improvements (Frankel et al. 2003). To be convincing, these visits must be consistent and sustained. When leadership starts to make rounds, staff often thinks that the visits are the "idea of the month" and expects them not to last, especially if previous initiatives in the organization have followed the same path. Senior leaders can have a powerful effect on safety by setting aside just one hour to make rounds and talk with staff, as long as they do so routinely and provide feedback. Some senior leaders have found these visits so beneficial that they have increased the amount of time they spend on this activity.

Changing culture and perceptions can take a long time and requires tremendous effort and attention. Leadership presence at the front line is essential but is only one piece of the package. The response to anything that occurs, whether an error, adverse event, or both, significantly affects staff beliefs. Acknowledgment that errors and adverse events are systems problems and not people problems is a crucial first step. Follow-through on that acknowledgment, with appropriate response when something happens, is critical. Many organizations have created nonpunitive reporting policies to encourage staff reporting of errors and adverse events without fear of reprisal, even if the reporter was involved in the event. These policies' success has been limited, especially at middle management levels. Many managers, trained in the old pattern of find and blame the individual, struggle with the concept of nonpunitive policies because they mistakenly conclude that no employee ever will be disciplined, especially their "problem employees." A true problem employee usually will accumulate enough offenses against other policies for the manager to take appropriate action. Even these individuals are as likely as all other employees to find themselves at the end of a system failure. This type of situation is not an opportunity to be rid of the problem employee. In a nonpunitive environment, every error or adverse event is analyzed as a system problem, and punitive action is not taken against anyone unless a policy was deliberately violated or there was intent to cause harm. Staff members will recall punitive action taken against anyone, even a problem employee, only as an example of how someone was punished for being involved in an error or adverse event. They will remember the incident far longer than a senior leadership round that occurred during the same week.

Punishment from an employee's perspective, and not just from a manager's, is important to consider. Managers sometimes consider formal disciplinary action, such as official written warnings, as the only type of punitive action. However, staff members feel penalized when they are criticized verbally in front of others, when errors or adverse events in which they were involved are discussed at a staff meeting with emphasis on how "someone" made a mistake (even if names are left out), or when details of reported errors or events are attached to their performance appraisals. Anytime staff members walk away from an event feeling that they may have been at fault or that management views them in such a way, a punitive environment is perpetuated and the likelihood that staff members will voluntarily report problems in the future decreases.

Dealing with Adverse Events

Handling an adverse event in a healthcare organization can be enormously complicated. Emotions add further complexity, particularly when a patient has been harmed. External pressures can escalate the intensity of the situation when media and regulatory agencies become involved. All of these contributing factors increase our natural tendency to blame someone. Leaders are pressured at such times to identify the responsible parties and report on actions taken. At such times, leaders and managers must work together with everyone involved and prevent a blame-focused or punitive response. Human factors expert James Reason (1997) provided wonderful resources on this subject in *Managing the Risks of Organizational Accidents*, such as an algorithm to analyze the sequence of events. With this tool, managers are prompted to consider key questions to determine whether a system failure occurred. Rather than assuming that an employee simply did not follow a policy, Reason (1997) suggests that an investigator evaluate aspects such as whether the policy was readily available, easily understandable, and workable. The investigator also should apply a substitution test to determine the likelihood that the same event would occur with three other employees with similar experience and training and in similar circumstances (e.g., hours on duty, fatigue, workload) (Reason 1997). If the same event is likely to occur, the problem is systems related.

Disclosure of harm to patients and families is another difficult aspect for hospital leaders and physicians to manage when an adverse event occurs. Traditionally, disclosure has not been handled well, resulting in public perception that those in healthcare cover up for each other. Punitive responses from regulatory agencies, accreditation bodies, insurers, and licensing boards discourage healthcare organizations and practitioners from reporting events, unless mandated by law. Lawyers dissuade practitioners from apologizing to patients when an adverse event occurs by advising that doing so would be considered an admission of guilt and would place themselves and the organization at risk for lawsuits, punitive damage awards, and loss of public trust, as well as market share. Fearful of lawsuits, practitioners and representatives of healthcare organizations stay silent, say very little, or speak vaguely about the event. This taciturnity causes frustration and distrust on the part of patients and families, who often know that something has gone wrong but are unable to obtain a straight answer, which increases the likelihood that they will file a lawsuit. Many who have filed malpractice lawsuits have reported that they were not motivated by the desire for retribution or a large financial settlement but that filing suit was the only way they felt they could discover the truth about what happened, obtain an apology, and ensure that the same event did not happen to other patients and families. Public concern about disclosure of events led The Joint Commission to add standards that now require accredited organizations to inform patients or their legal guardians of any unanticipated outcome, whether it be the result of an error or a known side effect of their treatment.

Involving patients and families in discussions about their care throughout the entire process is an essential element in cultural change. In the Institute of Medicine (2001) report *Crossing the Quality Chasm*, patient centeredness is one of the recommended changes. Every part of a patient's care should focus on the patient's needs first, not the needs of physicians, nurses, other clinical personnel, hospitals, or other healthcare agencies. Active participation by patients and families in rounds, goal setting, verification of identification before procedures, and verification of medications before administration are just a few examples of how their needs should be integrated into the process. A safety-focused culture must include patients, and open discussion in one area will encourage openness in other areas.

Reporting Adverse Events

A focus on reporting will increase reporting, but not substantially or for long. Organizations need to know more about the errors and adverse events that are occurring to be able to improve their systems. Most rely on voluntary reporting systems to gather this information, but as previously mentioned, these sources are not the most reliable and underreporting is a significant problem. To increase reporting, well-intentioned individuals in healthcare organizations try a variety of initiatives. They often include strategies such as education fairs, posters, safety hotlines, shorter reporting forms, and raffles or prizes for departments with the most reports. During the implementation of these strategies, heavy emphasis is placed on the guaranteed anonymity of the various reporting mechanisms and the assurance of nonpunitive approaches. For a short time, reporting increases result in celebration and excitement about the improved culture of safety and the new knowledge gained. However, over time, reporting declines and usually returns to where it was before, if not lower, leaving those who led the initiative feeling discouraged and disheartened. They may rally and try again, only to have the same cycle repeated.

Why does this decline occur? The focus has not addressed the core issue: the underlying culture. The heavy focus on reporting causes a temporary increase, but it does not become integrated into the daily routine, so eventually it is discussed less, unless someone attempts to keep the momentum going. Incentives also may help, but their effectiveness is highest when they are new, and over time, people either forget about them or are no longer motivated by them. The reporting system itself may be complicated and burdensome, requiring too much practitioner time to complete in a busy day. Also, the focus on guaranteed anonymity may cause the opposite of the desired effect. In a fair culture, one does not need to remain anonymous when reporting because there is no fear of reprisal. Reinforcing guaranteed anonymity may be important in the early stages but also may leave staff with the impression that potential for punitive action still exists.

Hospitals that have seen dramatic and sustained increases in voluntary reporting rates have not achieved these results by concentrating efforts on stimulating or improving reporting mechanisms. Rather, they have focused on their culture and on creating a safety-conscious environment. Leadership commitment to safety and strategies to improve teamwork among all levels is a fundamental first step. Once the dialog begins, feedback becomes critical. As frontline staff begins to alert management to safety issues and opportunities for improvement, its belief in the new system will be established only when management provides feedback about its suggestions. As these changes take root in the organization, the culture changes and voluntary reporting increases to levels not previously seen.

Even in a safety-conscious culture, errors will continue to occur, as will adverse events. Reason (1990) describes two types of errors: active and latent. In an active error, the effects or consequences occur immediately. An example is placing your foot on the gas pedal in a car, rather than on the brake, when engaging the shift out of park, and crashing through the garage wall (which is why automobiles now have a forcing function locking the shift in park unless your foot is on the brake). Latent errors, though, exist within the system for a long time, not causing harm until a situation arises where, in combination with other factors, the error becomes part of a chain of events resulting in disaster. The loss of the *Challenger* space shuttle was found to be the catastrophic result of latent errors, as have many other well-known disasters (Reason 1990). When an adverse event occurs in healthcare, retrospective review frequently reveals latent errors as contributing factors.

Each occurrence represents an opportunity for learning and sharing the lessons both internally and externally. In creating a safety-oriented culture, an organization must ensure that information about errors and action taken to reduce them are shared openly. Frontline employees can learn a great deal by hearing about the experiences of others, and organizations should provide mechanisms that encourage them to do so. Incorporating patient safety issues into change-of-shift reports and setting aside a regular time for staff to have safety briefings are just a couple of the ways that communication and teamwork can be enhanced. Organizations also should find ways for this information to transcend departments, units, and divisions. Sharing a safety lesson from one area across the entire organization is the only way to identify and change in other areas the same latent errors addressed in the lesson.

Learning from the external environment is also important. Fortunately, the most serious adverse events, such as removal of the wrong limb, are rare. Such an event may not have occurred at a hospital for years, but infrequency should not breed complacency. Every time a serious adverse event occurs at *any* hospital *anywhere*, the lessons learned from that event should be available to all hospitals so that all can analyze their own processes for improvement opportunities. Unfortunately, access to this information may not be easy to provide because legal issues from lawsuits and concerns about privacy prevent or hinder many organizations from sharing details. Organizations such as The Joint Commission and the Institute for Safe Medication Practices have disseminated newsletters with information they have obtained about serious adverse events, without including identifying information about the organization or people involved, as a way to facilitate learning and improvement. However, despite such worthwhile initiatives, the same events continue to occur.

Looking to Other Industries

Healthcare should look to other industries for ideas about how to implement safer practices. A common argument against looking at other industries is that in medicine, "we are not making widgets." Healthcare professionals carry a special and unique responsibility when rendering care to our fellow human beings. However, we still can learn from other industries. There are other industries in which an error can result in the loss of life, even hundreds or thousands at once; examples include aviation, air traffic control systems, nuclear power plants, and aircraft carriers. Despite enormous risks and extremely complex processes, these industries have safety records beyond anything in healthcare. In *Managing the Unexpected*, Weick and Sutcliffe (2001) describe organizations in these industries as *high reliability organizations*. The approach to daily work is an expectation and preoccupation with failure rather than success, which results in constant, early identification of errors and error-producing processes, with continuous improvement in processes and routines (Weick and Sutcliffe 2001). Healthcare leaders would be foolish not to learn more about how these organizations have achieved their safety records and which aspects are applicable in their own organizations.

One tool that was developed in the industrial setting and found application in healthcare is failure modes and effects analysis (FMEA). FMEA is a systematic, proactive method for evaluating a process to identify where and how it might fail and to assess the relative effect of different failures to identify the parts of the process that need the most revision. FMEA includes review of:

- steps in the process;
- failure modes (what could go wrong);
- failure causes (why would the failure happen); and
- failure effects (what would be the consequences of each failure).

An advantage to using this approach is the evaluation of processes for possible failures and the opportunity to prevent them by correcting the processes proactively rather than reacting to adverse events after failures have occurred. This approach is different from root cause analysis (RCA), which is conducted only after an event has occurred. Another significant difference is that RCA suggests that there is only one cause for an adverse event, which is rarely the case. FMEA, in contrast, looks at the entire process and every potential for failure, so the perspective is broader. FMEA is particularly useful in evaluating a new process before its implementation and in assessing the outcome of a proposed change to an existing process. Using this approach, organizations can consider many options and assess potential consequences in a safe environment before actual implementation in the patient care process.

FMEA emphasizes prevention to reduce risk of harm to both patients and staff. The use of forcing functions, such as oxygen flowmeters designed to fit only into oxygen outlets and not compressed air or vacuum outlets, is a prevention technique that works well for many processes. Although prevention is an important aspect in making practices safer, all errors cannot be prevented. When an error does occur, another important consideration is how visible the error will be. In conducting FMEA, a numeric value of risk should be assigned to the process, called a risk priority number (RPN), which is used to assess improvement, evident by its reduction. To calculate RPN, one asks three questions about each failure mode and assigns a value between 1 and 10, for very unlikely to very likely.

1. *Likelihood of occurrence*: What is the likelihood that this failure mode will occur?
2. *Likelihood of detection*: If this failure mode occurs, what is the likelihood that the failure will not be detected?
3. *Severity*: If this failure mode occurs, what is the likelihood that harm will occur?

The second question regarding detection relates directly to the issue of visibility. If an error is likely to occur, but likely to go undetected, then in addition to prevention strategies, one should look for methods to alert staff that an error has occurred. An example is the use of alert screens in computerized prescriber order entry (CPOE) systems. If a prescriber makes an error while ordering medications, an alert screen can notify a prescriber immediately that he or she needs to make a change.

Mitigation is a third and equally important aspect to making practices safer. Despite well-designed prevention and detection strategies, some errors will slip through and reach the patient. The ultimate goal in patient safety is not to cause harm. When an error does reach the patient, quick recognition and appropriate intervention can significantly reduce or prevent harm to the patient. Training staff in response techniques through the use of drills and simulations and ensuring that resources needed for interventions are readily available in patient care areas are strategies that can mitigate such events (Nolan 2000). A comprehensive patient safety approach requires that changes be made to improve all three areas: prevention, detection, and mitigation.

Using Technology to Improve Patient Safety

Technology often is seen as a solution to safer care, and although advances have offered many ways to improve systems and processes, each new technology also introduces new opportunities for error. A good basic rule before implementing a technological solution is never to automate a bad process. If frequent errors or process breakdowns reveal that a process is not working well, adding technology to it usually will not solve the underlying problems. Additions usually make the situation worse because even more process failures become evident; the technology is blamed as being "no good" and subsequently is abandoned or not used. CPOE is an example of a technological addition. Almost every hospital in the United States either has implemented or planned for this technology, which offers benefits such as decision support and elimination of illegible orders. Some hospitals have learned the hard lesson that implementation of CPOE should not coincide with the implementation of standardized processes that have not been used previously, such as order sets or protocols. These standardized tools work best when tested and implemented using paper systems first, if a hospital does not yet have computerized ordering. This initial testing provides physicians and staff with an opportunity to learn and become accustomed to the new processes, integrate them into their routines, and suggest improvements. When a CPOE system is introduced later, physicians will need to learn only the technical use and how to adapt the standard processes they already know to that environment. Introducing standardized ordering processes and CPOE simultaneously generally has been a recipe for failure of both.

Any new technology introduces new opportunities for error and failure. Technological solutions often are used in systems and processes that are already complex, and a change to one part of the system can produce unexpected effects in another (Shojania et al. 2002).

FMEA can serve as a useful resource for staff in evaluating the potential failures of the equipment and considering processes to prevent, detect, and mitigate those failures. The extra features of any technology must be used in a balanced manner. Overuse of any feature will diminish its effectiveness over time. For example, in a CPOE system, alerts and pop-up screens can provide critical prescribing information to users and even require the use of an override in certain high-risk situations. If too many alerts are used, users will begin to ignore them, and as a routine, they will proceed to the next screen without reading the alert information, which could cause a serious error to bypass the system. Audible alarms are another example, so their parameters should be set to alarm only when attention is required. If equipment alarms frequently, and for reasons that do not require immediate intervention, staff will become complacent to the alarms. This behavior often can be observed in a patient care unit where many ventilators are used and are alarming frequently and for long periods. Bypassing screens and not responding quickly to alarms are not failures of the people involved; they are the expected by-products of improperly designed systems. We are overloaded with the visual and auditory stimulation of technology, and our natural defensive mechanism is to shut some of it out. Other industries already consider this behavior in their safety designs, and healthcare also must.

Designing Safe Processes

To decrease the harm that occurs to patients, healthcare organizations must design patient care systems for safety. The underlying foundation for success in this journey is the creation and development of a safety-conscious culture. Organizations then must assess processes and systems for change using the following key elements.

1. Incorporate human factors knowledge into training and procedures. Expect and plan for error rather than react to it in surprise.

2. Design processes to be safely and reliably executed by staff with varying levels of experience, training, and environmental or personal stress. Is the process designed so that a nurse who is a recent graduate and performing it for the second or third time will be able do it as safely and reliably as a nurse with 20 years of experience who has done it hundreds of times? What about the pharmacist who is upset about personal problems and did not sleep well last night versus the pharmacist who is feeling physically and mentally fit today? Safeguards to account for these human factor variances must be designed into the system.

3. Design technology and procedures for end users, planning for failures (Norman 1988). Until all medical device manufacturers adopt this process, healthcare organizations, as purchasers, are responsible for seeking devices that incorporate safe designs and developing procedures to support safe use.

4. Decrease complexity by reducing the number of steps in a process whenever possible (Nolan 2000). As the number of steps in a process increases, the likelihood that it will be executed without error decreases. Periodically review all processes to determine whether they include steps that no longer provide value; all processes tend to change over time.

5. Ensure that safety initiatives address prevention, detection, and mitigation (Nolan 2000). A combination of all three is necessary to reduce harm. FMEA can ensure they are addressed.

6. Standardize processes, tools, technology, and equipment. Variation increases complexity and the risk of error. Technology can offer great benefits but must be applied to processes that already function well. Equipment may include features that decrease the need for reliance on memory, which is an important aspect of safety; however, if too many different types of equipment are in use, staff will find it difficult to move from one item to another. Imagine how difficult driving a rental car would be if every car manufacturer placed gas pedals, brake pedals, and shifts in different locations and used varying designs. Many medical devices introduce this same difficulty.

7. Label medications and solutions clearly and for each individual dose, including generic and trade names. Use extra alert measures for drugs

that have similar sounding names. (Unfortunately, healthcare organizations also are responsible for adding processes that address this safety issue because patient safety generally is not incorporated in the selection of drug names.)

8. Use bar coding. The Food and Drug Administration recently adopted bar coding requirements for all medications, which is a worthy but long-overdue measure. Supermarkets have been using bar code readers for years, and healthcare is shamefully behind in this regard, especially when one compares the difference in consequences of administering the wrong blood product to charging the wrong price for a grocery item. This technology will become a standard part of healthcare delivery.

9. Use forcing functions to prevent certain types of errors from occurring, but be sure to maintain a balance and not overdo them. Staff will find ways to work around too many constraints. Make things difficult that should be difficult (Norman 1988).

These elements are not new to quality improvement, industry, or in some cases, even healthcare; yet, healthcare has not adopted them widely. As we work toward decreasing and eliminating the unintended harm that our systems cause, we must realize that our industry *can* learn from non-healthcare industries. The analogies are not perfect, and there are some distinct and important differences in healthcare, but we must learn from them if we are to achieve significant improvement in safety within our lifetime. We are privileged to work in professions in which our interactions give us the opportunity to care for fellow human beings, hopefully to cure them when possible, but when not, to provide relief from their symptoms and ensure dignified deaths. This privilege obligates us to use every possible resource and tool at our disposal, whether or not created in our own industry, to ensure that this care is delivered in the safest manner possible and never causes unintended harm. Every patient has that right.

Clinical and Operational Issues

Patient Safety Research

Many of the greatest breakthroughs in medicine that have led to improvements in patient care have come about through research. As clinicians continue to discover improved methods and interventions for treating and curing disease, new research will provide results that will alter the delivery of care. Today, healthcare has best practices for many clinical conditions. Studies have demonstrated that these practices are reliable, and there is general consensus on them among clinical experts. Practices include diagnostic tests identifying disease and assessing severity and the interventions that improve patient outcome. Despite the amount of knowledge that has been accumulated on these practices and the general acceptance that they are best practices, however, huge variation in their adoption and use remains a problem (Kohn, Corrigan, and Donaldson 2000). A recent study found that most accepted best practices are documented as used in the treatment of only 50 percent of appropriate patients, at best (McGlynn et al. 2003). One could argue that failure to use a universally accepted treatment protocol is a planning error, unless clinically contraindicated.

Physician Objections

The objection that many clinicians raise to using known best practices, or evidence-based medicine, is usually one of two interrelated issues. First, they argue that the approach is "cookbook medicine" and an attempt to remove the clinician's expertise and judgment from the process. Evidence-based medicine, when used appropriately, does nothing of the kind. A clinician's training, skills, and expertise are essential in evaluating a patient, assessing the symptoms and results of diagnostic testing, and pulling all this information together to make a clinical diagnosis. Once the clinician has made a diagnosis, most patients will meet the criteria for a few evidence-based practices. Standard processes to ensure their application to all appropriate patients result in better quality of care. Clinicians should welcome these best practices, feel confident in the evidence, and determine whether there is any contraindication. Second, clinicians argue that their patients are different. Naturally, all patients are different in that they are unique individuals. Many patients, though, do not have contraindications for the evidence-based practices and still do not receive them. Clinicians must accept that evidence-based best practices take nothing away from their value and expertise but rather assist them in providing their patients with safe, high-quality care that may improve outcomes.

Limitations of Research

Research provides wonderful new knowledge, but it has some limitations. Insistence that complete and thorough research must be completed before implementing change hinders improvement and the adoption of safe practices. It is also an unrealistic expectation because complete evidence for everything never will exist (Leape, Berwick, and Bates 2002). Some practices to improve patient safety make sense and do not need research studies to prove their effectiveness; they simply should be implemented (Shojania et al. 2002). For example, how could anyone who has seen an illegible medication order claim that we need to conduct studies about the effectiveness of computerized systems that reduce or eliminate the need for handwritten orders before implementing them? Why would research need to be conducted on the need for verification of patient identification before a medical intervention? Research provides wonderful information, but we cannot research everything and should not allow it to become an obstacle that prevents us from adopting safer practices.

Effects of Fatigue

An area that researchers have studied, in healthcare and other industries, is the effect of fatigue on error and safety. Studies have shown that an individual who is sleep deprived demonstrates cognitive function at the ninth percentile of the overall population (Shojania et al. 2002). A person who has been awake for 24 hours often demonstrates actions and errors similar to those of a person who is under the influence of alcohol. Despite this knowledge, healthcare remains one of the only high-risk professions that does not mandate restrictions of hours (Leape, Berwick, and Bates 2002). No rest requirements exist for physicians who are not in training or other clinical personnel within the healthcare setting. Because many personnel work at more than one organization, no one has an overall perspective. The situation is not an easy one; with current shortages in most clinical professions and increasing numbers of hospitalized patients, most organizations rely on staff overtime to meet staffing levels, especially in states with mandated staffing ratios. All of these factors contribute to high workloads, increased work hours, and greater staff fatigue, circumstances that are known to contribute to the commission of errors.

Economics and Patient Safety

Healthcare is in turbulent times, and financial pressures weigh heavily on many healthcare leaders. In addition to staffing shortages, there are concerns regarding reimbursement, malpractice coverage, regulatory requirements, and access for the uninsured. Any healthcare CEO would agree that patient safety is important, but in actual practice it becomes a low priority at most organizations (Shojania et al. 2002). Distractions caused by the other aforementioned issues consume so much time that safety is easily bypassed. Ask any CEO which meeting he or she would be more concerned about missing—the finance committee or the patient safety committee—and he or she probably would choose the former.

Many factors affect healthcare, and economics is one of those factors—an important one, but not the only one (Kohn, Corrigan, and Donaldson 2000). Unsafe practices contribute to cost in many ways. These cost considerations include, but are not limited to, efficiency, increased length of stay, turnover, absorbed costs when an error or adverse event occurs, malpractice settlements, and increased premiums. The dollars lost to lack of safety every year are staggering, to say nothing of the consequences to the patients who are harmed, which cannot always be measured in financial terms. Patient safety must become a priority for healthcare leaders in action as well as in word. The current system is broken, and changing it requires the will to do so (Nolan 2000). In a safety-oriented organization, everyone takes responsibility for safety (Findlay 2000). All organizations should strive to function that way, all employees and clinicians should want to work in that kind of environment, and all patients should demand to be treated that way. Hopefully, in the near future, we will be able to claim that all of healthcare has achieved the safety record that anesthesia currently has. Hopefully, hospitals will be included in the list of highly reliable organizations. We must start working toward these ends so that all patients can access any part of the healthcare system confidently, without fear of harm.

Case Study: OSF Healthcare System

The OSF Healthcare System began its journey toward safer healthcare in earnest after release of IOM's (2001) *Crossing the Quality Chasm* report. OSF Healthcare System operates hospital facilities, various physician office practices, urgent care centers, and extended care facilities in Illinois, Wisconsin, and Michigan. Like many organizations, OSF took the call to action contained in the report seriously and has created some of the safest systems of care in the United States.

As is true of all organizations that create transformative and lasting change, OSF employed a top-down and bottom-up improvement strategy. The corporate office and individual hospital leaders made safer care a top strategic priority. They added muscle to that declaration by tying the executive compensation package to key safety indicators. OSF also began building the robust infrastructure needed to create and sustain change at the front line. It named physician change agents at the corporate office as well as physician change agents and patient safety officers at each hospital site. The change agents reported directly to senior leadership, and their role was designed to allow them to work at all levels of the organization and instigate improvement driven by strategic priorities.

To kick-start its safety journey, OSF enrolled St. Joseph Medical Center in the Quantum Leaps in Patient Safety collaborative with the Institute for Healthcare Improvement (IHI). St. Joseph Medical Center was one of 50 national and international teams that formed a learning community that would bring about unprecedented change in adverse drug event rates over the next year. An OSF team of early adopters representing administration, medical staff, nursing, and pharmacy was established and given the task of creating a strong and successful prototype. The team then used those successful changes to spread improvements throughout the organization. Leadership provided both human and financial resources and removed barriers so that the team could do its best work. OSF used the same successful process to reduce mortality and global harm rates as well, each time beginning with a prototype team that created successful, local change that was spread throughout each hospital within the OSF Healthcare System. The combination of fully engaged leadership, a creative and committed frontline team, the expectation of organization-wide spread coupled with explicit spread plans, and the development and use of a robust measurement capability was responsible for creating the unprecedented level of safety later witnessed.

To dramatically improve adverse drug event rates, OSF determined that the following changes needed to be made:

1. Improve the safety culture and maintain a cultural survey score that demonstrates that staff has a strong belief in the importance of safe practice and experiences the system of care in which it operates as respectful, empowering, and committed to learning and clear communication
2. Develop a medication reconciliation process to ensure that patients are on the correct medications at every point in their care
3. Use FMEA to reduce risk and improve the reliability of the dispensing system
4. Standardize the dosing and management of high-risk medications

All of these changes contributed to the overall goal: to reduce adverse drug events by a factor of 10. Industry measures defects as occurring in parts per 10, 100, 1,000, 10,000, and so on. Obviously, the aim is to reduce the rate to where 10,000 process events are needed to witness defects. The process event of interest in reducing adverse drug events is the number of doses of medication given to patients. At the start of the journey, medication events were occurring at rates that translated into the occurrence of adverse events in parts per 1,000 doses. The organization's goal was to decrease the number of adverse events so that they occurred in parts per 10,000, which would mean that nearly a full year would be needed to realize the same number of adverse events that, at the time, were occurring in a month.

Defining culture as "the predominating attitudes and behavior that characterize the functioning of a group or organization," OSF St. Joseph Medical Center initiated a comprehensive redesign of the culture and care systems to reduce the potential rate of harm to patients. In evaluating areas for improvement, the Center identified reduction of adverse events involving medications as the opportunity affecting the largest population of patients.

Reducing Adverse Drug Events

The drastic reduction in adverse drug events that OSF aimed to create required multifaceted changes in many processes. No single change or small combination of changes could take an organization to that level of safety.

OSF began by measuring the current rate of harm caused by medication using a trigger tool developed during the Idealized Design of Medication Systems sponsored by IHI. Trained clinicians sampled charts randomly and reviewed them to make an accurate assessment of the number and type of adverse drug events occurring in the hospital. They randomly selected 20 medical records and initially reviewed them using the adverse drug event trigger tool. The review indicated the hospital's adverse drug event rate to be 5.8 per 1,000 doses dispensed; the goal was to reduce this rate to 0.58 adverse drug events per 1,000 doses.

OSF learned a tremendous amount about the medication harm in its system. The organization also was concerned about the rate of reported actual and potential errors. Unreported errors may not have caused harm yet, but they represented a tremendous potential for learning and improvement. OSF came to believe that the incident-occurrence reporting system produced reports that revealed only the tip of the iceberg in identifying these events. To improve the rate and the organization's learning, OSF established an adverse drug event hotline. The hotline was located in the pharmacy, so a pharmacist was able to check it daily for reported events and proceed with an investigation into potential causes. This solution was win-win because the hotline identified the event for evaluation and trending, and the staff reported easily, quickly, and anonymously and saved time by avoiding paperwork needed to complete an occurrence report. The error reporting and potential error reporting rates improved markedly.

A key change in the reduction of adverse drug events was the use of a medication reconciliation process. Medication reconciliation is the act of comparing the medications the patient has been taking with the medications currently ordered. A patient's care often is fragmented and under the direction of multiple physicians. An orthopedist who admits a patient to the hospital may miss medications prescribed by that patient's cardiologist. The reconciliation process allows the caregiver to identify the correct medications, discover those that were missed, and identify those that need to be continued, discontinued, or adjusted for frequency on the basis of the patient's changing condition.

The comparison between ongoing and currently ordered medications is conducted in three phases: admission, transfer, and discharge. In *admission reconciliation*, the home medications are compared to the initial physician orders. In *transfer reconciliation*, the medications the patient was taking, as indicated by the previous nursing unit, are compared to the orders on the current unit. In *discharge reconciliation*, all current medications taken in the hospital are compared to those the physician orders for the patient at discharge. Variances between the lists should be reconciled by the nurse or pharmacist and the physician within 4 to 24 hours, depending on the type of medication. The addition of a physician signature line to the reconciliation form can turn it into a physician order sheet and thus save staff time and potential transcription errors.

Standardization of orders based on best known practices reduced the variability of individual clinician practices and dramatically reduced the number of adverse drug events. OSF used pharmacy-based services and order sets to accomplish this standardization. For example, to address dosing high-risk medications such as anticoagulants, a single, weight-based heparin nomogram was developed for use throughout the medical center. Additionally, the pharmacy offered both inpatient and outpatient Coumadin (an anticoagulant medication) dosing services. Renal dosing services were conducted on all patients with a creatinine clearance of less than 50 milliliters. Development of a perioperative beta-blocker protocol resulted in a dramatic and sustained reduction of perioperative myocardial infarctions and realized an unexpected benefit of reduced narcotic usage in patients receiving a perioperative beta-blocker.

One of the most fundamental and important changes was the availability of pharmacists on the nursing units to review and enter medication orders. Pharmacists were able to look at the orders firsthand and identify potential dosing errors and drug interactions.

Cultural Changes

The organization had to transform its culture while creating remedies for care processes and high-risk medications. This work, although less evident, was essential to create and maintain a culture that could sustain and improve safety over time. This work involved embedding safety into the very fabric of the organization—inserting safety aims into the organization's mission and corporate strategic goals, job descriptions, and meeting agendas. The transformation involved regular communication and reminders through meetings, conference calls, visits, and learning sessions. It was ever present and unrelenting.

In addition, specific changes made the importance of safety visible to frontline employees. The first change was the introduction of unit safety briefings. The staff gathered at a specified time for a five- to ten-minute review of safety concerns on the unit that day. Staff identified concerns involving equipment, medications, and care processes that posed a safety issue. The patient safety officer assigned the issues to the appropriate personnel for investigation and resolution. To close the communication loop, identified issues and their resolutions were summarized and presented to staff monthly.

The second change was the institution of executive walk-throughs. A senior leader visited a patient care area weekly to demonstrate commitment to safety by gathering information about the staff's safety concerns. The walk-throughs also served to educate senior executives about the type and extent of safety issues within their organizations. The issues were logged into a database, owners were assigned for resolution, and a feedback loop to the staff was established.

To measure the effect of all changes on the safety culture, a survey was conducted every six months to measure the cultural climate of the staff surrounding patient safety initiatives. The survey was a modified version of the J. Bryan Sexton/Robert Helmreich survey used by the aviation industry and NASA. Respondents included 10 percent of each hospital and medical staff. The survey was used as a tool for measuring the extent of a nonpunitive culture of reporting safety concerns and the effectiveness of safety initiatives, communication among team members, and overall teamwork.

Results

The drug-dispensing FMEA risk score was reduced by 66 percent in two years as a result of multiple action steps. Medication lists for discharged patients were retrieved hourly as pharmacy technicians made their rounds to deliver medications. Nursing unit stock medications were reduced by 45 percent, adult IV medications were standardized, and all nonstandard doses were prepared by the pharmacy. An IV drug administration reference matrix directed dosage, guidelines, and monitoring information for nursing staff, and the pharmacist compared lab values to orders to identify potentially inappropriate dosing. Anesthesia staff contributed to reducing potential dispensing events by assisting in standardization of epidural-safe pumps with the use of colored tubing.

OSF's hard work brought about the following results.

- Medication reconciliation was introduced in the summer of 2001; as of May 2003, admission reconciliation use ranged from 85 percent to 95 percent, transfer reconciliation was at 70 percent, and discharge reconciliation was at 95 percent.
- The organization completed the ordering FMEA, worked on reducing the risk at every step, and reduced its risk score from 157 to 103, a 34 percent reduction.
- Changes aimed at improving medication safety as well as specific interventions designed to improve the culture of safety were instituted. Culture survey results in the first year improved from a baseline score of 3.96 to 4.28 (out of a maximum score of 5).
- The organization continues to work hard at making progress every day. The proof of ultimate success came in the form of the most important outcome—the rate of adverse drug events that cause patient harm. In June 2001, that rate was 5.8 per 1,000 doses dispensed; by May 2003, the rate had been reduced to 0.72 per 1,000 doses, nearly a tenfold reduction in harm.
- Since 2004, OSF has collected adverse event rates, into which it subsumes the adverse drug events. The adverse event rate for all of OSF was

98 adverse events per 1,000 patient days in June 2004, and it was 31 adverse events per 1,000 patient days in March 2007.

- The all-OSF hospital standardized mortality rate (HSMR) was 103 for OSF in 2002 and 73 in 2006.
- The adverse event rate for St. Joseph Medical Center (the hospital within OSF referenced earlier) was 70 in June 2004 and 29 in March 2007.
- The HSMR for St. Joseph Medical Center was 120 in 2002 and 89 in 2006.

In summary, OSF created a culture of improvement by embracing an organized and corporate-wide method to improve patient care. It created small prototype teams of frontline clinicians who developed robust aims and measures in support of their strategic plan to reduce harm and improve care, first in regard to adverse drug events and later in service of reducing global harm and mortality rates. The teams used various small cycle tests to adapt evidence-based care processes on their units; they spread the learning and successful changes to all OSF organizations; and then they hardwired those changes into their corporate system. The level of commitment and amount of work that enabled OSF to achieve its successes cannot be overstated.

Conclusion

Healthcare should be safer than its current state, and we, as an industry, need to push for change at a faster rate. Every day, patients are harmed by healthcare processes and systems. We have a moral obligation to do better. Within healthcare organizations, leaders must demonstrate their commitment to safety visibly and set the example for establishing a safety-conscious culture. They must set the expectation that all members of the healthcare team are to work together, incorporating safe practices and awareness into daily operations.

Ultimately, the goal should be for every sector of healthcare to work together toward safety. Manufacturers should incorporate human factors into the design of medical devices. Educators of healthcare providers should include safety in their curricula. Reporting systems and legal processes should not assign individual blame for systems problems. Reimbursement systems should promote safe, quality care. Errors will continue to occur, but changes can be made to reduce their frequency and severity so that harm is eliminated. Healthcare has many people working hard to provide excellent, safe care to the patients they serve, and we should design systems and processes that enable them to do just that.

Study Questions

1. Describe how current reporting systems for medical errors and adverse events contribute to the issue of underreporting.
2. List three elements for designing safer processes and systems, and provide a real example of each (preferably healthcare examples).
3. Explain why the perspective of the patient is the most important determinant of whether an adverse event has occurred.
4. Provide an example of an error that can occur in a healthcare process and result in patient harm. Then, describe a strategy or several strategies that would accomplish each of the following objectives:
   a. Prevent the error from resulting in patient harm
   b. Detect the error when it occurs
   c. Mitigate the amount of harm to the patient

References

Blendon, R. J., C. Schoen, C. DesRoches, R. Osborn, and K. Zapert. 2003. "Common Concerns amid Diverse Systems: Health Care Experiences in Five Countries." *Health Affairs (Millwood)* 22 (3): 106–21.

Brennan, T. A., L. L. Leape, N. M. Laird, L. Herbert, A. R. Localio, A. G. Lawthers, J. P. Newhouse, P. C. Weiler, and H. H. Hiatt. 1991. "Incidence of Adverse Events and Negligence in Hospitalized Patients: Results of the Harvard Medical Practice Study I." *New England Journal of Medicine* 324: 370–76.

Findlay, S. (ed.). 2000. *Accelerating Change Today for America's Health: Reducing Medical Errors and Improving Patient Safety*. Washington, DC: National Coalition on Health Care and Institute for Healthcare Improvement.

Frankel, A., E. Graydon-Baker, C. Neppl, T. Simmonds, M. Gustafson, and T. K. Gandhi. 2003. "Patient Safety Leadership WalkRounds." *Joint Commission Journal on Quality and Safety* 29 (1): 16–26.

Gandhi, T. K., S. N. Weingart, J. Borus, A. C. Seger, J. Peterson, E. Burdick, D. L. Seger, K. Shu, F. Federico, L. L. Leape, and D. W. Bates. 2003. "Adverse Drug Events in Ambulatory Care." *New England Journal of Medicine* 348: 1556–64.

Hayward, R. A., and T. P. Hofer. 2001. "Estimating Hospital Deaths Due to Medical Errors: Preventability Is in the Eye of the Reviewer." *Journal of the American Medical Association* 286 (4): 415–20.

Institute of Medicine. 2001. *Crossing the Quality Chasm: A New Health System for the 21st Century.* Washington, DC: National Academies Press.

Kohn, L. T., J. M. Corrigan, and M. S. Donaldson (eds.). 2000. *To Err Is Human: Building a Safer Health System.* Washington, DC: National Academies Press.

Leape, L. L., D. M. Berwick, and D. W. Bates. 2002. "What Practices Will Most Improve Safety? Evidence-Based Medicine Meets Patient Safety." *Journal of the American Medical Association* 288 (4): 501–7.

McGlynn, E. A., S. M. Asch, J. Adams, J. Keesey, J. Hicks, A. DeCristofaro, and E. A. Kerr. 2003. "The Quality of Health Care Delivered to Adults in the United States." *New England Journal of Medicine* 348 (26): 2635–45.

Nolan, T. W. 2000. "System Changes to Improve Patient Safety." *British Medical Journal* 320 (March 18): 771–73.

Norman, D. A. 1988. *The Design of Everyday Things.* New York: Doubleday.

Pronovost, P., S. Berenholtz, T. Dorman, P. A. Lipsett, T. Simmonds, and C. Haraden. 2003. "Improving Communication in the ICU Using Daily Goals." *Journal of Critical Care* 18 (2): 71–75.

Reason, J. 1990. *Human Error.* New York: Cambridge University Press.

———. 1997. *Managing the Risks of Organizational Accidents.* Aldershot, UK: Ashgate.

Sexton, J. B. 2002. "Rapid-Fire Safety Ideas Minicourse." Presented at the Institute for Healthcare Improvement 14th Annual National Forum on Quality Improvement in Health Care, Orlando, FL, December 9.

Sexton, J. B., E. J. Thomas, and R. L. Helmreich. 2000. "Error, Stress, and Teamwork in Medicine and Aviation: Cross Sectional Surveys." *British Medical Journal* 320: 745–49.

Shojania, K. G., B. W. Duncan, K. M. McDonald, and R. M. Wachter. 2002. "Safe but Sound: Patient Safety Meets Evidence-Based Medicine." *Journal of the American Medical Association* 288 (4): 508–13.

Weick, K. E., and K. M. Sutcliffe. 2001. *Managing the Unexpected: Assuring High Performance in an Age of Complexity.* San Francisco: Jossey-Bass.

INFORMATION TECHNOLOGY APPLICATIONS FOR IMPROVED QUALITY

Richard E. Ward

Background and Terminology

The healthcare industry is facing increased complexity, escalating economic pressure, and heightened consumerism. These three trends drive an increased interest in finding ways to improve the quality and efficiency of healthcare processes and to apply information technology to meet this challenge.

Complexity

Healthcare involves the coordinated effort of professionals from multiple clinical disciplines and specialties, working in multiple settings. Patients with severe illnesses and chronic diseases in particular require such coordinated care. As life expectancy increases and the population ages, a greater proportion of patients face severe illnesses, often complicated with multiple comorbid conditions. New scientific discoveries and new medical technologies lead to constantly changing clinical processes. As medical knowledge grows, individual clinicians have increasing difficulty keeping up with it. As a result, healthcare has become more specialized, increasing the need for interdisciplinary coordination. Quality patient care is dependent on successful management of this complexity.

Healthcare organizations are poorly equipped to meet the challenge of complexity. Despite the inspiring dedication of talented, highly trained healthcare professionals on an individual level, the health system's collective track record is poor for many basic healthcare processes. The healthcare system can be confusing to patients and clinicians alike, leading to frequent errors and suboptimal care. Literature is full of studies exposing such problems. Table 12.1 provides a few examples.

The economic consequences of healthcare processes unable to meet the challenge of increasing complexity are severe. Healthcare expenditures in the United States represent 16 percent of the gross national product (U.S. Department of Health and Human Services and Centers for Medicare & Medicaid Services 2007). An analysis of care received by Medicare recipients with chronic conditions showed that almost 30 percent of the cost of care

TABLE 12.1
Examples of
Problems in
Healthcare
Delivery

Medication Errors	As new medications are developed and prescribed to patients with multiple comorbid conditions, the chance for unintended side effects grows. Because of poor processes and systems for managing this complexity, 106,000 fatal adverse drug reactions occur each year in the United States. This figure is equivalent to the number of casualties that would result from a Boeing 747 crashing every other day with no survivors (Lazarou, Pomeranz, and Corey 1998). The cost of fatal and nonfatal adverse drug events is estimated at $110 billion per year.
Failure to Receive Needed Interventions	A study assessed the quality of care provided to heart failure patients discharged from an Ivy League medical center (Nohria et al. 1999). Among the "ideal candidates" for ACE inhibitors (i.e., drugs proven to reduce mortality and rehospitalization rates), 28% were not prescribed the drug and another 28% were receiving doses lower than those recommended in large clinical trials. In the same study, 25% did not receive dietary counseling, 17% were not educated about exercise, 91% were not instructed to track their weight daily, and 90% of the smokers had no documented advice to quit.
Poor Follow-up	A study in a large Midwestern medical group found that 17% to 32% of physicians reported having no reliable method, not even a paper-based method, to ensure that they receive the results of all ordered tests (Boohaker et al. 1996). One-third of physicians do not always notify patients of abnormal results. Only 23% of physicians reported having a reliable method for identifying patients overdue for follow-up. Not unexpectedly, this lack of a follow-up process causes errors. Among women with an abnormal mammogram, which requires follow-up in four to six months, 36.8% had inadequate follow-up (McCarthy et al. 1996).
Unjustified Variation in Care	Numerous studies have shown that healthcare is delivered in a highly variable manner, unjustified by differences among patients. In a comparison of different geographic areas, rates of coronary artery bypass grafting, transurethral prostatectomy, mastectomy, and total hip replacement varied three- to fivefold across regions (Birkmeyer et al. 1998). Rates of surgical procedures for lower extremity revascularization, carotid endarterectomy, back surgery, and radical prostatectomy varied six- to tenfold across regions. This level of variation does not represent appropriate consideration of different patient situations. Rather, it demonstrates a fundamental lack of reliability and consistency in the process of implementing evidence-based best practices across the country.

was for services that may have been unnecessary (Center for the Evaluative Clinical Sciences and the Dartmouth Medical School 2006).

Economic Pressure on Physicians

Payers and employers are transmitting the economic pressure from this $2 trillion market to physicians and other healthcare professionals. In recent years, the U.S. Congress repeatedly has passed Medicare reimbursement cuts and failed to reverse the cuts as they wreaked havoc on the financial health of hospitals and medical groups. Private payers have followed suit, pressuring healthcare providers to reduce utilization and accept lower reimbursement rates. This pressure has been increasing for a long time, but only recently has it reached a sufficient intensity to motivate fundamental change. Hospitals and medical groups already have picked almost all of the "low-hanging fruit" available for cost savings. Facilities have closed, patient co-payments have increased, and inpatient length of stay has decreased to the point of becoming a public relations problem. To maintain income, clinicians are forced to see more patients with fewer resources and under externally imposed rules and regulations.

At the same time that reimbursement rates are falling, payers and employers are demanding evidence of improving quality and outcomes. To maintain their position on preferred physician lists and referral panels, physicians are challenged to produce data on quality, outcomes, satisfaction, utilization, and cost to prove they are offering a good value for the health-care dollar.

Healthcare organizations are ill prepared to respond to this pressure for accountability and economic efficiency. A few entrepreneurial clinicians have attempted to regain control of their practices by taking on financial risk in their agreements with managed care organizations, only to suffer financial losses because they were poorly equipped to manage this risk. Medical groups in competitive markets are being forced to lay off physicians or close down entirely. The groups that remain are highly motivated to find a better way.

Consumerism

In recent years, healthcare consumers have rejected a paternalistic approach to medicine and have lashed out against managed care. Consumers' loyalty to their doctors has declined. If consumers' needs are not met, they complain to their elected representatives or go straight to their lawyers to sue their healthcare providers. An increasing number of states are allowing such litigation against health plans. Consumers are demanding information, choice, control, and improved service from the healthcare industry.

A report commissioned by the Kellogg Foundation found that 65 percent of healthcare consumers felt that *they* should have the most control over healthcare decisions affecting them, 31 percent said that their physicians should have the most control, and less than 1 percent reported that insurance companies should control decisions. However, only 22 percent reported that they actually do feel in control of healthcare decisions, and only 15 percent said their physicians have control. As a result, one out of three respondents characterized the healthcare system as "in critical condition" or "terminally ill."

This gap between consumer expectations and current reality is widening as consumers experience precedent-setting improvements in customer service in other industries. They are exposed to 1-800 number call centers, web-based e-commerce, service guarantees, and higher levels of standardization and quality in products and services in general. Healthcare providers and administrators themselves are consumers and are beginning to express disdain at the lag in healthcare service quality. In larger healthcare organizations, members of boards of directors often are executives in companies involved in service quality improvements. As a result, healthcare organizations are coming to understand the need to make fundamental changes in the way they deliver their "product." Healthcare organizations are ready to make the commitment to take care process-improvement concepts that have been pursued on a pilot or demonstration basis over the past two decades and implement them on a large scale throughout their practices.

Taking a Lesson from Other Industries

The challenges of complexity, economic pressure, and heightened consumerism are not unique to healthcare. Over the last two decades, many other industries have faced similar challenges. Banking, insurance, retail, transportation, and manufacturing industries all have faced increased complexity from technology advancement. Many of these industries were redefined as a result of deregulation. Many faced intense economic pressures from international competition. All faced increased consumer expectations and demands.

In response, many companies in these industries turned to information technology to achieve fundamental transformation of key business processes for "enterprise materials management" and "customer relationship management," revolutionizing the way they complete their work and interact with their customers. These new applications enable companies to offer their customers increased access to information and services and a higher level of customization to meet their complex, individual needs. They also enable companies to improve retention of existing customers and to attract new business. At the same time, the new information technology applications increase companies' capacity to serve more customers and reduce the cost of providing each service.

Internet

Recent technology developments have led to an explosion of interest and investment in applications to redesign materials and customer relationship management processes in other industries. The most important of these technologies is the Internet. The Internet provides ubiquitous information access to service providers across geographic locations and traditional organizational boundaries. The Internet also provides access directly to customers. Internet technology permits applications to be provided as a service, like telephones and cable television, rather than as a software product that requires substantial up-front capital.

Business Process Applications

Sophisticated, flexible business process applications have benefited from recent improvements in the underlying technologies of database management, application integration, and workflow automation. The Workflow Management Coalition (Hollingsworth 1995) defines *workflow automation* as the "computerized facilitation or automation of a business process, in whole or in part." Workflow-enabled applications offer the flexibility to create and modify workflow process definitions that describe the sequence of tasks involved in managing production and providing customer service. A "workflow engine" uses these process definitions to track and manage the delivery of services to particular customers, routing tasks and information to the right person at the right time to perform the work smoothly, efficiently, and correctly. Workflow technology is being integrated with telephone devices, web application servers, and e-mail to establish "contact centers," bringing non-healthcare business process applications to an exciting new level.

Connectivity and Messaging

Connectivity and messaging standards have matured in recent years, including the common object-request broker architecture (CORBA), extensible markup language (XML), and, more recently, "web services" standards. Using such standards, business process applications can incorporate other third-party components, reducing the cost of development and maintenance.

Remarkably, the business process applications widely used in other industries have not penetrated the healthcare sector. The time to adapt the information technology tools and approaches to meet the unique needs of clinicians and patients has arrived.

The Emerging Field of Medical Informatics

Medical informatics is the scientific field concerning the storage, retrieval, and optimal use of biomedical information, data, and knowledge for problem solving and decision making (Shortliffe and Perreault 1990). Practitioners in this field include individuals with medical training who extend their knowledge of information technology, as well as individuals who begin as information technology professionals and later specialize in healthcare applications. As early as 1984, a report by the Association of American Medical Colleges identified medical informatics as an area for which new educational opportunities are required and recommended the formation of new academic units in medical informatics in medical schools. The National Library of Medicine (NLM) sponsors university medical informatics research training programs in institutions throughout the country. The NLM also holds week-long training courses and offers opportunities for advanced studies. With greater opportunities for training, the supply of qualified medical informatics professionals will increase, enabling more healthcare institutions to improve their capabilities for quality management by adding medical informatics skills to the mix.

Two Tiers of Clinical Information Technologies

Most healthcare organizations use information technology for clinical processes, and most consider clinical information systems to be of strategic importance. However, different organizations have different visions and different objectives for clinical information technology investments. On a high level, consideration of two tiers of clinical information technology is helpful: (1) information access and (2) care management.

Using Information Technology for Information Access

The information access tier centers on a vision of information technology that provides "fingertip access" to the right information at the right place and time. Organizations with an information access vision have a goal of achieving a paperless medical record. Such organizations primarily seek to solve information access problems, including the following:

- Paper chart at wrong location
- Paper chart used by only one person at a time
- Multiple paper charts, each incomplete
- Paper chart poorly organized
- Paper summary sheets not up to date
- Paper chart that takes up too much space

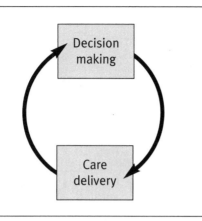

FIGURE 12.1
Two Core
Processes
Involving
Patients and
Clinics

- Hard-to-find clinical references, practice guidelines, and patient educational material
- Too much time spent on insurance eligibility, formulary, and so forth

In general, organizations focused on a vision of information access seek to achieve incremental benefits, with modest return on their investment. They do not apply information technology to achieve strategic imperatives. Such an information access vision is reasonable and perhaps prudent, given the long history of slow progress in clinical applications. Most of the current clinical information systems market is designed to address information access problems, even products from the newer e-health companies. However, an information access vision fails to address the need for the fundamental transformation of business processes that characterize the successful uses of information technology in other industries.

Using Information Technology for Care Management

The second tier of clinical information technology, which can be described as a care management vision, seeks to use information technology to enable successful continual improvements in the process of caring for individual patients and a patient population. Understanding the vision of information technologies for care management requires a clear definition of care management itself. On the most general level, all of healthcare can be conceptualized as a system involving two fundamentally different core processes: decision-making processes and care delivery processes, as illustrated in Figure 12.1.

Decision-making processes involve a clinician working with a patient to determine which, if any, healthcare interventions should be pursued at a given point in the patient's care. In this context, the term *healthcare intervention* is used broadly, encompassing everything from the components of a physical examination to the need for diagnostic testing or pharmaceutical

FIGURE 12.2
Healthcare
Management
System

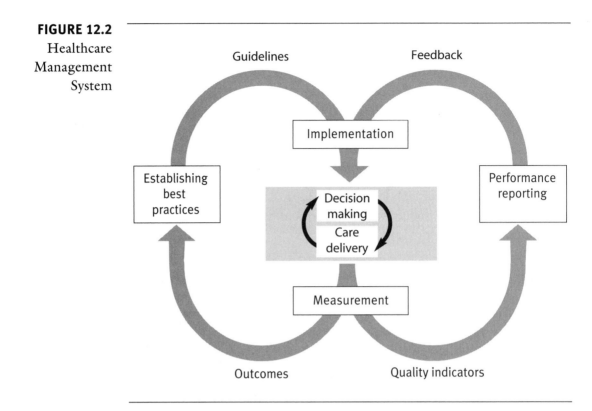

or surgical treatment. The output of this decision-making process is the patient's plan of care. The care delivery process, in contrast, involves the execution of the plan of care. The results of executed interventions, in turn, affect subsequent decisions. Even the most complex clinical processes can be broken down into cycles of deciding on a plan, executing the plan, and deciding on the next plan on the basis of the results achieved.

Quality is defined differently for decision-making and care delivery processes. For decision-making processes, *quality* means "doing the right thing"—identifying the alternatives and choosing the right one. For care delivery processes, quality means "doing it right"—carrying out the plan of care without making mistakes and without wasting resources. As illustrated in Figure 12.2, decision-making and care delivery processes interact with four important healthcare improvement sub-processes to form a general framework for the healthcare management system.

As shown in the bottom portion of Figure 12.2, the first important healthcare improvement sub-process is measurement. Given organizational commitment to measurement and the appropriate set of clinical information technology capabilities, data to support outcomes measurement and quality indicators can be collected as part of routine care delivery processes. Data needed for measurement include characteristics of patients, their risk factors, the medical interventions offered to them, and both immediate and long-term health and economic outcomes experienced by the population, including functional status, quality of life, satisfaction, and costs. Measurement, in turn, supports two other important healthcare improvement sub-processes: establishing best practices and performance reporting. Best practices include practice guidelines, protocols, care maps, appropriateness criteria, credentialing requirements, and other forms of practice policies. The process of establishing best practices involves clinical policy analysis, which is supported by scientific literature and available outcomes information. In addition, when these two sources of information are incomplete (as they often are), expert opinion is used.

Practice guidelines and other types of practice policies are meaningless unless they are used to influence clinician and patient decision making. The final important healthcare improvement sub-process is implementation, as shown at the top of Figure 12.2. Implementation involves the use of a variety of methods, including clinician and patient education; various decision aids such as reminders, alerts, and prompts; and incremental improvements or more extensive reengineering of care delivery processes. A particularly important method of supporting implementation is the use of feedback, with or without associated incentives. Over the past two decades, many healthcare organizations have attempted to implement clinical practice improvements without the benefit of an information technology infrastructure designed for that purpose. Many improvement efforts have achieved measurable success, at least on a small scale, during the time frame of the improvement project. In general, however, healthcare leaders have been disappointed with the success rate when improvements are rolled out to multiple settings, as well as with the durability of the changes. As attention turns to other processes and issues, gains from previous process improvements tend to evaporate.

Organizations with a "tier 2" vision seek to use information technology to enable healthcare management that is capable of large-scale, durable improvements in fundamental clinical processes, including decision-making and care delivery processes. The care management vision involves the use of information technology to solve problems such as the following:

- No affordable way to collect the clinically detailed data needed for quality and outcomes measures and research
- No way to incorporate up-to-date scientific evidence consistently into daily practice
- No feasible way to carry out multiple clinical practice improvement projects over time
- Inadequate tools to promote teamwork and a "do it once" approach to clinical and administrative tasks
- Too many intermediate parties and process steps required for care delivery processes (Documentation must be handled too many times, causing waste and errors.)

Healthcare organizations with a realistic vision of care management information technology realize that the goal of such technology is not to improve processes directly. Instead, such technology enables efforts to identify process problems, implement process changes, and assess whether such process changes represent improvements. In other words, clinical information technology is a tool, not a treatment. Organizations with a tier 2 vision focus on process improvement, not incentives. They focus not only on caring for individual patients with medical problems but also on prevention and disease management at a population level. They realize that different types of care processes involve different types of information technology solutions. This tier 2 vision is related to the concepts advocated by Wagner (1998) in his chronic care model and by various primary care professional societies in descriptions of the "patient-centered medical home" (American Academy of Family Physicians et al. 2007).

Technologies for Different Types of Clinical Care Management Initiatives

As illustrated in Figure 12.3, quality improvement, cost savings, or both can motivate care management initiatives. Initiatives can be focused on simple clinical processes involving the delivery or avoidance of specific medical interventions to specific cohorts of patients, or they can be focused on complex processes involving the coordination of many different clinicians from different disciplines to deliver a series of interventions over time. For simple processes, effective improvement methods include evidence-based guidelines, reminders, alerts, ticklers, and feedback of performance measures based on process variables (e.g., the percentage of two-year-olds who are up to date on all needed immunizations). The most important information technology capabilities supporting such process improvements include reminders integrated into medical records and physician order entry applications, and access to an analytic data warehouse with comparative quality measures.

For more complex processes, such as management of diabetes and heart failure, typical methods include practice policies in the form of consensus-based algorithms, protocols, and care maps. Other methods applied to complex processes include improving the knowledge base of clinicians through continuing medical education, engaging patients in their own care through patient education, and using care managers—typically nurses who aggressively track patient status and coordinate care for complex cases. The types of enabling technologies suitable for such complex processes include the use of workflow automation technology to support protocol-driven, team-based care (described more fully in the sections that follow). In addition, complex processes are best measured on the basis of overall outcomes achieved. Therefore, data collection systems that administer outcome surveys to patients

FIGURE 12.3
Different
Types of Care
Management
Initiatives Call
for Different
Methods and
Technologies

	Types of Care Management Initiatives	
	Simple Processes	**Complex Processes**
Improve quality	Improve HEDIS rates • Mammography • Pap smears • Immunizations	• Improve survival rates for cancer or AIDS • Improve control of blood sugar for mild- to moderate-risk diabetics • Primary prevention of CAD events by reducing cardiovascular risk profile

Improve quality and reduce cost	Improve HEDIS rates
	• Beta-blockers for patients who had a heart attack
		• Improve management of patients at high risk for hospital admission
		  • High-risk asthmatics
		  • Class III or IV heart failure
		  • First six months after heart attack
		  • Patients meeting "frail elderly" criteria
		• Discharge planning for hospitalized patients

Reduce cost	• Increase use of generic and in-formulary drugs • Avoid unneeded referrals and radiology studies • CT, MRI during first month of acute low back pain	• Attempts to attract only healthy members • Attempts to provide physicians with incentives to order and refer less
Typical methods	• Evidence-based guidelines • Reminders, alerts, ticklers • Performance measurement with process variables	• Consensus-based algorithms and protocols • Continuing medical education • Patient education • Care managers
Enabling technologies	• Reminders integrated into medical records and ordering process • Analytic data warehouse with comparative quality measures	• Protocol-driven, team-based care supported by workflow automation technology • Outcomes data collection systems, including survey and structured documentation and access to comparative outcomes data

(Left margin label: Drivers)

and structured documentation (template charting) tools that support the acquisition of data from clinicians are critical to providing the feedback loop needed to drive continual improvements in complex care processes.

Requirements and Architecture Framework for Clinical Information Technology

According to the Institute of Medicine (2003), electronic records should support the following high-level functions:

• Physician access to patient information, such as diagnoses, allergies, lab results, and medications
• Access to new and past test results among providers in multiple care settings
• Computer order entry

FIGURE 12.4

Architecture Framework for Clinical Information Systems

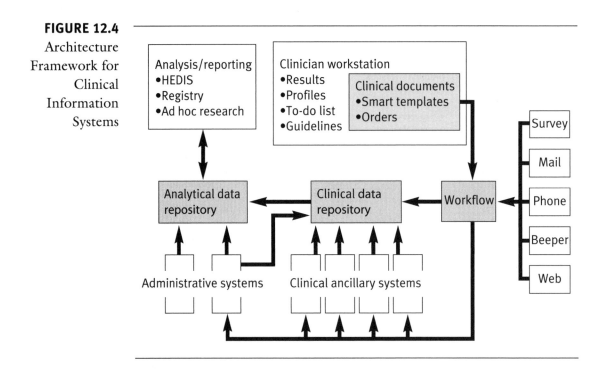

- Computerized decision-support systems to prevent drug interactions and improve compliance with best practices
- Secure electronic communication among providers and patients
- Patient access to health records, disease management tools, and health information resources
- Computerized administration processes such as scheduling systems
- Standards-based electronic data storage and reporting for patient safety and disease surveillance efforts

As illustrated at the bottom of Figure 12.4, most healthcare provider organizations have an existing portfolio of administrative and clinical information systems. Administrative systems include ambulatory practice management and inpatient admit/discharge/transfer systems, and associated systems for appointment scheduling, registration, charge capture, patient accounting, and claims management. Additional administrative systems may include financial accounting, budgeting, cost accounting, materials management, and human resources management. Clinical systems include various applications used by clinical ancillary departments such as laboratory, radiology, and cardiology. These systems are capable of entering requisitions, tracking tests to completion, and capturing and communicating results.

Data Repositories

Some healthcare organizations expand on this core of administrative and clinical systems by developing data repositories. Analytical data repositories and associated data analysis and reporting applications take data primarily from administrative systems and make them available for routine and ad hoc reporting and research. Such systems go by many names, including *decision support systems, data warehouses, data stores, executive information systems*, and *business intelligence systems*. Such systems should include provisions for statistical analysis, including risk and severity adjustment, graphical analysis, and statistical modeling. Analytic data repositories are more useful if attention is paid to the quality of the data going into the repository, including the consistency of coding of procedures and diagnoses and the correct matching of all data for a single patient based on the use of an enterprise-wide patient identifier or probabilistic matching algorithms.

A smaller percentage of healthcare organizations (less than half) have implemented clinical data repositories, which take results data from various clinical ancillary systems, store the information in a database, and make the information accessible through some front-end application used by clinicians. Such systems are called *clinician workstations, electronic medical records, computerized patient records*, and *lifetime patient records*. In addition to displaying results data, clinician workstation applications often maintain patient profile information, including medical problem lists; medication lists; drug allergies; family and social history; and health risk factors such as smoking status, blood pressure, and body mass. Clinician workstations also may include a clinical to-do list; secure clinical messaging; and access to online medical reference materials such as internal practice guidelines, the hospital or health plan formulary, scientific articles indexed in MEDLINE, the *Physicians' Desk Reference*, and a collection of medical textbooks.

Template Charting

A small percentage of clinicians have access to template charting, an important feature of advanced clinician workstations. *Template charting* is the acquisition of unstructured and structured data as a single process carried out by a clinician during or immediately following a patient encounter to provide medical record documentation while simultaneously supporting other data needs, such as billing, research, and quality and outcomes measurement. Template charting applications also are known as *clinical documentation, note-writing*, and *charting* applications. They permit a clinician to create clinical notes efficiently by incorporating material from previously prepared templates and then modifying the note as needed for a patient. Templates not only speed up the documentation process but also remind the clinician of the data items that should be included, resulting in more complete and standardized notes. Such notes are better for patient care and produce, as a by-product, computer-readable, analyzable data that can be used for orders, requisitions, referrals, prescriptions, and billing. Indirectly, documentation that is more complete can generate increased revenue by supporting higher-level encounter and management (E&M) codes, leading to higher reimbursement for clinical visits. Structured documentation that is more complete can provide the data inputs for clinical alerts, reminders, and order critique features. For example, by documenting drug history, drug allergies, and body mass, the system can analyze a new drug added to a patient's plan of care to determine whether it interacts with other drugs the patient is taking, whether the patient is allergic to the drug, whether the dose is inappropriate in relation to the patient's body mass, and whether there are other drugs that are more cost-effective or in greater compliance with hospital or health plan formulary policy. Finally, notes based on structured data, when more complete, can be used to support clinical research, quality assurance, and outcomes measurement, enabling evidence-based clinical process improvement.

As noted above, template charting applications are used to acquire both unstructured and structured data. Unstructured data include handwritten notes incorporated into a computerized patient record through document imaging or captured through voice dictation (followed by manual transcription or electronic voice recognition). Unstructured data also can take the form of a clinical diagram, such as a diagram showing the anatomic location of a breast lump or showing the distribution of low back pain. In contrast, structured data are captured as a number or code that a computer can read. Structured data include procedure codes, diagnosis codes, vital signs, and many physiologic parameters such as range of motion of a joint and visual acuity. Structured data also may include outcomes survey data collected from patients or clinicians.

As illustrated in Figure 12.5, a fundamental trade-off must be made between the quantity and quality of structured data that can be collected because of physicians' limited tolerance to being "fenced in" by template charting systems that seem to keep them from expressing themselves as

FIGURE 12.5

Template Charting Trade-Off: Quantity Versus Quality of Structured Data

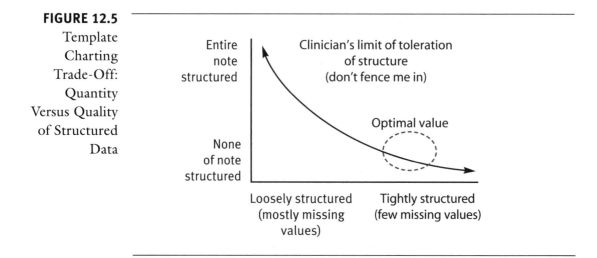

they wish. In practice, clinicians who use systems that attempt to capture the entire clinical note as structured data express frustration and demand that the structure of the data be loose. In this context, "loose" structure means that the system cannot demand that specific data elements be provided. Therefore, the resulting structured note represents a collection of computer-readable facts only for patient aspects that the clinician documented, with no data on a large number of other patient aspects documented for other patients. This loose form of structured data is analogous to a database table with a large number of fields but many missing values.

On the other hand, tightly structured data are characterized by rigorous, complete collection of specified elements. In practice, clinicians using template charting applications that include tightly structured data tend to be unwilling to use the system unless the number of required data elements is small and their short-term use is clear. Experts in medical vocabulary traditionally have advocated for the use of standardized vocabulary for as much of the chart as possible, reasoning that whatever is collected using standardized codes can be pooled with data from a great number of patients and analyzed, and that the resulting large sample size will lead to conclusive results. However, biostatisticians, epidemiologists, and health services researchers know that missing values severely limit the usefulness of data sets in ways not corrected by large sample sizes. This insight applies not only to population research studies but also to the use of the data for more immediate purposes, such as to drive reminders, alerts, and other decision aids. The logic rules used for such decision aids tend to require complete data for a small number of variables and often cannot be applied reliably when data inputs have missing values. Therefore, both research and decision aids, two of the most important tools for clinical practice improvement, need complete data. The philosophy should be to "start with the end in mind"—define the use of the data first, then characterize the requirements of the data, and finally design a data acquisition approach to meet those requirements. Therefore, when selecting a template charting approach, a solution that emphasizes the tight structuring of specified data elements, rather than a loosely structured model, is preferable.

Template charting applications also may include integrated decision support. By creating templates of orders that represent standing order sets, healthcare organizations can increase the standardization of testing and treatment. For example, a postoperative order set can help busy surgeons remember all the services they should consider ordering after every surgical procedure. In addition, "smart templates" can incorporate clinical logic to include or exclude items within templates conditionally. For example, in a medical history template, gynecologic history items may be excluded automatically from templates for men, and an order for a screening mammogram may be offered automatically in the template applied to a note for a woman who needs a mammogram. Finally, template charting applications are especially powerful if they are linked to reminders, alerts, and order critique rules that are processed immediately. For example, if a drug is included in a patient's plan of care and the patient is allergic to the drug, the template charting application would alert the clinician by displaying that drug in red or displaying an appropriate alert message. In this manner, template charting can reduce medical errors.

Such examples illustrate the importance of the functional integration of template charting applications and order entry applications. Many healthcare organizations fail to recognize this issue and implement separate applications with separate user interfaces for capturing orders and unstructured clinical notes using dictation. Many even implement separate devices for different kinds of orders. For example, many organizations are implementing handheld personal digital assistant devices for use in capturing prescriptions (drug orders) while using a full-sized computer for capturing laboratory or radiology orders. This approach offers important short-term benefits, including reductions in medication errors, but it risks being shortsighted if the long-term goal is to integrate the process of developing a plan of care into the process of creating a clinical note.

Workflow Automation Technology Applied to Clinical Processes

As shown on the right side of Figure 12.4, a general framework for clinical information technology to support clinical practice improvement includes a role for "workflow automation technology." Workflow systems generally provide a capability for entering workflow specification data that describe the sequence of tasks or activities in a work process, the resources required to execute each task, and the data needed to manage the flow of activities and to execute each task. Workflow systems generally also include a component that manages the execution of individual workflows, such as a workflow to track the execution of a single medical order. This component is called a *workflow engine,* a *workflow automation server,* or a *workflow enactment service.* It tracks the status of each workflow, determines which task is needed next and the human or system resources needed to execute the task, and communicates with those resources to transport the needed data to and from the resources. In these systems, completion of a computer-based form provides the data required to initiate the workflow.

Improvements in Processes of Care

Workflow systems increase the efficiency of service delivery because they are able to route the right task to the right person or machine at the right time. They increase the consistency and quality of service delivery because they track work according to workflow specifications that can define best practices. They also increase the reliability of services because bottlenecks and errors can be identified and managed. Some workflow systems provide a generic framework that can be adapted to a wide variety of service delivery processes.

In the context of healthcare, workflow automation provides the ability to encapsulate other information technologies and services and make them available for incorporation into processes of care. Such services include surveys; outbound recorded telephone messages; outbound e-mail messages; printing and mailing of generic or tailored educational materials; outbound faxes; electronic pager or short text messaging; and requests for third-party telemonitoring, care management, and disease management programs. Clinical workflow systems also can provide an interface for insurance eligibility and preauthorization transactions and for ancillary departmental systems for orders and order status checking.

Improvements in Change Management

Workflow automation technology offers the promise of improving teamwork and coordination across the continuum of care, including clinicians in different clinic locations, inpatient facilities, ancillary service providers, home healthcare, call centers, and other settings. It promises to coordinate care over time, ensuring follow-up with each needed test or treatment, and it ensures that a sequence of healthcare interventions happens consistently according to a predetermined clinical protocol or care map. It enables clinicians to take charge of cycles of process improvement because it provides tools that permit changes to workflow specifications without always requiring changes to software. As a result, a team of clinicians can make a decision about a clinical process change and implement the change in the workflow system without having to write proposals, obtain capital funding, and wait until the change makes it to the top of overcommitted programmers' priority lists. When even small changes in care processes require the navigation of frustrating capital and information technology development processes, clinicians leading such changes often resort to non-information technology methods to implement changes. They use racks of paper forms, rubber stamps, guidelines printed on pocket cards, signs taped to exam room walls, symbols marked on whiteboards, decks of cards as tickler files, and various other low-tech alternatives. These approaches may prove effective in the short term at the local setting, but they tend to break down over time and at different locations, resulting in medical errors. By reducing the burden of making scalable, durable process changes, clinical workflow automation technology promises to be a powerful tool for reducing medical errors and improving the efficiency and quality of clinical processes.

Other Clinical Information Technology Components

Telemedicine

In large, geographically distributed healthcare organizations, telemedicine capabilities allow clinicians to care for patients in remote locations. Such capabilities include a variety of technologies, including multimedia telecommunications (e.g., video conferencing) that allow clinicians to interact with patients or other clinicians. Remote sensors allow physicians to extend their ability to observe patients. For example, in a home setting, remote sensors may include devices to capture and communicate body weight, blood glucose, or peak expiratory flow, or to count pills. In a clinic setting, a remote sensor can provide the capabilities of a stethoscope or ophthalmoscope. In the inpatient or intensive care setting, remote sensors allow the real-time viewing of vital signs, electrocardiogram tracing, ventilator outputs, and other devices. Finally, digital radiology allows radiographic images to be communicated remotely for interpretation by experts in another setting.

Rules Servers

Sophisticated clinical information systems include one or more rules server components that apply clinical logic to healthcare data. These components are described as *inference processors, expert systems, artificial intelligence, knowledge-based systems, smart systems, real-time decision support*, and various combinations of these terms, such as *network-based real-time rules servers*. In general, the role of such components is to increase the performance and decrease the maintenance cost of applying clinical logic as part of various features of a clinical information system. Such rules servers improve response-time performance by placing logic processing in close proximity to the clinical database and using high-powered processors optimized for such mathematical calculations. Rules servers decrease maintenance cost by avoiding the "hard coding" of clinical logic throughout many different applications and by providing a single tool and syntax for creating, maintaining, and protecting clinical logic. By improving the standardization of the syntax used to represent clinical rules, these servers enable rules to be shared more easily across different parts of a healthcare organization or even across healthcare organizations. In this manner, centralized rule processors can help healthcare organizations treat their clinical logic as valuable intellectual property to be protected and leveraged.

Although inference processing may seem like an esoteric function, it is surprisingly ubiquitous within clinical information systems. For example, to load data into a clinical data repository, an "integration engine" component is often used, which includes logic for routing data, reformatting and transforming data, and determining how data are to be inserted into database tables. In clinician workstation applications, clinical logic is applied to displays of abnormal values and intelligent summarization of clinical data for specific medical problems. In template charting, rules are applied to support "smart template" features that determine when specific parts of templates are to be included or activated.

Clinical Vocabulary Servers

Another important component of sophisticated clinical information systems is a clinical vocabulary server. This component, also known as a *lexical mediation component*, is responsible for translating codes, terms, and concepts to permit rule processing. For example, in a centralized rules server, rules optimally are stated in terms of standard medical concepts, even though these rules may act on data collected using many different nonstandard codes. A vocabulary server is a special kind of rules server that applies rules that take nonstandard codes and determines how they relate to standardized concepts, as well as how standard concepts relate to each other. For example, the International Classification of Disease (ICD) 9 diagnosis code "864.12" corresponds to the concept "minor laceration of liver with open wound into abdominal cavity." A vocabulary server determines that the Systemized Nomenclature of Medicine (SNOMED) vocabulary represents this same concept as "DD-23522." In rule processing applications, this specific clinical concept is part of a more general concept of "laceration of liver," represented in the ICD-9 as "864.05" and in SNOMED as "DD-23502." Such logic is a prerequisite to a rule that may suggest an appropriate diagnostic algorithm for evaluating suspected laceration of liver. Vocabulary servers are included as part of the infrastructure of clinical software suites; some vendors also offer them as stand-alone components. A good vocabulary server includes up-to-date content regarding various standardized code sets for clinical use, such as the Logical Observation Identifiers Names and Codes (LOINC) and SNOMED. A vocabulary server also offers standardized codes for administrative uses, such as ICD, Current Procedural Terminology (CPT), and National Drug Codes (NDC). A good clinical vocabulary offers concepts that are specific enough to support clinical decision rules but also practical for busy clinicians' use. A vocabulary server should provide a classification hierarchy to facilitate term searches and handling generalization, and routine maintenance and timely updates should be made to it to keep current with continuously changing vocabulary.

Patient Surveys

A complete clinical information system designed to support clinical practice improvement also should include patient survey components to facilitate the acquisition of data directly from patients. A variety of technologies and methods are used for this purpose, including:

- preprinted paper-based surveys or tailored surveys printed at the point of care (with subsequent data capture through manual data entry, scanning, or optical mark reading);
- fax-based survey systems;
- systems that allow a patient to directly enter information in a clinical facility using a touch screen or handheld device;
- web-based survey applications that allow a patient to enter data from home; and
- telephone-based interactive voice response systems that use touch-tone entry or voice recognition technology.

Evaluation of Systems

Important features to consider in evaluating such systems include the ability to deliver surveys to the patient at home, in a clinic waiting room, or in a hospital bed. Ideal systems reduce the risk of loss and breakage of valuable equipment. Survey systems should be suitable to deal with patient limitations (for example, they should offer larger type size for patients with poor eyesight, voice or pictures for patients who cannot read, and translations or pictures for patients who do not speak the predominant language). Patient survey systems should be adaptable to meet the changing needs of the healthcare organization (for example, they should permit local customization of surveys to meet internal needs without requiring programming). Ideally, they should reduce the burden of patient data entry (for example, they should offer automated patient-level customization of surveys to avoid unneeded or duplicate questions and offer branching logic for survey items that do not apply to all patients). Finally, the flow of information in good patient survey systems is bidirectional, combining patient education with data acquisition. For example, shared decision-making systems combine interactive video technology to educate patients about the pros and cons of alternative treatment options while collecting data to assess the patient's comprehension of the information, documenting the patient's utilities and preferences, and collecting additional data items to support patient care and research.

Study Management Capabilities

To support outcomes research and clinical research essential to implementing a care management vision of clinical information systems, such systems also should include study management capabilities. Study management systems handle the processes of identifying patients eligible for enrollment in a study, handle enrollment and disenrollment of patients into or out of one or more study protocols, and determine which study subjects need which data collection forms at any given point in time. A good study management system should be able to handle multiple study protocols as a single process and track the status of data collection forms through the entire life cycle to a final disposition. This administration of data collection instruments should integrate with patient survey systems (described above) and facilitate the details of printing forms; cover letters and mailing labels for mailed surveys; reminder letters for overdue surveys; and physician referral letters, chart notes, and other reports based on completed surveys. Such systems also should facilitate the process of preparing the data to be analyzed or sent to an external research center for incorporation into a multi-institutional database. They should be able to produce appropriately formatted data files for transmission to the data center, check data integrity, and accept feedback regarding rejected records.

Study management capabilities can take the form of a separate application dedicated to this purpose, leading to efficiencies in managing outcomes research and clinical studies. However, this approach is inconsistent with the overall vision of tier 2 clinical information systems to support care management. The kinds of capabilities that would be part of a study management system—the ability to identify patients who need a service, track the delivery of the service to completion, and collect the structured data needed to support the goals of the process—are the same fundamental capabilities needed for clinical decision making and care delivery. The additional requirements of outcomes research and clinical studies should be integrated seamlessly into the routine clinical processes, enabling the healthcare organization to learn and innovate as a by-product of caring for patients. Only a small fraction of healthcare organizations have articulated and incorporated such a vision in their strategic plans, and, unfortunately, it has been achieved in a frustratingly small number of settings.

Data Analysis and Reporting Capabilities

A complete clinical information system should provide data analysis and reporting capabilities. Data analysis tools should not only support the needs of statisticians and data analysis professionals but also provide "canned" graphical and tabular outcomes analysis of patient populations for healthcare leaders and other occasional users. Such tools also may provide predictions and formatted reports for individual patients to support informed medical decision making.

Information Needed for Practice Improvement on a National Level

Although such data analysis and reporting capabilities are useful within the healthcare organization, the sample size available within one organization may not be sufficient to support analysis of treatment effectiveness, practice patterns, medical errors, disease progression, and other topics of interest. Also, the feedback of performance and quality measures is more effective if other institutions and settings provide comparative data. To achieve this comparison, access to data pooled across healthcare organizations on a regional, national, or international level is required.

As illustrated in Figure 12.6, the deepest and most rigorous source of information supporting research and practice improvement is randomized clinical trials, which involve careful collection of specific data items by dedicated study personnel under controlled conditions. The U.S. Food and Drug Administration mandates such trials for on-label uses of drugs and certain biomedical devices. Unfortunately, the high expense of clinical trials has precluded their use in many types of clinical practices and protocols. Prospective outcomes studies, typically involving nonrandomized study designs and often involving data collection as part of the routine care process, are less expensive but also less rigorous and conclusive. On the other end of the spectrum, large Medicare databases, employer-based claims processing, and pharmacy benefit managers often are used for analysis and reporting.

A third source of data is a *collaborative data warehouse*, created as part of a consortium of like-minded healthcare organizations that pool their data to meet their common needs for comparative data and large sample sizes. Depending on the type of collaborator, the resulting data may center on hospital stays or may be more comprehensive, including both inpatient and outpatient activity and clinical data such as laboratory results and

FIGURE 12.6

Sources of Information for Practice Improvement

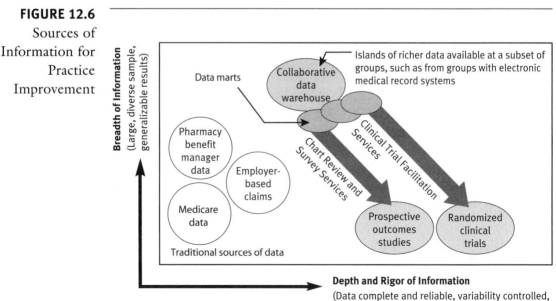

electronic medical records data. In many community practice settings, the creation of a collaborative data warehouse may be logistically and politically difficult because data describing different aspects of a patient's health and medical care reside in different systems in different organizations using different patient identifiers. In certain settings, however, such as the military health system, the Veterans Administration, and large multi-specialty group practices or hospital chains, the data-pooling process is easier. Such organizations "own" a greater portion of the complete healthcare picture for their patients, usually have systems centralized in one facility and under one leadership structure, often have common identifiers, and sometimes have existing analytic databases they can leverage.

Even in such organizations, creating a collaborative data warehouse may be difficult in face of various types of apprehension by the prospective collaborators. For example, leaders of such organizations may worry that competitors will access and use the data against them, that suppliers will use the data for target marketing, that patient privacy will be compromised, or that the healthcare organization may be embarrassed if unflattering performance data were made public. Pooling and analysis through a trusted intermediary, such as a trade organization, a purchasing cooperative, a common parent company, or a government agency that oversees all the prospective collaborators, may help them overcome their apprehension. Furthermore, clear legal agreements that set limits to uses of data (consistent with the interests of collaborators) and organizational structures and policies that allow for collaborator input and control may reduce the level of worry.

Case Examples

Flu Immunization Reminder Letters

One example of the use of information technology to drive improvement in a simple care process involves a project to increase compliance with guidelines for adult influenza immunization at a large integrated delivery system in the Midwest. In the project, the team used information technology along with other approaches to guideline implementation, including staff training, patient education, and continuous quality improvement methods. To increase the medical staff's knowledge, the team created and disseminated a memorandum describing the flu guideline and included the guideline in a preventive services handbook, bound in a soft cover and designed to fit into lab coat pockets. The team also incorporated the flu guideline into a course on preventive services in its "managed care college" program, a continuing medical education program involving approximately 85 staff members in a series of lectures and mentored improvement projects. The team increased patients' knowledge by including an article about flu immunization in the magazine distributed by the organization's HMO and by displaying in clinic locations posters and tent cards featuring a cartoon character explaining the benefits of flu immunization. The team developed institution- and physician-level performance measures based on analysis of billing data present in the analytic data repository. The team did a small-scale study to validate the measures by calling a random sample of patients and asking them about flu immunizations they received within the clinic and in other community locations such as churches, shopping malls, and senior centers. They found that 15 to 20 percent of all immunizations were administered by locations outside the scope of the organization's billing data. Therefore, the team decided to use the institutional performance measure as a way to measure improvement over time and to compare performance of interventions to increase performance. However, the team decided to forgo dissemination of physician-level performance measures to avoid subjecting the overall performance measurement program to criticism as a result of inclusion of a measure known to be pessimistically biased.

The team then implemented Saturday flu shot clinics during the flu season, placing them close to lobby entrances to create the quickest possible visit for patients. To support these clinics, the team performed an analysis of the analytic data repository to prepare reports that listed patients who were known to have received the immunization previously and the date of service, along with a listing of patients' primary care physicians. Finally, to encourage patient immunization, the team created computer-generated reminders. To evaluate the effectiveness and cost-effectiveness of such reminders, it conducted a trial that randomized 24,743 patients to one of three interventions and included a control group that received only the benefit of other aspects of the flu shot improvement program described above. The intervention media of the trial included (1) a generic, non-tailored postcard, (2) a postcard with a tailored message, and (3) an automatically generated tailored letter from the patient's primary care physician, mentioning risk factors present in the patient's records that put the patient in a risk category requiring a flu shot.

As shown in Figure 12.7, there was a "dose-response" relationship with expected performance increases as additional reminder features were added. Overall, the tailored letter increased compliance with flu shots by about 5 percentage points. Although this increase may seem small, it represents an important improvement at a population level. The letters cost 42 cents to produce and send through an outside service with expertise in mass mailing. The vaccine itself cost $4.09. According to studies published elsewhere, the expected annual hospital cost for influenza care is reduced from $355 to $215 when patients receive flu shots. On the basis of the size of this institution's population and the prevalence of influenza, a cost-effectiveness model calculated the net savings to be $118,000 in a nonepidemic year and $268,000 in an epidemic year. Furthermore, the team perceived

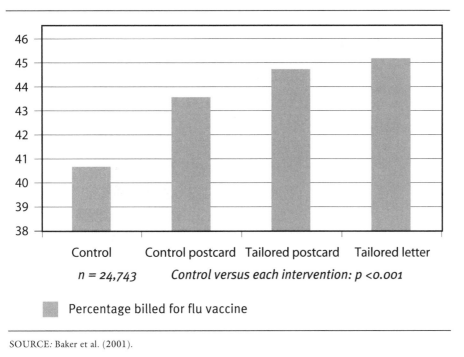

FIGURE 12.7
Results of Randomized Trial of Alternative Reminders for Adult Influenza Immunization

SOURCE: Baker et al. (2001).

the program to have achieved additional noneconomic benefits for the organization in the form of patients' satisfaction with the attentiveness of their primary care provider and the organization in general to their personal health needs.

Diabetes Care Management

An example of information technology application to complex care processes is the use of a web-based population management tool to support the management of diabetes (Baker et al. 2001). As with the flu immunization project described above, the diabetes care management team used a multimodal approach to improving diabetes care. The team created a practice guideline for various diabetes-related interventions and made it available in paper form and through a link from an intranet diabetes care management application. This application was accessible through a web browser anywhere within the organization and could be reached through a link included as a drop-down menu within the main window of the clinician workstation application. In addition to displaying the diabetes practice guideline, this care management application provided statistics describing the characteristics of the diabetes patient population for an individual care provider, a local clinic setting, or larger aggregations such as "region" and "institution-wide." See Figure 12.8.

The care management application also offered a diabetes patient registry, including the ability to generate lists of diabetes patients. These reg-

FIGURE 12.8

Screen Shot of Performance Graph in Diabetes Care Management System

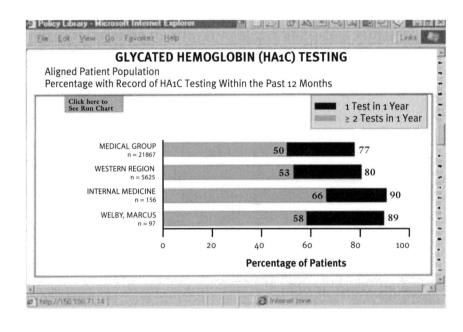

istry lists took the form of a grid with rows for each diabetes patient and columns displaying key variables related to diabetes care, including the date and value of the last glycated hemoglobin (HA1C) test; whether the patient received two HA1C tests the previous year; whether the patient received a dilated eye exam the previous year and the date of the last eye exam; whether the patient received a microalbumin test during the last year; and the date and values of the last lipid profile test, including total cholesterol, LDL, and triglycerides. This care management application allowed the clinical staff to view a preliminary risk stratification, generating lists of patients who require diabetes services such as a primary care visit, HA1C testing, and eye exams. These lists included patient contact information. The application also provided practice feedback and comparative benchmarking. It presented feedback in the form of graphs that showed the percentage of patients who had good, intermediate, and poor control of blood glucose (as indicated by average HA1C test results), comparing an individual care provider to the average for the local practice setting as well as to regional, institutional, and national averages. Other graphs showed the trend line of the percentage of diabetes patients who had received needed diabetes services.

An evaluation of the diabetes care management application revealed that, during the first year of use, 29 percent of primary care physicians initiated a session and that these physicians used the system eight times on average. More important, nonphysician staff from 94 percent of the primary care clinics initiated at least 1 session, averaging 30 sessions per year. The team developed a statistical model to evaluate the effect of the system on guideline performance related to 13,325 diabetes patients, adjusting for patient sociodemographic and clinical characteristics and the testing history of the patient, primary care physician, and primary care clinic. As a result of using the system, compliance with diabetes practice guidelines improved. Among the patients of physicians who used the system at least eight times, 17 percent were more likely to do two HA1C tests, 12 percent were more likely to do a cholesterol test, and 4 percent were more likely to do a retinal exam. Among the patients of clinics that had staff use the system at least 30 times, 34 percent were more likely to do two hemoglobin tests.

The diabetes care management team then applied the knowledge it gained from evaluation of the first-generation improvement program to drive the next cycle of improvements. From the evaluation, the team learned that 10 percent of diabetes patients were not seen in the clinic during the past 12 months. The team concluded that an outreach intervention was needed to engage patients in their care. Subsequently, the team implemented computer-generated, tailored letters from primary care physicians to the diabetes patients who had not visited the clinic. The team also learned from the evaluation that 50 percent of the patients seen in the clinic during the past 12 months did not receive necessary tests and exams. Therefore, the team developed a system using workflow automation technology to track receipt of diabetes-related tests and exams (along with a number of preventive services) and to prompt the clinician for these services. It incorporated this reminder system into the user interface for the clinician workstation. This reminder system now provides clinicians with health maintenance reports through which they can track diabetes interventions (and other interventions) and reminds them of due dates.

Overall Return on Investment of Clinical Information Systems

To assess the effect of various clinical information technology investments on cost savings and revenue enhancement, a return on investment (ROI) model can be used. The model includes assumptions based on a review of studies providing evidence of cost savings or revenue enhancement, including MEDLINE, vendor materials, and analyses published by information technology consultants. Each identified benefit is categorized and associated with a functional area that corresponds to a type of information technology investment, as shown in Figure 12.9.

Assumptions are made on the basis of institution-specific input regarding such variables as personnel costs, costs of software and associated imple-

FIGURE 12.9
Clinical
Information
Technology
Benefit
Categories
and Associated
Functional
Areas

Benefit Category	Functional Area
Information access	Clinical data repository
Improve decision making	Physician ordering with alerts
Information capture	Clinical documentation
Improve process	Workflow automation and disease management
Improve market share*	Patient/community access

*No literature measuring market share outcomes of clinical systems offering patient/community access was identified, so this functional area was not included in this generation of the ROI analysis.

mentation, volume of activity, and payer mix. For each assumption, an unbiased best estimate is made, along with a range of uncertainty bounded by a pessimistic estimate and an optimistic estimate. In addition, for each calculated cost or revenue effect, an assessment of the strength of evidence is assigned, judging both general and institution-specific assumptions underlying the estimated effect. These strength-of-evidence assessments are coded as "Strong Evidence," "Medium Evidence," "Poor Evidence," and "Educated Opinion."

The results of the model are dependent on institution-specific variables. For example, the bottom-line impact of using disease management to reduce the rate of hospitalization is to reduce revenue from fee-for-service patients and to reduce cost for globally capitated patients. Therefore, the same result has a different financial effect depending on payer mix. The model is highly sensitive to other institution-specific variables such as the assumed speed of implementation, the order in which functional areas are implemented, and the compensation levels of different types of personnel. Nevertheless, Figure 12.10 includes model results for a hypothetical healthcare organization to illustrate the general structure of such ROI calculations and to provide a high-level perspective on the relative benefits of different clinical information technology investments and the sensitivity of the estimates to the desired threshold for evidence. The hypothetical healthcare organization has 300 physicians across all specialties, a teaching hospital, and a payer mix that includes 50 percent capitation.

As shown in Figure 12.10, the model for a hypothetical healthcare organization assumes a six-year implementation period, beginning with implementation of a clinical data repository, followed by implementation of physician ordering, clinical documentation, and finally workflow automation and disease management.

As shown in Figure 12.11, the "uptake" of the clinical information system components by clinicians and other personnel is assumed to take some time following the initial implementation of the component. Full utilization of all components is expected to take a total of ten years.

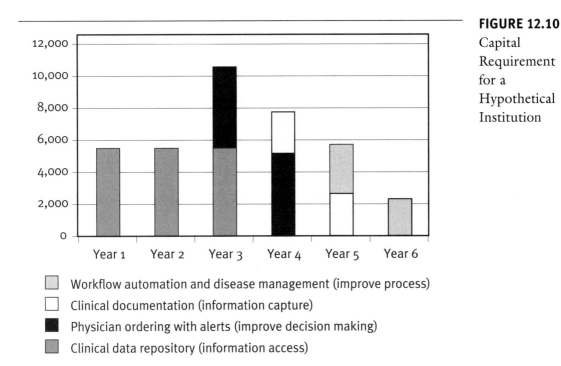

FIGURE 12.10

Capital Requirement for a Hypothetical Institution

☐ Workflow automation and disease management (improve process)
☐ Clinical documentation (information capture)
■ Physician ordering with alerts (improve decision making)
▨ Clinical data repository (information access)

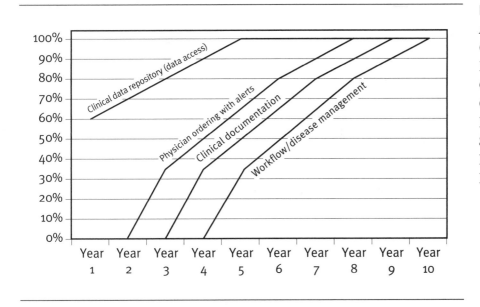

FIGURE 12.11

Assumed Gradual Deployment of Components of Clinical Information Systems for a Hypothetical Institution

As shown in Figure 12.12, clinical information systems may have many different effects on a healthcare organization's net income. The greatest effects, based on the assumptions used for this hypothetical organization, are (1) the increased revenue generated from more outpatient visits and from the use of high-quality documentation capable of supporting higher E&M billing codes and (2) the cost savings in the population of

Source of Change in Net Income	Change in Net Income at Full Implementation (Thousands)
Revenue from improved visit capacity	18,445
Disease management—all diseases other than congestive heart failure, asthma, and diabetes	14,331
Decrease in "down coding" behavior for E&M coding	12,726
Congestive heart failure disease management in clinic	4,278
Reduced unnecessary inpatient lab utilization	4,050
Reduced unnecessary inpatient drug utilization	3,403
Diabetes disease management	2,373
Quicker prescription refill by clinic nurses	1,913
Increase in claims acceptance from improved coding	1,818
Reduced need for transcription	1,521
Reduced preventable adverse drug events	1,511
More efficient NP/RN/clerical support task allocation	1,316
Decrease in lost charges from improved coding	1,260
Quicker information access by clinic nurses	918
Reduced inpatient lab utilization for fee-for-service patients	668
Reduced need for chart pulls	600
Reduced inpatient drug utilization for fee-for-service patients	561
Asthma disease management in emergency room	515
Quicker visit preparation (support staff)	426
Reduced need for lab result filing	108
Reduced need for medical record supplies	40
Reduced need for chart copies	0
Reduced outpatient drug utilization for capitated patients	?
Outsourcing enabled by workflow tools	?
Decrease encounter preparation errors	?
Physician-to-RN/PA/NP task allocation	?
Savings from demand management of capitated patients	?
Revenue from new patients	?

? = Insufficient information to estimate

capitated patients resulting from disease management interventions and efforts to reduce unneeded utilization of inpatient drugs and laboratory tests. Note that the different effects have different levels of evidence supporting them. One large benefit category is the $7.5 million net income effect (net of revenue losses from fee-for-service inpatients) of reducing unnecessary inpatient lab and pharmacy utilization. One institution (the

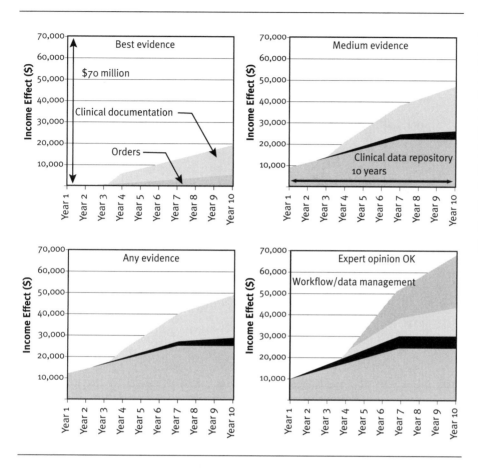

FIGURE 12.13

Net Income
Effect of
Different
Clinical
Information
System
Investments
for Different
Thresholds for
Required
Strength of
Evidence

University of Indiana, Regenstreif) had effects of similar magnitude across all categories of inpatient charges (not assumed for this model). If true, the effect would increase from 2.3 percent to 13 percent of inpatient net revenue, creating an additional $29 million benefit for the hypothetical institution.

As shown in Figure 12.13, the overall annual effect on the healthcare organization's bottom line (net income) ranges from just over $20 million to almost $70 million, depending on whether the decision maker demands the best evidence before considering a specific cost or revenue effect to be trustworthy or whether less certain effects should be considered and counted. The best evidence is available for certain categories of benefits, particularly related to order entry and clinical documentation. Intermediate quality of evidence is available for various categories of benefits related to the use of a clinical data repository. The literature includes many studies documenting dramatic benefits from disease management interventions, including many disease management interventions using supportive information technologies. Most such studies focus on common conditions such as asthma, congestive heart failure, and diabetes. However, there is little evidence of the

FIGURE 12.14

ROI for Clinical Information Systems Investments in Hypothetical Institution Varies on the Basis of Standard of Evidence and Degree of Optimism of Estimating Assumptions

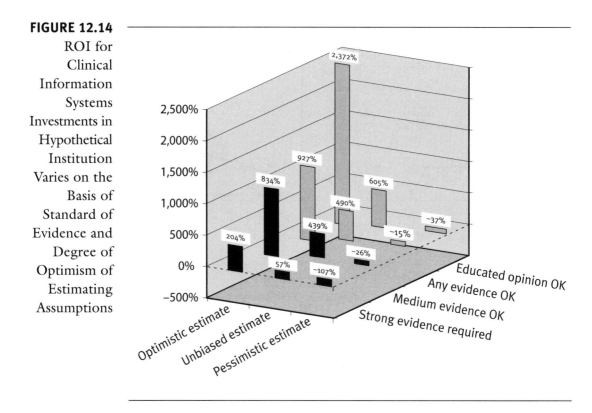

effect of implementation of disease management approaches more broadly across a larger number of clinical conditions. Furthermore, few studies directly assess the contribution of clinical information systems to disease management effectiveness. Such studies would attempt to compare the same disease management approach in settings with and without various supporting information technology capabilities and would track the effect over a long enough period to determine when the manual processes begin to break down as the initial enthusiasm over a new disease management process wanes and staff turn their attention to other priorities. Over longer periods, disease management processes incorporated seamlessly into clinical information systems seem likely to suffer less breakdown. Such comparative studies have not been done, however, so this model rates evidence of disease management effects of clinical information technology investments as supported by educated opinion only. The magnitude of benefits from disease management capabilities also is dependent on the assumed proportion of patients for whom reimbursement is based on capitation or disease-specific sub-capitation arrangements. In settings where reimbursement is predominantly fee for service, disease management interventions, which are usually uncompensated, reduce the need for subsequent care. In such settings, disease management leads to increased cost and decreased revenue.

Figure 12.14 shows that the calculated ROI over a ten-year period ranges from extremely favorable (2,372 percent) to negative (–107%), depending on the range of uncertainty (from pessimistic to optimistic) and the degree of evidence required to count a specific effect. These results underscore the need for more rigorous clinical trials and effectiveness studies of clinical information system components, and of careful collection of institution-specific data to support ROI calculations needed for planning and investment decision making.

Key Strategy Debates

Waiting Versus Tier 1 Versus Tier 2

The biggest strategic debate within healthcare organizations regarding investments in clinical information systems is between those who want to minimize clinical information technology investment, those who want to pursue a tier 1 vision of clinical information technology to improve information access, and those who advocate a tier 2 vision of implementing clinical information technology to transform care management processes.

Those for minimizing clinical information technology investment argue that rigorous studies have not proven such investments to be effective and, more importantly, that the low proportion of healthcare organizations that have implemented clinical information technology on a large scale is evidence that such investments are not yet mainstream. Healthcare leaders are often risk averse and may prefer to wait until most of their peers have pursued a strategy before doing so themselves. Furthermore, declining revenue, poor capital reserves, and a long list of other priorities competing for limited dollars support the argument to wait to invest in large-scale clinical information technology.

The argument for pursuing a tier 1 information access vision is based on a "walk before you run" philosophy and on the realization that the clinical data repository components at the heart of the information access vision are also prerequisites to more ambitious tier 2 care management strategies. The arguments for information access are the easiest to articulate. Information access requires the least amount of potentially controversial clinician process changes and can be implemented by information technology staff members who do not understand the details of clinical processes and the methods of clinical practice improvement. Finally, the community of information technology vendors has developed products with features that focus on the information access vision, so the majority of peer references from institutions that have pursued clinical information technology investments are those focusing on a tier 1 vision.

The argument for pursuing a tier 2 care management vision is that the potential for gaining sustainable competitive advantage for the organization is greatest in this area. Rather than worrying that clinical information technology may *require* clinician process changes, advocates of the care management vision describe a proactive goal of *enabling* clinician process changes. They point out that process improvement is the whole point of information technology deployment in other industries and that evidence-based improvement in clinical processes is consistent with the mission and vision of healthcare institutions and with clinicians' professionalism. Clinical leaders best articulate the vision for clinical information technology investments to support care management because they understand and are able to describe clinical decision-making and care processes and the methods of biomedical research and quality improvement. Proponents of the tier 2 vision are most successful in competitive markets, especially those with active, vocal, organized purchasers and consumers—including business coalitions, local payers, and patient/consumer advocates. In such markets, the need to make changes to create a noticeably different experience for patients and to decrease waste and cost is foremost in leaders' minds, and there is a greater sense of urgency.

Balancing the Needs of Clinicians and the Organization

When making decisions about tier 1 or tier 2 clinical information systems investments, leaders should balance the goals of healthcare organizations making the financial investment and the goals of the individual clinicians making the investment in process change and learning to use the new systems.

As illustrated in Figure 12.15, the organization balances costs and benefits to the organization, whereas the clinician balances the benefit to the user and the burden of use. Organizational costs include not only the cost of software and hardware but also other costs, such as the disruption that implementing new systems and processes causes within facilities. The organizational benefits include better management of utilization, cost, risk, and quality. On the clinician side, user benefits include time savings and improvements in coordination and effectiveness of care. The burden of use includes confusion, tediousness, and decreased productivity during the learning process, as well as a more general concern that the use of systems that structure documentation and integrate practice guidelines and protocols may erode clinicians' sense of autonomy and professionalism. Organizational and clinician decision making are inextricably linked because the potential to make clinicians satisfied or angry is part of the calculus of the organization, and the effect of improved care processes on the organization's financial health and competitive advantage is in clinicians' interest as well.

Investment Pathways in Geographic Regions

Another strategy debate is taking place on a community level within regional areas across the country. This debate involves the organization, funding, and prioritization of investments for clinical information technologies

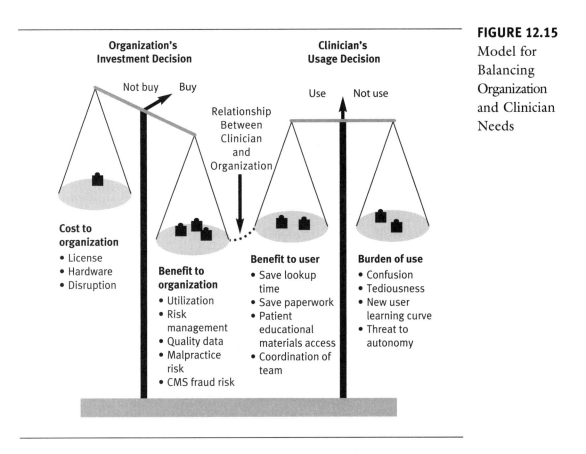

FIGURE 12.15

Model for Balancing Organization and Clinician Needs

intended to serve the needs of multiple constituencies within a geographic area. These initiatives are called *regional health information organizations, health information exchanges, community health information networks,* and *collaborative data warehouses.* As illustrated in Figure 12.16, different parties pursue such community-level initiatives for different reasons and use different data management approaches.

Investment Pathways Within Integrated Settings

Another strategy debate taking place within many healthcare organizations relates to defining the optimal pathway and sequence for making investments in clinical information technology. As illustrated in Figure 12.17, settings that have preexisting "legacy" clinical systems (often mainframe applications used in the inpatient environment) must choose a pathway for migrating from such systems to using a clinical data repository and associated inpatient clinician workstation applications. Because the legacy applications included features beyond clinical processes, investment in a comprehensive integrated suite of applications that cuts across clinical and administrative processes, instead of in separate clinical systems, is key. Within the domain of clinical systems, organizations must decide to pursue a unified

FIGURE 12.16
Community-Level Initiatives to Improve Healthcare Data

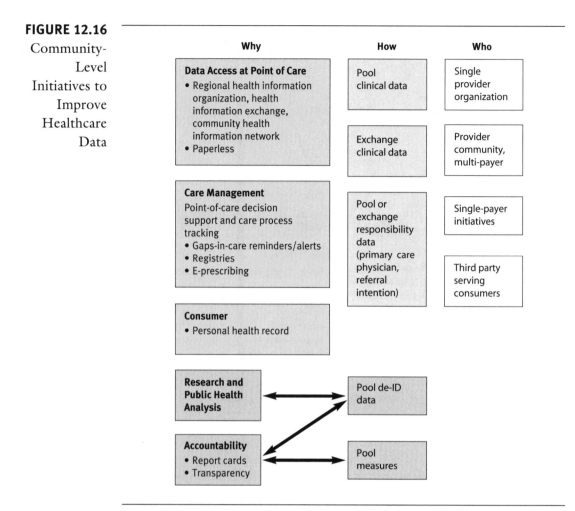

FIGURE 12.17
Debate About Optimal Pathway for Clinical Information Technology Investments

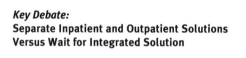

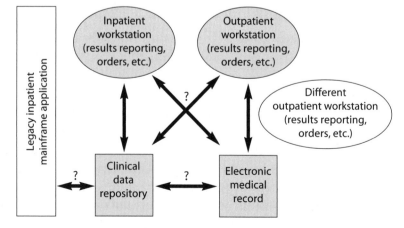

clinical system instead of separate "best of breed" applications for different clinical areas, such as laboratory, radiology, and intensive care.

Settings with both inpatient and outpatient facilities must decide whether to purse an inpatient clinical data repository separate from an ambulatory electronic medical record application or to pursue a single integrated clinical system that cuts across inpatient and outpatient settings. Although major clinical information technology vendors promote their respective systems as fully capable across inpatient and outpatient settings, different products have distinct advantages in one setting over the other, making this strategy decision difficult.

The Role of Departmental Care Management Systems

Another debate going on within many healthcare organizations relates to the role of departmental solutions versus enterprise-level solutions. As illustrated in Figure 12.18, this debate can be characterized as an "ice versus spikes" problem. Information technology leaders with responsibility at the enterprise level, such as a chief information officer, typically place the highest priority on developing applications that offer benefits to the greatest number of users. Because they have limited financial and human resources to dedicate to clinical systems, they focus on deploying simple technologies that apply across the enterprise—analogous to a thin layer of ice across an entire pond. Such simple technologies include laboratory results retrieval, e-mail, clinical dictation, note writing (template charting), and workflow enhancements related to billing and other administrative processes that apply to all settings. Information technology leaders desire to make such investments in the context of a longer-term strategy to offer deeper, richer capabilities, such as specialty-specific results reporting, clinical reminders and alerts, protocol-based care, population and disease registries, and tools that support quality and outcomes measurement and process improvement. In the short term, they focus on the "practical" and "first things first"— and tend to demote deeper functions from the current funding cycle.

In contrast, clinical leaders at the level of specialty departments or centers of excellence such as cancer centers and heart and vascular centers hold a different view. They believe themselves to have a mandate to transform clinical processes to improve care processes dramatically. They recognize that achieving large-scale, durable success in these efforts will require deeper clinical information technology capabilities. They salute the long-term strategies for deploying such capabilities enterprise-wide but express frustration with the slow pace of progress toward these goals. They would characterize the "ice layer" as one that is thickening at a glacial pace, and they do not want to wait that long. Therefore, they pursue deeper "spikes" of function within their own clinical domains, seeking to deploy systems that offer them the ability to transform their own clinical processes. Their

Key Debate:
Ice Versus Spikes: Enterprise Level Versus Departmental Level

clinical leadership position in a clinical domain of manageable size enables such leaders to drive the cultural change and attend to the details of the process changes to achieve success. The ensuing debate about whether such spikes of departmental information technology capabilities are desirable or undesirable can be fierce, however. The enterprise information technology leaders argue that the spikes are really "weeds" demanding support, which distracts them from making more rapid progress on enterprise-level goals. They actively resist proposals for such departmental capabilities. On the other hand, the departmental leaders argue that clinical process transformation is urgent and that the lessons learned in their department will be important and will apply generally across other departments. They argue that the technology investments for such changes are small in comparison to the investment in cultural and process change, and that even if they eventually discard department-specific technology as enterprise capabilities advance, the organization will be better off from having progressed on the cultural and process changes that take time to achieve.

The Challenge

Over the past two decades, the healthcare field has made some progress in establishing a tradition for evidence-based medicine, quality improvement, and care management—and to develop clinical information technologies that support these traditions. A number of important challenges remain, however. Overall healthcare quality is the sum of the quality of thousands of decision-making and care delivery processes. The examples described above compose a tiny slice of overall healthcare quality. Most organizations could not apply the level of resource intensity and leadership attentiveness in these examples simultaneously to more than a few dozen of their processes. Therefore, implementation of practice improvements should be a critical, integral part of all clinicians' overall practice. Only then will these methods scale up to the enormous task of improving thousands of healthcare processes.

Three fundamental changes in the healthcare environment are required to support clinical process improvement on a large scale: (1) incentives, (2) clinical education, and (3) information technology.

Incentives

Healthcare organizations and individual clinicians need increased incentive for improvement. The growing interest in external performance measurement, such as with HEDIS measures, is a step in the right direction. Overall quality improvement, however, requires a market structure in which healthcare organizations face competition based on quality rather than only price competition and in which individual clinicians' compensation is driven by quality measures rather than by work effort only. However, clinician-level quality measurement is a difficult proposition. Patient variation makes clinician-to-clinician comparisons difficult, even for the most common clinical practices. The measurable subset of practices represents a small fraction of all clinical practices. As a result, providing clinicians with incentives to focus on improving measurable processes is similar to encouraging students to "study for the test," calling into question the validity of measure generalization to assess overall practice quality. Furthermore, some warn that the use of quality measurement to drive clinician incentives or as a basis of identifying "bad apples" for remedial attention is counterproductive to the use of measurement for learning and improvement.

Clinician Education

The second fundamental change needed is the education of clinicians in the methods and tools of quality improvement and medical informatics. Changes of greater substance are needed in medical school curricula, residency training, board exams, and the criteria used for medical school admissions.

Information Technology

As described above, the third necessary change is a substantial investment in information technology to support clinical practice. Although healthcare organizations have applied information systems to their administrative processes, the sophistication of systems to support patient care and quality improvement is inadequate. Other industries, such as financial services and manufacturing, invest a substantially larger portion of their budgets to information technology.

FIGURE 12.19

Barriers to
Adoption of
Information
Technology

- Consumer knowledge and culture
  - Consumers think they want choice and low out-of-pocket cost
  - Consumers never experienced truly integrated care
  - Current measures are constrained by widely available data
- Too much government intrusion
  - Concern over fraud and abuse is stronger than desire to transform healthcare system
  - Stark laws inhibit care integration
- Too little government intrusion
  - Token "demonstration"- or "evaluation"-level funding for Agency for Healthcare Research and Quality and other agencies
  - State budgets too tight to permit healthcare information technology investments
- Too little investment by nongovernmental payers
  - Many-to-many relationship between payers and providers adds complexity to value proposition

In the healthcare industry, barriers have inhibited the adoption of clinical information technology. These barriers are summarized in Figure 12.19.

Scalable, durable quality improvements will require systems that offer three important capabilities. First, information systems must permit the acquisition of structured data on patients, healthcare interventions, and outcomes as part of the routine care delivery process. Second, information systems must offer decision aids such as reminders, alerts, and prompts to clinicians at the moment they make a clinical decision. Third, information systems must facilitate the complex logistics of coordination of care, involving many disciplines in many settings, according to protocols and guidelines. The tide is beginning to change in this regard. When the Leapfrog Group promoted computerized physician order entry (CPOE) adoption as a patient safety initiative in 1999, survey data indicated that fewer than 2 percent of hospitals already had installed such a system. More recently, surveys indicate that 25 percent of hospitals have implemented the technology (Robert Wood Johnson Foundation 2006), but less than 10 percent are using a system with comprehensive functionality that includes collection of patient information, display of test results, entry of medical orders and prescriptions, and decision support. Only 5 percent of the United States' 6,000 hospitals have adopted CPOE systems. Nevertheless, industry experts agree that CPOE technology continues to build momentum as it moves from academic medical centers and government facilities to community hospitals, and all major vendors now emphasize CPOE in their marketing strategies (Hobbs, Bauer, and Keillor 2003).

In addition to providing care to individuals and improving evidence-based clinical practice (working to improve the care of populations), clinicians and healthcare leaders have a responsibility to advocate and drive change in their environments to enable large-scale, durable improvement. In a world with incentives, education, and technology to support quality improvement, the public can expect dramatic, measurable improvements in the overall effectiveness of our healthcare system.

Study Questions

1. Describe a framework for care management and clinical practice improvement, and explain why information technologies are needed to support it.
2. What different types of clinical information technology capabilities are needed to support efforts to improve simple versus complex clinical processes?
3. What types of problems do clinical information systems address?
4. What are the essential components of clinical information systems, and what types of benefits are associated with these components?
5. When deciding on clinical information technology investments, what are the arguments for pursuing systems aimed to enhance data access versus systems designed to enable care management?
6. What are the common differences in the priorities and perspectives of enterprise-level information technology leaders versus department-level clinical leaders?
7. What are the barriers to creating a national collaborative data warehouse, and what are the strategies to overcome them?
8. What are the different perspectives regarding the degree of structure in data collected through template charting applications?

References

American Academy of Family Physicians, American Academy of Pediatrics, American College of Physicians, and American Osteopathic Association. 2007. "Joint Principles of the Patient-Centered Medical Home." [Online information; retrieved 4/11/08.] www.medicalhomeinfo.org/Joint%20Statement.pdf.

Baker, A. M., J. E. Lafata, R. E. Ward, F. Whitehouse, and G. Divine. 2001. "A Web-Based Diabetes Care Management Support System." *Joint Commission Journal of Quality Improvement* 27 (4): 179–90.

Birkmeyer, J. D., S. M. Sharp, S. R. Finlayson, E. S. Fisher, and J. E. Wennberg. 1998. "Variation Profiles of Common Surgical Procedures." *Surgery* 124 (5): 917–23.

Boohaker, E. A., R. E. Ward, J. E. Uman, and B. D. McCarthy. 1996. "Patient Notification and Follow-up of Abnormal Test Results, A Physician Survey." *Archives of Internal Medicine* 156: 327–31.

Center for the Evaluative Clinical Sciences and the Dartmouth Medical School. 2006. "Executive Summary: The Care of Patients with Severe Chronic Illness: A Report on the Medicare Program by the Dartmouth Atlas Project." [Online information; retrieved 8/12/08.] www. aspeninstitute.org/site/c.huLWJeMRKpH/b.3920369/k.E7E/Value_a nd_quality_in_care_are_paramount.htm.

Hobbs, G., J. Bauer, and A. Keillor. 2003. "New Perspectives on the Quality of Care: Reducing Medical Errors Through Cultural Change and Clinical Transformation." *Medscape Money & Medicine* 4 (2).

Hollingsworth, D. 1995. *Workflow Management Coalition: The Workflow Reference Model.* Hampshire, UK: Workflow Management Coalition.

Institute of Medicine. 2003. National Academy of Sciences press release, July 31.

Lazarou, J., B. H. Pomeranz, and P. N. Corey. 1998. "Incidence of Adverse Drug Reactions in Hospitalized Patients: A Meta-Analysis of Prospective Studies." *Journal of the American Medical Association* 279 (15): 1200–05.

McCarthy, B. D., R. E. Ward, Y. M. Ulcickas, M. Rebner, E. A. Boohaker, and C. Johnson. 1996. "Inadequate Follow-up of Abnormal Mammograms." *American Journal of Preventive Medicine* 12 (4): 282–88.

Nohria, A., Y. T. Chen, D. J. Morton, R. Walsh, P. H. Vlasses, and H. M. Krumholz. 1999. "Quality of Care for Patients Hospitalized with Heart Failure at Academic Medical Centers." *American Heart Journal* 137 (6): 1028–34.

Robert Wood Johnson Foundation. 2006. *Health Information Technology in the United States: The Information Base for Progress.* Princeton, NJ: Robert Wood Johnson Foundation.

Shortliffe, E. H., and L. E. Perreault (eds.). 1990. *Medical Informatics: Computer Applications in Health Care.* Reading, MA: Addison-Wesley.

U.S. Department of Health and Human Services and Centers for Medicare & Medicaid Services. 2007. "National Health Expenditure Projections 2006–2016." January. [Online information; retrieved 4/11/08.] www.cms.hhs.gov/NationalHealthExpendData/03_NationalHealthAcco untsProjected.asp.

Wagner, E. H. 1998. "Chronic Disease Management: What Will It Take to Improve Care for Chronic Illness?" *Effective Clinical Practice* 1 (1): 2–4.

LEADERSHIP FOR QUALITY

James L. Reinertsen

Leadership is essential to quality improvement, whether at the level of a small team of clinicians working to improve care for a particular condition or at the level of an entire organization aiming to improve performance on system-level measures such as mortality rates or costs per capita.

Background

A useful general definition of *leadership* is "working with people and systems to produce needed change" (Wessner 1998). Every system is perfectly designed to produce the results it gets, so if better results are to be expected, systems (and the people in them) must change. Studies of leaders and leadership have produced many theories and models of what is required to "work with people and systems to produce needed change" (Bass 1990). This complex mix of theories can be considered at two levels: individual leadership and organizational leadership systems.

Individual Leadership

This set of leadership ideas is about what people must *be*, and what they must know how to *do*, if they are to influence others to bring about needed changes. Examples of these two aspects of individual leadership are described in Table 13.1. Having strong personal leadership attributes without knowing how to use them is not enough. Similarly, knowing the leadership toolbox without authentically embodying the characteristics required of leaders is insufficient for successful leadership. Both being and doing are needed, especially when the changes required for quality improvement involve reframing core values (e.g., individual physician autonomy) or remaking professional teams (e.g., the power relationships between doctors and nurses). Many improvements in healthcare will require these kinds of deep changes in values. These changes sometimes are labeled *transformational changes* to distinguish them from *transactional changes*, which do not require changes in values and patterns of behavior.

TABLE 13.1

Individual Leadership: Being and Doing

What Leaders Must Be (Examples)	What Leaders Must Know How to Do (Examples)
• Authentic embodiment of core values • Trustworthy: consistent in thought, word, and deed • In love with the work, rather than the position, of leadership • Someone who adds energy to a team, rather than sucks it out • Humble, but not insecure; able to say, "I was wrong" • Focused on results, rather than popularity • Capable of building relationships • Passionately committed to the mission	• Understand the system context in which improvement work is being done • Explain how the work of the team fits into the aims of the whole system • Use and teach improvement methods • Develop new leaders • Explain and challenge the current reality • Inspire a shared vision • Enable others to act • Model the way • Encourage the heart (Kouzes and Posner 1987) • Manage complex projects

Organizational Leadership Systems

The ideas and theories at this second level of leadership are not about individual leaders and what they must be and do but rather about creating a supportive organizational environment in which hundreds of capable individual leaders' work can thrive. This environment is at the system-of-leadership level. One way to view this level is as a complex set of interrelated activities in five broad categories.

- *Set direction.* Every healthy organization has a sense of direction, a future self-image. A leader's job is to set that direction. The task can be thought of as something like the creation of magnetic lines of force running through the organization that pull people toward a future they find attractive and push them out of a status quo they find uncomfortable.
- *Establish the foundation.* Leaders must prepare themselves and their leadership teams with the knowledge and skills necessary to improve systems and lead change. They must choose and develop future leaders wisely and build a broad base of capable improvers throughout the organization. Often they must take the organization through a painful process of reframing values before they can set forth toward a better future.
- *Build will.* The status quo is usually comfortable. To initiate and sustain change takes will, especially in healthcare organizations, which seem to be highly sensitive to discord and often grind to a halt because of one loud voice opposing change. One way to build will for quality improvement is by making logical and quantitative links, including financial links, between

improvement and key business goals. Will also can be greatly enhanced when boards of directors pay attention to quality and hold senior leadership accountable for performance improvement.

- *Generate ideas.* Many healthcare quality challenges require innovation if they are to be successfully met. Excellent organizations have well-developed systems for finding and rapidly testing ideas from the best performers, other industries, and other cultures and nations. They also find and use the thousands of ideas latent within the organization itself. Encouraging and developing ideas are key aspects of the leadership system. Ideas are particularly important for achieving depth of change.
- *Execute change.* The best improvement ideas will fail to have much effect if they cannot be implemented across the organization. Good leadership systems adopt, teach, and use a good change leadership model and consistently execute both small- and large-scale changes. System-level measurement of performance is an important element in executing change, as is the assignment of responsibility for change to line managers rather than quality staff. This organizational system is particularly important for achieving breadth of change.

Figure 13.1 provides a visual representation of the leadership system with additional examples.

The model outlined above is one general version of a leadership system for quality transformation. A number of excellent organizations have established leadership systems that fit their own business contexts and missions (Tichy 2002). Any individual leader's work is set into the context of the leadership system of a specific organization. Some aspects of that leadership system (e.g., compensation, performance measurement) may support the leader's improvement work, and other aspects (e.g., human resource policies, budgeting processes, or information systems) may be barriers to that work. Leaders will not achieve large-scale performance changes simply by improving their own leadership skills; they also need to work on improving the system of leadership in their organizations. Deming (1986) referred to this approach when he stated that "Workers work in the system. Leaders work on the system."

Important Leadership Concepts and Definitions

The following terms are helpful to understand when considering how to improve leadership.

- *Leadership*: working with people and systems to produce needed change.
- *Management*: working with people and systems to produce predictable results. (Note that management is not inferior to leadership; both are important for quality. Leadership, however, is somewhat more hazardous than management because it involves influencing people to change.)

FIGURE 13.1

Leadership System for Transformation

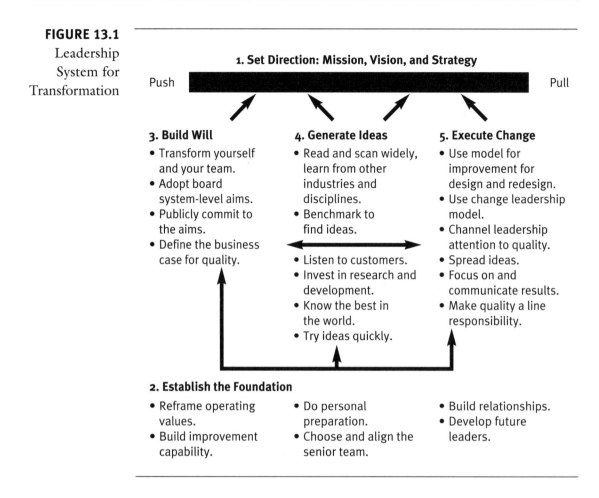

1. Set Direction: Mission, Vision, and Strategy

Push   Pull

3. Build Will
- Transform yourself and your team.
- Adopt board system-level aims.
- Publicly commit to the aims.
- Define the business case for quality.

4. Generate Ideas
- Read and scan widely, learn from other industries and disciplines.
- Benchmark to find ideas.
- Listen to customers.
- Invest in research and development.
- Know the best in the world.
- Try ideas quickly.

5. Execute Change
- Use model for improvement for design and redesign.
- Use change leadership model.
- Channel leadership attention to quality.
- Spread ideas.
- Focus on and communicate results.
- Make quality a line responsibility.

2. Establish the Foundation
- Reframe operating values.
- Build improvement capability.
- Do personal preparation.
- Choose and align the senior team.
- Build relationships.
- Develop future leaders.

- *Governance*: the process through which the representatives of the owners of an organization oversee the mission, strategy, executive leadership, quality performance, and financial stewardship of the institution. The owner's representatives usually are structured into a board of directors or board of trustees. (In the case of not-for-profit institutions, the owner is the community, usually through a state-chartered process monitored by the state's attorney general.)
- *Technical leadership challenges*: change situations in which there is a high degree of agreement about the nature of goals as well as a high level of certainty about how to achieve the goals (i.e., the problem has been faced before, and a method of solving it is known).
- *Adaptive leadership challenges*: change situations that require new learning, resolution of value conflicts, and resolution of deep differences in goals and methods of achieving the goals (very common in healthcare quality improvement work).
- *Boundaries of the system*: leaders must choose the boundaries of the system they wish to improve (e.g., for physicians, is the target system their individual practices, the group of physicians in which they work, the

entire medical staff of the hospital, the entire community of physicians, or the entire profession?). As Deming (1995) said, "The larger the boundary chosen, the greater the potential impact, and the greater the difficulty of achieving success."

- *Change leadership*: a framework or method for planning and executing major change (Kotter 1996).
- *Leadership development*: the processes by which an organization identifies, improves, evaluates, rewards, holds accountable, and promotes leaders.
- *Transformation*: change that involves fundamental reframing of values, beliefs, and habits of behavior, along with radical redesign of care processes and systems, to achieve dramatic levels of improvement.
- *Vision*: a statement describing a future picture of the institution or care delivery system. Good visions are usually specific enough that individual staff members easily can see themselves, and what their workday would be like, in that future picture. A quality vision for a hospital, framed in terms of the Institute of Medicine (IOM) quality dimensions, could be: "A place with no needless deaths, no needless pain, no needless helplessness, no needless delays, and no waste, for everyone we serve."
- *Mission*: a statement of the purpose of the institution; the reason it exists. This statement usually rests on the core needs of the institution's customers and on the core values of its people. In the case of hospitals, for example, a general statement of mission could be: "To cure when cure is possible; to heal, even when cure is not possible; and to do no harm in the process."
- *Strategic plan*: the organization's hypotheses about the causative relationship between a set of actions (e.g., capital investments, new structures, process redesigns, new staff capabilities) and achievement of system-level, mission-driven aims (e.g., reduced costs of care, improved levels of safety, lower mortality rates).
- *Budget*: the operational and financial expression of the strategic plan, usually for a defined period such as the next fiscal year.

Scope and Use of Leadership Concepts in Healthcare

The introduction makes obvious that effective leadership—at both the individual and system of leadership levels—is essential to quality improvement. If improvement did not require people and processes to change, leadership would not be needed. However, change—often deep, transformative change—is a part of virtually every quality improvement activity, whether at the level of a small project within an office or department or a massive improvement effort involving entire communities. Leadership is therefore necessary.

We are tempted to think of leadership as the responsibility of those at or near the top of organizations, departments, and other structures. This hierarchical view of leadership is natural and, to a certain extent, useful. The CEO does have a larger system view and can accomplish some improvements that an individual nurse, administrator, or physician cannot. The CEO's leadership opportunities to influence the system are greater, and so are his or her responsibilities for system-level results.

To think that the term *leadership* applies only to those in formally designated senior positions of authority, however, is incorrect and often harmful. Healthcare organizations are large, complex systems and cannot be led effectively by a few senior executives. These senior leaders do not have a deep understanding of the quality issues that frontline staff faces every day. Facing, understanding, and improving performance at the critical interface between clinicians and patients is work that must be done by hundreds of capable individual leaders throughout the organization, supported by a well-aligned leadership system.

Finally, there is no simple formula for successful healthcare leadership or for specific strategies that, if carried out, will result in organizational quality transformation. Care delivery systems are "complex adaptive systems" (Zimmerman, Lindberg, and Plsek 1998) and therefore behave unpredictably, in large part because of the powerful influence of the professional, community, and macrosystem (regulation, policy, markets) context of each organization and care system.

For this reason, leaders within organizations would be presumptuous to believe that by working within their organizations alone, they can transform those organizations to a dramatically higher level of quality performance. The example vision given earlier ("a place with no needless deaths . . .") describes an organization so different from the ones in which we now work that realization of the vision requires a fundamental state change, like going from water to steam. This sort of state change in healthcare will not be evolutionary, but revolutionary. To put it into *Crossing the Quality Chasm* terms (Corrigan, Donaldson, and Kohn 2001), the gap between our current organizations and this vision is a chasm that cannot be crossed in two steps.

All of these ideas—state change, revolution, crossing a chasm—suggest that when healthcare transformation does occur, it will be an emergent event—a surprise, something that comes about in this complex adaptive system not as a result of a detailed leadership plan but because of the convergence of multiple factors, some planned, others completely unplanned. The roads that lead to that convergence could come from multiple directions. Leaders of hospitals and healthcare delivery systems can build and travel these roads, but these leaders alone can neither design nor build other roads that might be required. The most robust plan to achieve transformation requires healthcare leaders to work on a plan to achieve things within their control and simultaneously influence as much of their context as possible, even though that context is out of their direct control. Healthcare organizational leaders should be aware of at least four routes to the transformational "surprise," only one of which (route 3) is more or less within their direct control.

Route 1: Revolution (Leadership from Below)

One critical factor in the transformation of organizations is a dramatic change in the culture of the professional workforce. The central themes of that cultural change are:

* from individual physician autonomy to shared decision making;
* from professional hierarchies to teamwork; and
* from professional disengagement in system aims to "system citizenship."

Why label this route to transformation *revolution*? If these changes were to occur in the health professions, particularly in medicine and nursing, and the organizations in which those nurses and doctors worked did not change responsively, the tensions between the workforce and its organizations eventually would kindle a "peasants at the gates with torches" sort of revolution, with healthcare professionals demanding dramatic change from the leaders of healthcare organizations. For example, imagine 15 years of profound cultural changes taking place in newly trained physicians because of the new American Council on Graduate Medical Education requirements (Leach 1999), without a corresponding change in the way hospitals and group practices function. The new generation of physicians likely would revolt against the old systems and constitute a powerful force for dramatic change in all types of healthcare delivery.

Route 1 is particularly important for two of the three principal strategies of the *Crossing the Quality Chasm* report: use all the science we know, and cooperate as a system. Health leaders cannot simply wait for this cultural change to move through medicine but should be aware of it and take steps both within and outside their organizational boundaries to support and accelerate that cultural change. When possible, hospital and physician leaders should harness the energy from this slow shift in the culture of medicine and use it to drive needed changes inside their organizations. Route 1 is clearly one of the main highways to the emergent surprise called *transformation*.

Route 2: Friendly Takeover (Leadership from Outside)

The example mission statement given earlier depicts another sort of cultural change, the impetus for which could come from outside the healthcare organizational culture: a profound shift in power from the professional and organization to the patient and family. In many ways, healthcare is already well down route 2. For example, patients and families have broken into the medical "holy of holies," the special knowledge that has defined physicians' source of professional power. They watch open-heart surgery on television and bring printouts of the latest scientific articles to office visits. Patients now can see various reports on the performance of nursing homes, hospitals, and physicians and soon will see many more such reports. The power of information is already in the hands of the public.

This shift in power is positive and needs to drive a broad range of changes, from how the aims of care plans are defined to radical redesign of how care is delivered, paid for, measured, and reported. Ultimately, this power shift to patients and families will give them as much control of their care as they wish to have. They will lead the design of their own care and make important decisions about resources. We must go down route 2 to implement the patient-centeredness strategy of the *Crossing the Quality Chasm* report.

As for route 1, healthcare leaders cannot make travel down route 2 happen by themselves, but they can be aware of its importance, its necessity in the transformation of their own organizations, and its power to help leaders drive needed change. A lot of patients are driving down route 2 right now, and the job of healthcare leaders is to find them and use their energy and leadership to invite a friendly takeover of their hospitals and clinics.

Route 3: Intentional Organizational Transformation (Leadership from Above)

This route to transformation should be the one most familiar to CEOs and other senior executives. This set of leadership strategies, implemented with constancy of purpose over some years, would be likely to drive organizational transformation. To reiterate, because transformation is an emergent property of a complex adaptive system, leaders should not assume that a well-built, well-traveled route 3 will get them to the vision without some convergence from the other routes, which are not entirely within the control of leadership.

Why *leadership from above*? Route 3 contrasts with route 1 in that route 1 sees the principal drive for change coming from those working at the front lines, whereas route 3 envisions the push coming from visionary leaders who want to place their organizational change agendas at the leading, rather than trailing, edge of transformation. From a traditional hierarchical organization perspective, these leaders are from above.

Route 4: Intentional Macrosystem Transformation (Leadership from High Above)

The fourth route does not begin with diffused, perhaps even unorganized, cultural changes in professions and patients as in routes 1 and 2, nor does it arise from within healthcare delivery organizations as an intentional act of leadership. Route 4 is a way to transformation that arises out of intentional acts of policymakers, regulators, and others in positions of authority outside the healthcare delivery system. Many of the characteristics of the example mission would be accelerated by, and perhaps even dependent on, such macrosystem changes.

For example, organizations do not naturally disclose data publicly on their performance, especially when the performance is suboptimal. Without public policy that requires disclosure, widespread transparency would not be the norm in healthcare, aside from a few brave pioneers. In general, measurement, payment, and accountability regulations that would encourage and reward those who demonstrate evidence-based practices, patient centeredness, and cooperation would be powerful drivers of deep organizational change. Healthcare delivery system leaders cannot design or travel this policy/regulation highway (route 4) directly, but they could influence it and harness its power to accelerate the changes they want to realize in their organizations. The role of delivery system leaders in route 4 is analogous to the military situation of "calling in fire on your own position." If such regulatory fire could be guided sensibly by what healthcare executives are learning and trying to accomplish, it might be exceptionally powerful in getting their organizations through some difficult spots on their own routes to transformation.

These routes make up the large arena for the application of leadership principles in healthcare: at the individual and system-of-leadership levels within care delivery organizations, and in the professions, communities, and macrosystems that make up the broad context for our work. The best leaders will be able to work effectively across this arena.

Clinical and Operational Issues

Within healthcare delivery systems, some unusual quality improvement leadership challenges present themselves. These challenges are briefly described below.

Professional Silos, Power Gradients, and Teamwork

Physicians, nurses, pharmacists, and other clinicians go through separate and distinct training processes. This separation often persists in the way work is organized, information is exchanged, and improvement work is done. This *professional silo* problem is compounded by a power gradient issue, namely that all other professionals' actions are ultimately derivative of physicians' orders. The net effect is to diminish teamwork and reduce free flow of information, both of which are vital for safety and quality. Quality improvement leaders must be capable of establishing effective multidisciplinary teams despite these long-standing challenges.

Physician Autonomy

Physicians are taught to take personal responsibility for quality and have a highly developed attachment to individual professional autonomy. This cultural attribute has an enormous negative effect on the speed and reliability with which physicians adopt and implement evidence-based practices. As a general rule, physicians discuss evidence in groups but implement it as individuals. The resulting variation causes great complexity in the work of nurses, pharmacists, and others in the system, and it is a major source of errors and harm. Quality improvement leaders will need to reframe this professional value. Perhaps the best way to frame it is: "Practice the science of medicine as teams, and the art of medicine as individuals" (Reinertsen 2003).

Leaders and Role Conflict in Organizations

The clinicians who work in healthcare organizations tend to see the organization as a platform for their individual work and seldom feel a corresponding sense of responsibility for the performance of the organization as a whole. As a result, they expect their leaders (e.g., department chairs, VPs of nursing) to protect them from the predations of the organization rather than help them contribute to the accomplishment of the organization's goals. This expectation puts many middle-management leaders in an awkward quandary. Are they to represent the interests of their departments or units to the organization, or are they to represent the interests of the organization to their departments? The answer to both questions—yes—is not comforting. Both roles are necessary, and leaders must be able to play both roles and maintain the respect and trust of their followers. This sense of role conflict is especially acute among, but not unique to, physician leaders (Reinertsen 1998).

Keys to Successful Quality Leadership and Lessons Learned

Transform Yourself

A leader cannot lead others through the quality transformation unless he or she is transformed and has made an authentic, public, and permanent commitment to achieving the aims of improvement. Transformation is not an accident. You can design experiences that will both transform and sustain the transformed state. Examples include the following actions.

- Personally interview a patient who has experienced serious harm in your institution, along with the patient's family members, and listen carefully to the impact of this event on that patient's life.
- Personally interview staff at the sharp end of an error that caused serious harm.

- Listen to a patient *every day*.
- Read and reread both IOM reports: *To Err Is Human* (Kohn, Corrigan, and Donaldson 2000) and *Crossing the Quality Chasm* (Corrigan, Donaldson, and Kohn 2001).
- Learn and use quality improvement methods.
- View and discuss the video *First, Do No Harm*[1] with your team.
- Perform regular safety rounds with your care team.

Adopt and Use a Leadership Model

Literature is replete with useful models and frameworks for leadership. Heifetz's model (1994) is particularly valuable when you are facing adaptive leadership challenges, which tend to be marked by conflict, tension, and emotion and by the absence of clear agreement about goals and methods. Many other models are available; as leaders learn them, they often reframe the models into ones that work well for their specific situations (Joiner 1994; Kouzes and Posner 1987; Northouse 2001).

Grow and Develop Your Leadership Skills

Good leaders in healthcare engage in three activities that help them continually grow and develop as leaders.

1. *Learn new ideas and information*. Read about, talk to, and observe leaders. Take courses (including courses outside the healthcare context) and find other means of importing information.
2. *Try out the ideas*. Growing leaders take what they learn and use it in the laboratory of their practices, departments, and institutions. They use the results to decide which ideas to keep and which to discard.
3. *Reflect*. Truly great leaders tend to have maintained a lifelong habit of regular reflection on their leadership work. The method of reflection (e.g., private journaling, private meditation, written reports to peers, dialog with mentors and coaches) is not as important as the regularity, purpose, and seriousness of the reflection.

Avoid the Seven Deadly Sins of Leadership

The following list details behaviors and habits that are not predictive of success as a leader.

1. *Indulging in victimhood*. Leaders initiate, act, take responsibility, and approach problems with a positive attitude. They do not lapse into victimhood, a set of behaviors typified by "if only" whining about what could be accomplished if someone else would improve the information technology system, produce a new boss, or remove querulous members

of the team. Leaders do not say "tell me what to do, and I'll do it." They do not join in and encourage organization bashing. To paraphrase Gertrude Stein, when one arrives at leadership, there is no "them" there. Leaders face the realities before them and make the best of their situation.

2. *Mismatching words and deeds.* The fastest way to lose followers is for leaders to talk about goals such as quality and safety and then falter when the time comes to put resources behind the rhetoric. Followers watch where their leaders deploy their time, attention, and financial resources and are quick to pick up mismatch between words and these indicators of the real priorities in the organization.

3. *Loving the job more than the work.* As leaders rise in organizations, some become enamored of the trappings of leadership rather than of the work of improving and delivering high-quality health services. They divert their attention to signs of power and status such as office size, reserved parking, salaries, and titles, away from the needs of their customers and staff members. This path does not lead to long-term leadership success. Leaders should be focused on doing their current job, not on getting the next job.

4. *Confusing leadership with popularity.* Leadership is about accountability for results. Leaders often must take unpopular actions and courageously stand up against fairly loud opposition to bring about positive change. In a leadership role, being respected is better than being liked.

5. *Choosing harmony rather than conflict.* In addition to popularity, leaders also are tempted to seek peace. Anger and tension, however, are often the markers of the key value conflicts through which leaders must help followers learn their way. By avoiding the pain of meetings and interactions laden with conflict or soothing it with artificial nostrums, leaders can miss the opportunity for real creativity and renewal that lies beneath many conflicts.

6. *Inconstancy of purpose.* Nothing irritates a team more than when its leader flits from one hot idea to the next without apparent long-term constancy of aim and method. An important variant of such inconstancy is when the leader's priorities and actions bounce around like the ball in a pinball arcade game because the leader is always responding to the last loud voice he or she has heard.

7. *Unwillingness to say "I don't know" or "I made a mistake."* The best leaders are always learning, and they cannot learn without recognizing what they do not know or admitting mistakes. Good leaders are secure enough to admit that they do not have the answer and are willing to bring the questions to their teams.

Case Study of Leadership: Interview with William Rupp, MD[2]

Luther Midelfort-Mayo Health System (LM), in Eau Claire, Wisconsin, although small, has gained a reputation as a successful innovator and implementer of quality and safety ideas. This fully integrated healthcare system includes a 190-physician multi-specialty group practice, three hospitals, two nursing homes, a retail pharmacy system, ambulance services, a home care agency, and a partnership with a regional health plan. In a unified organizational structure with a single CEO and a single financial statement, LM provides 95 percent of all the healthcare services needed for the majority of the patients it serves.

The record of LM's quality accomplishments over the past decade is broad and deep and includes significant advances in medication safety, access to care, flow of care, nurse morale, and nurses' perception of quality. LM has been a highly visible participant in many of the Institute for Healthcare Improvement's (IHI) Breakthrough Series[3] and is now deeply involved in implementation of Six Sigma process management[4] (Nauman and Hoisington 2000) as well as the development of a culture to support quality and safety. William Rupp, MD, a practicing medical oncologist, became chairman of the LM board in 1992 and CEO of LM in 1994. He led the organization's drive to innovate in quality and safety. Dr. Rupp stepped down as CEO in December 2001. In the following interview, conducted in February 2002, he discusses the leadership challenges and lessons he learned during his tenure.

JR: Under your leadership, LM has become known as a quality leader among organizations. Are you really that good?

WR: LM is making progress in quality, although we're clearly not as good as we'd like to be. What we *are* really good at is taking ideas from others and trying them out, quickly. For example, we heard about a red/green/yellow light system for managing hospital flow and nurse staffing at a meeting I attended. We tried it out within two weeks and refined it within three months. We believed that this traffic light system was a tool for managing the flow of patients through the hospital and for directing resources to parts of the hospital that needed them. But when we tried it out, the traffic light system turned out to have little to do with managing our flow. Rather, for us, it has been an extraordinary system for empowering nurses, communicating across nursing units, improving nurse morale, and avoiding unsafe staffing situations [Rozich and Resar 2002]. Our nurse vacancy rate is now *very* low. It was a great idea, but not for the purpose we originally thought.[5]

JR: How did you get interested in safety?

WR: At an IHI meeting in 1998, our leadership team heard Don Berwick talk about medication errors. We had 20 LM people at the meeting, and our reaction was, "We can't be that bad, can we?" When we came home, we interviewed some frontline nurses and pharmacists about recent errors or near misses and were amazed at the sheer number of stories we heard. So we reviewed 20 charts a week on one unit for six weeks and found that the nurses and pharmacists were right—we were having the same number of errors as everyone else. We also identified the major cause of most of the errors in our system: poor communication between the outpatient and inpatient medication record systems.

We then took our findings from the interviews and the chart reviews and went over them with the physician and administrative leadership. The universal reaction was surprise and shock, but the data were very convincing, and everyone soon agreed we needed to do something about the problem. We put a simple paper-and-pencil reconciliation system in place for in/outpatient medications, and adverse drug events decreased fivefold.[6]

JR: What was your role as CEO in driving these sorts of specific improvements?

WR: I couldn't be personally responsible for guiding and directing specific projects like the traffic light system, medication safety, and implementation of evidence-based care systems for specific diseases. But I could make sure the teams working on these problems knew that I was interested in them, and that I wanted results. I met monthly individually with the project leaders, even if only for 15 minutes, to hear about progress. And I also made sure that my executive assistant scheduled me to "drop in" for a few minutes on the meeting of each team at least once a month so that all the members of the team knew that the organization was paying attention to their work. I know this sort of attention must be important because when specific projects didn't go well (and we had a few), they were projects to which I didn't pay this sort of attention.[7]

JR: Trying out new ideas and changes all the time must cause a lot of tension for your staff. How did you handle this?

WR: You're right—innovation and change are sources of tension. I found it exceptionally useful to have a small number of people working directly for me whose only role was to be a change agent. Roger Resar, MD, is a great example. His job was to find and try out new ideas, and when he did, I inevitably got calls from doctors, nurses, and administrators saying, "We can't get our work done with all these new ideas coming at us. Get Dr. Resar off our backs." At that point, my job was to support Roger, especially if the resistance was based simply on unwillingness to change. But I also listened carefully to the content and tone of the resistance. If I thought there really was a safety risk in trying out the idea, or if there was genuine meltdown under way, I would ask him to back down, or we might decide to try the idea on a much smaller scale.

For example, when we first tried open-access scheduling in one of our satellite offices, we didn't understand the principles well enough and the office exploded in an uproar. Rather than pushing ahead, I went to the office and said, "We really didn't do this very well. We should stop this trial. I still think open access is a good idea, but we just haven't figured out how to implement it yet." After we learned more about implementation, we tried it out elsewhere and are now successfully putting open access in place across virtually the entire system (except for the office in which the uproar occurred). I shudder to think what would have happened if we had bulled ahead.

So, I'd say my change leadership role was to push for needed change, support the change agents, listen carefully to the pain they caused, and respond.

JR: That must be a hard judgment to make—when to back down on change and when to push ahead.

WR: The right answer isn't always obvious. In some cases the decision is easy, especially when the resistance conflicts directly with a broadly supported organizational value or is in opposition to a strategic approach that the organization has adopted after a lot of debate. For example, we are now well along in our adoption and implementation of Six Sigma process management. If an administrative vice president, or a prominent physician, or a key nurse manager were to come to me and say, "This process management stuff is baloney, I'm not going to do it," my response would be to say, "Well, process management is a major strategy of this organization, and if you can't help to lead it, then you'll have to leave."

JR: How do you deal with resistance to important initiatives, such as clinical practice guidelines, if the resistance is coming from doctors?

WR: We are fundamentally a group practice. Once we have made a group decision about a care process and have designed a system for implementing that process (e.g., our insulin sliding-scale protocol or our choice of a single hip or knee prosthesis), we expect our physicians to use the protocol. We monitor protocol usage and always ask those who aren't using the protocol to tell us what's wrong with the protocol. Sometimes they point out problems with the design. But most of the time, they simply change their behavior to match the protocol. One way or another, we don't back down on our commitment to evidence-based practice of medicine.

JR: During your tenure, did you ever have to face a financial crisis? Were you ever pressured to cut back on your investment in quality and safety?

WR: In 1998/99, we sustained financial losses for the first time in our history, due to the effects of the Balanced Budget Act. I received a lot of pressure from parts of the organization to reduce our investment in innovation and quality. They said, "Cut travel costs. Don't send the usual 20 people to the IHI National Forum." And the physicians said, "Put those physician change agents back into practice, where they can do real work and generate professional billings." I resisted both pressures. I felt that during rough times we needed more ideas, not fewer. So we sent 30 people to the IHI Forum. And we showed the doctors that for every dollar invested in change agents' salaries, we had generated ten dollars in return. The financial results have been good. Last year, we had a positive margin—3.5 percent.[8]

JR: I've heard of your work on culture change and "simple rules." What is all this about?

WR: In 1997, we realized that the rate of change in LM was not what it needed to be and that the biggest drag on our rate of improvement was our culture. We went through an organization-wide exercise in which we discussed our cultural "simple rules" with people from all levels of our organization. A leader cannot significantly change a culture until he or she can describe it and outline it on paper and the staff agrees with the description of the current culture. Only then can you begin to describe what you want a new culture to look and feel like, what you want it to accomplish for patients.

JR: What rules did you find were in place in your culture?

WR: We think the main characteristics of our old culture were embedded in six rules.

1. Success is defined by quality.
2. Physicians give permission for leaders to lead (and they can withdraw it).
3. Physician leadership means "I'm in charge."
4. Results are achieved by working hard.
5. Compliance requires consensus.
6. Conflict is resolved by compromise.

We will keep the first rule, but the others are up for redefinition. We will not get to our long-term goals if these rules define our culture. How can we reach for exceptional levels of quality if we resolve all conflicts by compromise? How can we design and implement systems of quality and safety as our primary strategy if deep in our hearts we still believe that individual effort is what drives quality?

JR: How would you sum up the main lessons you have learned about the CEO's role in leadership for quality and safety?

WR: I don't think there's a prescription that works for every CEO, in every situation. This is what I have learned from my work at LM:

1. The CEO must always be strategically searching for the next good idea. On my own, I come up with maybe one good idea every two or three years. But I can recognize someone else's good idea in a flash, and my

organization can get that idea implemented.

2. The CEO must push the quality agenda. He or she must be seen to be in charge of it and must make it happen. There are many forces lined up to preserve the status quo, and if the CEO doesn't visibly lead quality, the necessary changes won't happen.

3. The CEO doesn't make change happen single-handedly. The leader does so through key change agents, and his or her job is to protect and support those change agents while listening carefully to the pain they cause.

4. This whole experience has profoundly reinforced for me the concept of a system of quality. The professional culture that focuses responsibility for quality and safety solely on individuals is dead wrong. The vast majority of our staff is doing the best they can. Asking them to "think harder next time," or telling them, "Don't ever do that again," will not work.

Conclusion

Leaders play a critical role in improvement. They create an organizational climate in which improvement teams can be effective. Leaders are responsible for the overall structures, systems, and culture in which improvement teams function. Good leaders create environments in which quality can thrive.

However, leaders do not make healthcare improvements alone. The "atomic units" of improvement are projects at the frontline or microsystem level that are carried out by nurses, doctors, and managers who know how to run rapid tests of change, measure results, respond, and then start the cycle again.

Study Questions

1. What aspects of individual leadership (being and doing) does William Rupp demonstrate?

2. Examine Figure 13.1 and describe the elements of this organizational leadership model evident in the LM organization.

Notes

1. For more information, see the Partnership for Patient Safety's website at www.p4ps.org.

2. William Rupp, MD (former CEO, Luther Midelfort-Mayo Health System), in discussion with the author, March 2004.

3. See IHI's website at www.ihi.org.

4. Six Sigma refers to an approach to performance improvement in which

the organization's strategic goals are traced directly to certain key processes; those key processes are then managed toward a high standard of quality—3.4 defects per million opportunities, or "six sigma." For example, most hospitals' medication systems currently produce three or four medication errors per 1,000 doses, or three sigma. *Sigma* is a statistical term used to describe the amount of deviation from the norm, or average, in a population—the more sigmas, the greater the deviation (Kouzes and Posner 1987).

5. One of the most important tasks of leaders is to be on the lookout for good ideas. Leaders have more than an academic interest in ideas, however; they know that simply accumulating interesting ideas from other organizations, industries, and innovators is not sufficient. Good leaders apply ideas to their work environment and establish ways to test many ideas on a small scale, discarding those that fail.

6. Another task of leaders is to marshal the will to take action. Data about the problem, collected in a credible fashion, can create discomfort with the status quo, often a vital factor in developing organizational will.

7. The "currency" of leadership is attention. Choosing how and where to channel attention is one of the most important tasks of leadership.

8. Healthcare leaders often state that the business case for quality is weak, in that investments in quality and safety do not produce the same kinds of business returns as investments in expensive technologies and procedures. In the case of safety, however, the professional case overwhelms concerns about the business issues; courageous healthcare leaders understand this case. When Paul O'Neill was CEO of Alcoa, he refused to allow anyone to calculate Alcoa's business returns from workplace safety improvements. He treated worker safety as a fundamental right of employment. If "first, do no harm" is a fundamental value of our profession, can healthcare leaders play dollars against patient harm?

References

Bass, B. M. 1990. *Bass and Stogdill's Handbook of Leadership.* New York: Free Press.

Corrigan, J. M., M. S. Donaldson, and L. T. Kohn (eds.). 2001. *Crossing the Quality Chasm: A New Health System for the 21st Century.* Washington, DC: National Academies Press.

Deming, W. E. 1986. *Out of the Crisis.* Cambridge, MA: MIT Press.

———. 1995. *The New Economics for Industry, Government, and Education,* 2nd ed. Cambridge, MA: MIT Press.

Heifetz, R. 1994. *Leadership Without Easy Answers.* Cambridge, MA: Belknap Press.

Joiner, B. 1994. *Fourth Generation Management: The New Business Consciousness.* New York: McGraw-Hill.

Kohn, L. T., J. M. Corrigan, and M. S. Donaldson (eds.). 2000. *To Err Is Human: Building a Safer Health Care System.* Washington, DC: National Academies Press.

Kotter, J. 1996. *Leading Change.* Cambridge, MA: Harvard Business School Press.

Kouzes, J., and B. Posner. 1987. *The Leadership Challenge: How to Get Extraordinary Things Done in Organizations.* San Francisco: Jossey-Bass.

Leach, D. 1999. "ACGME Outcome Project." [Online information; retrieved 5/24/04.] www.acgme.org/outcome/comp/compFull.asp.

Nauman, E., and S. H. Hoisington. 2000. *Customer Centered Six Sigma: Linking Customers, Process Improvement, and Financial Results.* Milwaukee, WI: ASQ Quality Press.

Northouse, P. G. 2001. *Leadership Theory and Practice.* Thousand Oaks, CA: Sage.

Reinertsen, J. L. 1998. "Physicians as Leaders in the Improvement of Health Care Systems." *Annals of Internal Medicine* 128 (10): 833–88.

———. 2003. "Zen and the Art of Physician Autonomy Maintenance." *Annals of Internal Medicine* 138 (12): 992–95.

Rozich, J., and R. Resar. 2002. "Using a Unit Assessment Tool to Optimize Flow and Staffing in a Community Hospital." *Joint Commission Journal of Quality Improvement* 28: 31–41.

Tichy, N. 2002. *The Leadership Engine.* New York: HarperCollins.

Wessner, D. 1998. Personal communication, May.

Zimmerman, B., C. Lindberg, and P. Plsek. 1998. *Edgeware: Insights from Complexity Science for Health Care Leaders.* Irving, TX: VHA Press.

14

ORGANIZATIONAL QUALITY INFRASTRUCTURE: HOW DOES AN ORGANIZATION STAFF QUALITY?

A. Al-Assaf

My favorite definition of quality is simple: incremental improvement. Fulfillment of this definition, however, is a major task. The term *quality* is being transformed rapidly to *performance improvement (PI)*. Therefore, for our above definition of quality, current performance must be measured as a baseline for judging whether improvement has occurred. A system also should be in place to monitor progress toward improvement on a regular, continous basis to verify whether improvement is actually happening. This type of system requires an adequate and effective infrastructure, a process for data gathering, a process for data analysis and reporting, and a process for identifying and instituting improvements. Management must have a strong commitment to these processes, and the organization must have high intentions to improve its performance.

Quality Assurance, Quality Improvement, Quality Control, and Total Quality Management

What is the difference between quality assurance (QA), quality improvement (QI), monitoring/quality control (QC), and total quality management (TQM)? According to the Quality Management Cycle (see Figure 14.1), each of these activities has certain steps that must be followed to achieve the desired objectives.

QA includes all activities toward proper planning (operational and strategic) as well as pre-assessment and self-evaluation. In addition, QA is the process of ensuring compliance with specifications, requirements, or standards and implementing methods for conformance. It includes setting and communicating standards and identifying indicators for performance monitoring and compliance with standards. These standards can come in different forms (e.g., protocols, guidelines, specifications). QA, however, is losing its earlier popularity because it resorts to disciplinary means and blames human error for noncompliance.

FIGURE 14.1

Quality
Management
Cycle

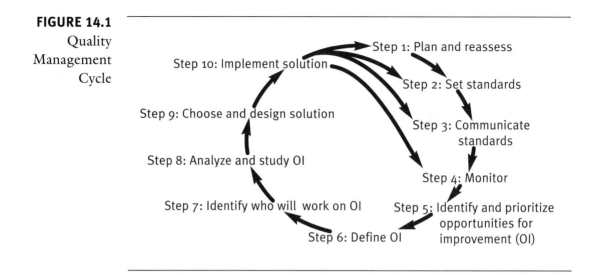

QC, on the other hand, is defined by Brown (1994) as "a management process where actual performance is measured against expected performance, and actions are taken on the difference." QC originally was used in the laboratory, where accuracy of test results dictates certain norms and specific (and often rigid) procedures that do not allow for error and discrepancy. Thus, an effort must be made to reduce variation as much as possible. In this stage, organizations are drafting indicators and using them to measure their performance against benchmarks.

QI efforts and processes complement QA and QC and sometimes overtake them. QI is defined as an organized, structured process that selectively identifies improvement teams to achieve improvements in products or services (Al-Assaf 1997). It includes all actions to identify gaps (opportunities for improvement), prioritize and select appropriate gaps to study, analyze them, and narrow or close them.

TQM, or quality management in general, involves all the above three processes: QA, QC, and QI. It involves processes pertaining to the coordination of activities related to all or any one of the above three as well as the administration and resource allocation of these processes. Administration may include training, education, organization of committees and councils, building of infrastructure, resource acquisition and allocation, and so on. Quality management is the umbrella encompassing all processes and activities related to quality. Quality management also may encompass such terms as *continuous quality management* and *total quality leadership/improvement*.

Management Commitment

There are not enough words to describe how important management commitment is to the success of quality, at least in other industries. Time and again, experts have demonstrated the value of management commitment to the quality process. Management can open doors, facilitate interventions freely, and coordinate resources easily. In most cases, management has the final say on activities and makes the final decision. Therefore, management support of activities and encouragement of professional involvement can enhance the implementation of quality in healthcare.

According to Deming (1986), if an organization does not have the commitment of top management, the odds of successful quality implementation are severely jeopardized. He further tells the prospective leader that "if you can't come, then send no one." Commitment to a cause means being involved, supportive (in words, actions, and resources), active, and participatory in that cause. Commitment also means leading the efforts, facilitating activities, participating in tasks, and providing the necessary and adequate resources to make quality improvement a reality and a success. Commitment to a process or a program means taking pride and joy in supporting it. It includes taking enthusiastic initiative to learn more about it. It certainly is not just rhetoric and oral support, although even that is better than no support at all.

You cannot be committed without understanding what you want to commit to and for what reason. Therefore, paramount to this step are increased knowledge and awareness of the subject/field that needs your commitment. Management's unequivocal commitment to healthcare quality is difficult to procure without demonstrating results. Managers are usually quick to say, "show me that it works or it has worked." Healthcare quality must be based on data and should be driven by outcomes. With adequate planning and process design, commitment will be cultivated and positive results can be achieved.

The Role of the Coordinator of Healthcare Quality

Once commitment is achieved, the person in charge of the organization, usually the CEO, needs to identify a coordinator/director of healthcare quality. This position is usually a full-time, authoritative position and may be filled by an experienced person with leadership skills and a clinical background. A direct link is necessary between this individual and the CEO or his or her designee for maintaining credibility and authority.

This position is so important that in some organizations, CEOs themselves assume the role of quality council chairman. This approach, however, has advantages and disadvantages. A prominent person like the CEO would give instant recognition and support to the quality department. He or she would establish commitment from day one, which sends a clear message to the rest of the organization that quality is important and everyone must concur. The disadvantage, on the other hand, is that often the CEO is not a permanent person, thus causing possible process discontinuity once he or she resigns.

Regardless of who the QA/QI coordinator/director is, once identified, this individual should be trained extensively in healthcare quality techniques and must prepare to organize the quality council. The roles and responsibilities of the quality coordinator are numerous, including:

- advocate and speaker for healthcare quality;
- facilitator of the quality council;
- builder of the infrastructure and necessary resources in healthcare quality;
- designated liaison with outside agencies related to quality activities;
- coordinator of the strategic and operational planning for healthcare quality activities and the allocation of resources;
- developer and updater of the quality/PI program and plan documents;
- ensurer of organizational compliance with accreditation standards;
- monitor of performance measurement activities;
- member and coordinator of the organization's quality/PI committees;
- initiator of process improvement teams;
- coordinator of key quality personnel selection;
- coordinator of the healthcare quality training plan; and
- facilitator of healthcare quality intervention strategies.

The Role of the Quality Council

The quality council or similar entity is formed to act as the body that will direct the healthcare quality process at the facility. It works as a committee to coordinate individuals representing the different aspects of healthcare delivery, disciplines, and departments/units in the organization as they formulate policies on healthcare quality.

Organization of a quality council is not imperative but recommended. The membership of the council is important, and careful selection of these individuals should rest with the top official of the organization (CEO), supported by advice and assistance from the quality coordinator and the consultant (if any). Members should be prominent individuals representing different disciplines and units of the organization. Membership may be broadened to include other individuals from other units of the organization and may benefit from inclusion of some frontline workers.

Once members are identified, the council must develop a *charter* (a description document) that delineates roles and responsibilities. The role of the council is somewhat similar to the role of the quality coordinator: give the organization collective perspective and act as the central resource in healthcare quality to which the organization may refer when necessary. Similarly, quality council members need to be adequately prepared for their roles and should be exposed to the concept of healthcare quality and its principles at an early stage.

Mission and Vision

Once the quality council forms its charter, each member should be made aware of his or her roles and responsibilities as outlined in it. Members should involve themselves actively in the revision and redrafting of the charter to reflect "ownership" in the council. The council also needs to address the development of mission and vision statements for the organization, which should reflect the desire for healthcare improvement. The council members should draft both statements with input from all key personnel. These statements establish the organization's constancy of purpose and serve as a constant reminder of the organization's direction as well as a map for its future. Mission and vision statements should be concise, clear, and realistic and should reflect the true desire of the organization, which is why real input from other key individuals is necessary. A mission statement should answer the following questions.

- Who are we?
- What is our main purpose as an organization?
- Who are we serving?
- What are the needs of those we serve, and how do we meet those needs?

Vision statements are futuristic (visionary) and should project what the organization is striving to be in the future (in three, five, or ten years). Once these statements are finalized, the council should communicate them to the rest of the organization actively and consistently. Some organizations post the mission and vision statements in prominent places throughout the organization and even print them on the back of personnel business cards. In this way, all activities of the organization will be guided by the organization's mission and designed to achieve the organization's vision.

Allocation of Resources

Resources are needed for quality training and to increase healthcare professionals' awareness of the concept of healthcare quality. Additional resources are required to monitor compliance with standards; to draft, test, and enforce compliance with policies and procedures; to identify opportunities for improvement; to initiate and coordinate improvement projects; and to disseminate the concept of quality and PI at the grassroots level. Funds also should be set aside for future improvements. Some organizations use funds to acquire reference material and create a resource library on healthcare quality. Others allocate funds to hire reviewers and quality coordinators, and some use funds to publish a newsletter on quality and hold seminars on the subject. As incentives, funds may be allotted to offer support to units or individuals who have demonstrated substantial quality improvements.

In addition to a council, organizations also allocate resources to establish a central healthcare quality department/unit. This unit should include a number of health professionals, be headed by the quality director, and be linked directly to the CEO or his or her designee. This unit is responsible for setting standards (in hospitals, they usually are standards established by The Joint Commission or the American Osteopathic Association, but organizations such as HMOs and ambulatory care facilities have a choice of accrediting organizations, each with its own standards). This unit also is responsible for communicating these standards to the rest of the organization, disseminating information related to healthcare quality, monitoring the quality of care delivered, and acting on opportunities for improvement.

The organization's CEO and board provide financial and political support to the unit and grant it broad authority to survey and monitor the performance of any healthcare or service department in the organization. The quality unit's objectives are to coordinate quality for the entire organization—supported by direct input and participation of every unit—and to institutionalize and ensure sustainability of quality.

Organizational Structure

What is the organizational structure of this quality unit? To answer this question, one should outline the main and customary functions of this unit and then decide where to place the unit in the organization's hierarchy. One also should consider the support this unit should receive from the organization's committee structure.

This unit's responsibilities may include the following functions:

- Initiate planning for quality initiatives
- Set organizational standards for quality (including the development of essential policies and procedures and ensuring proper documentation of processes and activities in the organization)
- Communicate standards to the organization's employees
  - Organize seminars to increase awareness
  - Disseminate information on standards
  - Discuss mechanisms for compliance with standards
  - Deliver workshops and lectures on standards
  - Provide training on quality skills and methods

- Monitor compliance with standards
  - Identify measurable indicators of performance

- Collect data on indicators
- Analyze data on indicators
- Perform periodic audits
- Review medical records
- Review care processes retrospectively
- Measure outcomes of patient care
- Measure satisfaction of customers, employees, patients, and providers
- Collect data on patient complaints and concerns
- Assist in meeting accreditation standards
- Review and update policies and procedures
- Identify and draft new policies and procedures

- Identify opportunities for improvement in care and services
- Initiate and coordinate improvement projects
- Facilitate performance and productivity measurement and improvements
- Facilitate documentation of essential processes and activities and provide guidelines for proper and adequate documentation, including medical record entries, risk management, patient safety issues, staff education and training, and personnel files
- Coordinate all committees related to quality and PI
- Identify and acquire necessary resources for quality and PI
- Develop the organization's quality program document and annual plan
- Evaluate the organization's quality program annually
- Develop the annual quality report for the organization's board of directors
- Coordinate all functions and activities related to the optimum use of resources
- Coordinate all functions and activities related to prevention, control, and management of risks to organization's customers, both internal and external
- Coordinate an effective system for credentialing and re-credentialing the organization's practitioners
- Act as a liaison with all of the organization's units to facilitate the improvement of their performance

This unit should have access to the data the organization collects on patient care and the services the organization provides internally and externally. It therefore should work closely with the organization's information technology unit.

There is considerable variation as to what constitutes a typical organizational structure of such a unit. There is variation as to who reports to this unit and to whom this unit should report. Traditionally, it has been placed under the medical staff affairs section of the organization, although new trends suggest that it should be moved to a higher level, where it reports directly to the CEO. As to who reports to this unit, some organizations include both administrative and clinical functions, whereas others narrow the scope to only the clinical functions. Some hospitals add more, including infection control, utilization, case management, risk management, and credentialing.

Other functions of this unit usually are handled through the informal structure of the organization (i.e., the committees). Again, there is considerable variation as to which committees belong to quality and which belong to medical staff affairs. In general, however, the credentialing, peer review and clinical services management, utilization and case management, patient safety, risk manangement, infection control, and medical record review committees usually report to the quality unit. In addition, the organization's quality council (or similar) is directly related to the quality unit (although it does not report to it), and the quality unit staff usually coordinates the quality council's activities. Other committees such as pharmacy, therapeutics, facility management, and information technology may be a part of the quality structure.

Increasing Awareness of Healthcare Quality

Healthcare quality is a concept that has different facets, principles, skills, techniques, and tools. A vast amount of literature has been written about it. Therefore, early on, the members of the quality council should participate in a seminar on healthcare quality. This seminar should be followed by intellectual discussions with a designated facilitator on the application of this concept to that organization, taking into consideration the available resources, the culture, and the current healthcare status and structure. A similar activity should be organized to present healthcare quality to other key personnel to obtain further support and to increase dissemination of the concept. Certainly, the facilitator's services could be used to present a number of short sessions with other key personnel and middle managers to discuss healthcare quality. These sessions, to be repeated at least annually, should be attended by at least the quality coordinator and some members of the quality council and can serve as focus group sessions to gather feedback on quality implementation and applications in healthcare. Information and feedback gathered at these sessions can be used in the next planning phase at the operational level and in launching improvement projects and initiatives.

Mapping Quality Improvement Intervention

In collaboration with the quality council and with information collected during the planning phase, the quality coordinator may identify areas in the system where opportunities for improvement exist. Identified areas should be selected carefully to include the projects that require the least amount of resources and have the highest probability of success, yet benefit a large population. Examples of such projects include:

- improving the reception area of the organization;
- improving the aesthetics of the organization;
- improving the timeliness of tests and services to patients;
- identifying and improving patient safety in areas such as infections, falls, complications, and medication errors;
- initiating a campaign to improve reporting on sentinel events and their management efforts;
- selecting a few areas that receive numerous complaints from external customers and trying to improve them;
- initiating a campaign to promote health awareness to the public; and
- leading an informational campaign on improvement initiatives with participation of all units.

Of course, the council is not limited to these projects. It can identify other opportunities for quality improvement and initiate improvements with an interdisciplinary team from the affected departments. When a project is completed, the quality council should analyze the lessons learned and prioritize services and organizational areas for further implementation of improvements. For example, services selected for intervention could be those that are:

- high volume;
- problem prone;
- high risk;
- high impact; or
- high cost.

On the other hand, other criteria used for selection of venues and units for intervention may include:

- availability and accessibility of necessary data;
- size and homogeneity of the "study" population;
- simplicity of the infrastructure;
- definition and focus of the proposed intervention;
- stability and supportiveness of leadership;
- level of need for improvement;
- ability to complete the intervention with available resources;
- willingness of health professionals to participate; and
- feasibility of demonstrating improvements.

Using the above criteria, the quality council will be able to choose the specific area or service and decide what resources are needed to implement the intervention. The use of objectivity in selecting a system or an area for intervention is crucial to successful outcomes.

Quality/PI Program Document

One of the most important documents the quality unit must develop is the program description document, which is required for accreditation of the organization. An organization that lacks this document never will be accredited.

This document should provide a description of the different activities of the quality unit and an outline of the scope of work in which this unit or the organization's quality program is engaged. It also should describe the functions of the different individuals and committees associated with the quality program. This document should serve as the basis for evaluating the organization's quality performance. The following list provides suggestions for the outline of a program description document.

Quality Program Document

- Purpose of document
- General program description and overview
- Statements of mission, vision, and values of the organization and the quality unit
- Goals and objectives of the quality program
- Strategies for PI
- Organizational structure supporting PI
- Formal structure
- Committee structure
- Roles and responsibilities of the PI program (narrative of roles and responsibilities of each below)
    - Board of directors
    - CEO and executive team
    - Quality council
    - Quality/PI unit
        - Quality director
        - Quality coordinators
        - Quality reviewers/specialists
    - Quality committees
    - Project teams
    - Departmental, section, and other unit leaders
    - Staff responsibilities and involvement in PI
- Scope of work and standards of care and service
- Authority and accountability
- Reporting mechanisms
- Criteria for setting priorities on PI monitors and projects
- List of indicators for monitoring PI
- Methods of monitoring compliance with standards and measuring performance
- Confidentiality of information

- Mechanism/model for improvement interventions
- Education and awareness activities on quality/PI
- Rewarding results program
- Annual evaluation of QI/PI
- Audits and reviews
- Credentialing and re-credentialing
- Peer review
- Utilization management
- Risk management and patient safety

This document should be reviewed, rereviewed, and approved at least once annually by appropriate staff of the QA unit.

Evaluation, Monitoring, and Continuous Quality Improvement

Evaluation

The 1990s were dubbed the "period of performance measurement." Providers, consumers, and purchasers were looking for ways to satisfy one another through measuring and reporting on care outcomes. Several third-party organizations attempted to produce certain measures to report on these care outcomes. As a result, a number of national indicators were developed and are now in use by healthcare organizations. Report cards are being assembled on the nation's healthcare organizations. Benchmarking efforts are under way to identify and emulate excellence in care and services. All these activities are being carried out in an effort to measure and improve performance in healthcare. In the international arena, the World Health Organization (WHO) organized and facilitated a number of activities related to quality assessment, performance improvement, and outcomes measurements (see work coordinated by the Centers for Medicare & Medicaid Services [CMS] at www.cms.gov and the Agency for Healthcare Research and Quality at www.qualitymeasures.ahrq.gov). A large number of countries and institutions participated in these activities and initiatives. In the end, all agreed that there has to be an organized mechanism to account for quality and continuous measure and to improve performance in healthcare organizations (see 2000 WHO report on health systems rankings at www.who.int/whr2001/2001/archives/2000/en).

Performance measurement includes the identification of certain indicators for performance. Data are collected to measure those indicators and then compare current performance to a desired performance level. Several systems of measurements and indicators already have been developed. The Healthcare Effectiveness Data and Information Set (HEDIS) is one example (www.ncqa.org/tabid/59/Default.aspx) of a system of measurements and indicators. This set has over 50 measures primarily for preventive health services against which organizations can measure their performance, compare their performance with the performance of their peers, and trend their progress toward improvement. Other systems include the U.S. Public Health Service Healthy People 2000 and 2010 list of indicators (www.healthypeople.gov), The Joint Commission's ORYX clinical indicator system for hospitals (www.qiproject.org/pdf/2008_QI_Project_Indicators.pdf), the Canadian Council on Health Services Accreditation hospital indicators (www.cchsa.ca), and the CMS QISMC indicator system for managed care (www.cms.gov).

Monitoring

Monitoring is based on specific and measured indicators related to standards. It is a process of measuring variance from standards and initiating processes to reduce this variance. Monitoring is a necessary step for proper selection of and consideration of quality improvement projects and studies. It also can provide the organization with an indication of the status of care and services provided.

In advanced healthcare systems, elaborate and comprehensive systems of monitoring have been developed that use the patient's medical record for the abstraction of specific data, which in turn are fed into a central database for analysis and monitoring. Each organization then receives a periodic report showing aggregate data of national healthcare indicators compared to their specific set of data for the same indicators. Variance from the mean is then studied and acted on using the QA/QI process described above.

Continuous Quality Improvement

Improvements are not onetime activities. When a team has worked on a process and improvement has been accomplished, it should not abandon this process and move on to the next one. Improvement is a process, and a process is continuous. Monitoring should continue, and improvements should be initiated every time they are needed. Once compliance has been achieved, incremental improvements in the standards also are important. If high or even perfect compliance with a specific standard has been documented, upgrading this standard is the next step to take. Otherwise, the organization will stay in the status quo and further improvement will not occur.

Challenges, Opportunities, and Lessons Learned for Sustaining QA/QI

A Quality Culture

Establishing a quality culture is the next milestone. A hospital that combines high-quality standards with a quality culture institutionalizes quality.

Institutionalization is achieved when appropriate healthcare quality activities are carried out effectively, efficiently, and on a routine basis throughout a system or an organization (Brown 1995). It is a state of achievement whereby healthcare quality is practiced and maintained without additional outside resources. In such a state, expertise is available within and commitment is fully integrated and maintained.

A quality environment or culture is achieved when quality activities become day-to-day activities. Such activities are not separate from the normal activities carried out daily by the system and its personnel. It is a state in which each employee is aware of the quality concept, believes in it, practices its principles, and makes it part of his or her responsibility and not the responsibility of a department or another individual. In such a culture, each individual is responsible for his or her task's own quality structure, process, and outcome. Employees make every effort at that level to ensure that the processes of QA are maintained (i.e., planning, standard setting, and monitoring). Employees also practice QI—they identify variance from standards and select opportunities for improvements to be acted on individually or in collaboration with others. It is also a situation in which employees are empowered to achieve their goals, which are in turn aligned with the organization's mission and vision statements.

Lessons in Institutionalization

- *Planning* for quality should be done systematically and thoroughly. Delineation of responsibility, identification of scope of involvement, allocation of resources, and anticipation for the change should be completed before activities in QA or QI begin.
- Securing *commitment* from management is helpful and can make the process of implementation move rapidly. The involvement of top managers in early planning activities is essential.
- Develop a *policy* for quality at the central level as early and as solidly as possible. A policy that is well prepared and developed in collaboration with senior staff will have a much better chance of survival, even with its expected high turnover.
- Identification of a *leader* or *champion* (local cadre) to lead this movement is highly recommended. A local person with authority, credibility, enthusiasm, and interest can be an asset to the acceleration of healthcare quality implementation. This individual can act as facilitator and cheerleader for healthcare quality initiatives.
- Organization of a steering committee or *council* of local/internal representatives gives the healthcare quality process credibility, sustainability, and momentum.
- Formation of the *structure* for healthcare quality should be gradual, cautious, and based on progress and understanding of the concept and

practice. Early organization of large committee and council structures may shift the focus to organization and away from the actual mission of healthcare quality, which is improvement. At the beginning of implementation, staff should concentrate more on learning and understanding the concept and practice it daily to achieve positive results. Too many committees with too many meetings and tasks distract from focus on expected goals.

- Always have an *alternative plan* in case one is slowed down because of staff changes. Don't rely on a single individual when trying to implement healthcare quality effectively. Train a number of individuals, and prepare several qualified staff members simultaneously. This practice will allow for wider selection of coordinators and will enhance sustainability efforts.

- Prepare to answer questions related to *incentives* for staff to participate. As long as healthcare quality activities are not required as integral parts of their jobs, employees will question their role in participation. A system of employee rewards and recognition based on healthcare quality achievements is necessary.

- *Document improvements* by measuring pre- and post-status. Always have quantitative data available for comparisons and measurements of effectiveness. Calculation of cost savings is useful in measuring efficiency. Providing measurable parameters gives credibility and sustainability to the process of healthcare quality.

- Actively *disseminate achievements* and healthcare quality awareness information to as many individuals in the system as possible. Make sure participation is voluntary and open to everyone as opportunities for improvement are identified. Do not make it a private club. Keep everybody informed and involved as much as possible.

- Resist the temptation of *expansion* to other regions or sectors early. Building an effective process in one area is more important than starting several incomplete processes in different locations and areas. Keep the implementation process focused.

- Always keep *adequate funding* available for the development of new projects and activities not originally planned. Doing so also will give you the flexibility of shifting additional funds to areas where improvements are taking place more effectively. Adequate funds will increase the likelihood of sustainability.

- Finally, encourage and foster an environment of *learning, not judgment*. In particular, rely on data and facts in making judgments. Avoid the antiquated disciplinary method of management.

Remember that, according to Deming (1986), "Every system is perfectly designed to meet the objectives for which it is designed." Therefore, ensuring that the quality infrastructure is designed effectively is essential, and monitoring its performance regularly is even more important.

Case Example

It was only 8 p.m. when Jerry, an intern, wheeled the new EKG machine into Ms. Smith's room, but Jerry could sense he was in for another sleepless night. Ms. Smith, who was 68 years old, had been admitted earlier in the day for an elective cholecystectomy. She now appeared acutely ill. She was pale and sweaty, her pulse was 120, her respiration was shallow and rapid, and her blood pressure was 90/60.

Jerry quickened his attempts to obtain the EKG. He momentarily considered asking a nurse for help but reasoned that the night shift would not have received any more training on the use of these new EKG machines than he had.

He had read an article in the hospital's weekly employee newspaper that the new EKG system was great. It featured a computerized interpretation of the cardiogram, which was tied to data banks containing previous EKGs on every patient. The chief of cardiology spearheaded the effort to purchase the system, believing it would provide sophisticated EKG interpretations during off hours and solve growing data storage problems. Technicians operated the EKG machines during the day, but they had long since gone home.

After affixing the EKG electrodes to the patient, Jerry looked at the control panel. He saw buttons labeled STD, AUTO, RUN, MEMORY, RS, and TIE. Other buttons, toggles, and symbols were attached, but Jerry had no clue as to what they meant. He could not find an instruction manual. "Totally different from my old favorite," Jerry thought as he began the process of trial and error. Unfortunately, he could not figure out how to use the new machine, and after 15 minutes he went to another floor and fetched his favorite machine.

"Admitted for an elective cholecystectomy," Jerry remarked to himself on reading the EKG, "and this lady's having a massive heart attack! She came to the floor at 4 p.m.; I hadn't planned to see her until 9 p.m.!" He gave some orders and began looking through the chart to write a coronary care unit transfer note.

Jerry's eyes widened when he came across the routine preoperative EKG, which had been obtained at 1 p.m. using the new computerized system. It had arrived on the floor four hours earlier, along with Ms. Smith. It showed the same abnormalities as Jerry's cardiogram, and the computer had interpreted the abnormalities appropriately.

Jerry returned to Ms. Smith's room. On direct questioning, she volunteered that her chest pain had been present since late morning, but she didn't want to bother nurses or physicians because they appeared too busy.

Jerry then discussed the case with the CCU team. They decided with some regret that Ms. Smith would not qualify for thrombolytic therapy (an effective treatment for myocardial infarction) because the duration of her symptoms precluded any hope that it would help her. They initiated conservative therapy, but Ms. Smith's clinical condition steadily deteriorated overnight, and she died the next morning.

Jerry reflected on the case. Why had he not been notified about the first abnormal tracing? He called the EKG lab and found that a technician had noticed the abnormal cardiogram coming off the computer. However, he assumed the appropriate physicians knew about it and, in any event, did not feel it was his duty to notify physicians about such abnormalities.

Jerry assumed the new EKG system would notify him about marked abnormalities. When Jerry first read about the new system, he thought it would serve a useful backup role in the event he did not have time to review EKGs himself until late in the evening.

1. What is the main problem in this scenario?
2. What should be done about it?
3. How should this hospital organize for quality?

Study Questions

1. If you were assuming the chief executive position in a hospital and the chief quality officer position was vacant, what type of person would you seek to fill the position? Background? Experience?
2. How do accreditation and adherence to standards mix with quality/performance improvement activities? Is there an optimal percentage of time a group should spend on one or the other?
3. What are the cultural barriers and enablers to achieving a successful quality improvement program?

References

Al-Assaf, A. 1997. "Strategies for Introducing Quality Assurance in Health Care." In *Quality Assurance in Health Care: A Report of a WHO Intercountry Meeting*, 33–49. New Delhi, India: World Health Organization.

Brown, J. A. 1994. *The Healthcare Quality Handbook*. Glenview, IL: National Association for Healthcare Quality.

Brown, L. D. 1995. "Lessons Learned in Institutionalization of Quality Assurance Programs: An International Perspective." *International Journal of Quality in Health Care* 7 (4): 419–25.

Deming, W. E. 1986. *Out of the Crisis*. Cambridge, MA: MIT Press.

Suggested Reading

Al-Assaf, A. 1997. "Institutionalization of Healthcare Quality." *Proceedings of the International Association of Management* 15 (1): 55–59.

Al-Assaf, A. F. 1998. *Managed Care Quality: A Practical Guide.* Boca Raton, FL: CRC Press.

———. 2001. *Health Care Quality: An International Perspective.* New Delhi, India: World Health Organization–SEARO.

Al-Assaf, A. F., and J. A. Schmele. 1993. *The Textbook of Total Quality in Healthcare.* Delray, FL: St. Lucie Press.

Juran, J., and K. F. Gryna. 1988. *Juran's Quality Control Handbook.* New York: McGraw-Hill.

Nicholas, D. D., J. R. Heiby, and T. A. Hatzell. 1991. "The Quality Assurance Project: Introducing Quality Improvement to Primary Health Care in Less Developed Countries." *Quality Assurance in Health Care* 3 (3): 147–65.

IMPLEMENTING QUALITY AS THE CORE ORGANIZATIONAL STRATEGY

Scott B. Ransom, Thomas J. Fairchild, and
Elizabeth R. Ransom

The changing paradigm of competition in healthcare over the past decade has caused providers to put an increased premium on implementing change focused on improving healthcare quality. Although many of the initiatives described in this text are supported in the literature, make sense, and appear to be practical approaches that can be implemented, identification of organizational leaders who have successfully executed a strategy that focuses on lasting improvement in healthcare quality remains a challenge.

Volumes have been written about the value of healthcare quality improvement frameworks, such as continuous quality improvement. Many organizations and foundations, such as the Institute of Medicine (IOM),[1] Leapfrog Group,[2] Institute for Healthcare Improvement (IHI),[3] National Quality Forum (NQF),[4] National Commission for Quality Long-Term Care,[5] Brookings Institution,[6] Commonwealth Fund,[7] Robert Wood Johnson Foundation,[8] RAND Corporation,[9] and Center for Health Transformation,[10] have focused their energy and resources on improving healthcare quality. In addition, prestigious awards, such as the Malcolm Baldrige National Quality Award, have been offered for 20 years as a way to encourage quality. These organizations have engaged numerous experts and spent countless hours and millions of dollars to examine and encourage quality.

Despite these continuing efforts, our healthcare system is faced with more challenges related to quality improvement today than ever before. One key link in the healthcare system that has seen little improvement is hospitals. Regina Herzlinger, in her thought-provoking book *Who Killed Health Care?* (2007), points out that "the hospital is an increasingly dangerous place for a sick person." *Adverse events*, bureaucratese for mistakes that gravely injure patients, affected nearly 400,000 cases in 2004. Between 1998 and 2004, tens of thousands died because of hospitals' "failure to rescue" and 32,000 had an "infection due to care."

The tidal wave of quality improvement efforts unfortunately has resulted in, at best, minimal improvements in this country's healthcare system, and the quality of healthcare that Americans receive remains largely unchanged. Porter and Teisberg (2004) argue:

	AUS	CAN	GER	NET	NZ	UK	US
TABLE 15.1 Medical, Medication, and Lab Errors in Seven Countries, 2007							
Percentage of patients with two or more chronic conditions reporting either a medical, medication, or lab test error	26	28	16	25	22	24	32

SOURCE: Schoen et al. (2007).

The U.S. Health Care System has registered unsatisfactory performance in both costs and quality over many years. While this might be expected in a state-controlled sector, it is nearly unimaginable in a competitive market—and in the United States, health care is largely private and subject to more competition than virtually anyplace else in the world.

As an example, the 2007 Commonwealth Fund International Health Policy Survey comparison of seven countries found that "among adults with multiple chronic conditions, patient-reported error rates ranged from 16 percent in Germany to 32 percent in the United States" (Schoen et al. 2007). See Table 15.1.

Error rates and other quality challenges continue to plague our healthcare system despite the large amount of money spent on it. The latest numbers from the Agency for Healthcare Research and Quality (Andrews and Elixhauser 2007) show that in 2005, the nation's hospital bill reached a record high of $873 billion—nearly double the 1997 spending, adjusted for inflation. State and federal governments and providers have spent millions of dollars to improve performance and the experience of patients, yet few lasting improvements have been realized.

Implementing a culture that has quality improvement at its core is an important goal for providers who want to serve patients better, gain the support of healthcare providers, stay ahead of government regulation, meet consumers' demands for transparent information on quality and cost, and gain a competitive advantage in the marketplace. However, recent history suggests that only a few of these quality improvement efforts have been successful; many efforts have not resulted in the sustainable quality improvements that the leaders who designed the change had hoped to see.

Incorporating quality as a central element of an organization's culture and strategy must begin with leadership from the board of trustees, the CEO, and the executive team. Despite best intentions, developing a focus on improving quality is a challenge for most healthcare organizations because of the many internal competing agendas; the rapidly changing competitive environment shaped by providers, employees, and policymakers; and the often underappreciated impact of organizational culture on quality improvement. Daily conflicts confront healthcare providers and can disrupt a quality focus. Conflicts include declining revenues and market share, union difficulties, electronic medical records, Health Insurance Portability and Accountability Act requirements, review by The Joint Commission, malpractice concerns, employee recruitment and retention, physician relations, and community expectations. Every governing board and CEO supports healthcare quality improvement, but few are able to establish a culture that will support the execution of a sustainable strategy.

Successful organizations that have visionary leaders who are willing to take calculated risks have approached their journey to quality with a realization that the first step is to establish an organizational culture that will support this excursion. The starting point for this effort is leadership, which must be aligned with and fully support a cultural perspective of quality.

Many of these leaders have expanded their view of quality to include a more balanced vision that reflects the ideas embedded in the performance management tool developed by Kaplan and Norton (2001) called the Balanced Scorecard. Some healthcare providers have embraced this tool fully, whereas others have used the ideas of the Balanced Scorecard more loosely to shape their strategies. The Balanced Scorecard approach includes the perspective of the patient and family, internal processes such as clinical pathways, learning and growth opportunities that focus on employees, and financial performance. By adapting this broader and more balanced view, these organizations show an understanding of the wide range of interdependent factors that they must address on their journey to implementing a change strategy that will focus on quality of care. Leaders in these organizations ask financial questions about market share, margins, and quality implications of purchasing multimillion-dollar equipment, such as a DaVinci robot to maintain the cutting edge of surgical innovation. They raise questions related to the satisfaction of their internal and external customers and the way in which business processes must change to improve and sustain quality. Deliberate primary focus on this broad range of organizational measures is essential to creating a culture of quality. This approach ensures not only that the journey toward quality improvement is grounded in financial metrics, but also that the organization develops the capabilities and skills it will need to carry out the quality improvement strategy productively.

The Baldrige National Quality Program (2007) criteria for performance excellence best describe the role of leadership and the interdependence of the elements of an organization that has a culture of performance excellence. Figure 15.1 presents a slightly modified version of this structure by including the all-encompassing role of culture in creating and sustaining performance excellence. As the figure suggests, the change toward quality starts with leadership that creates and drives a system of excellence that will bring about sustainable results.

FIGURE 15.1

Health Care
Performance
Excellence
Framework

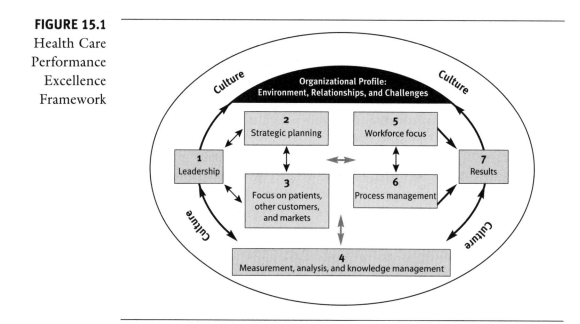

SOURCE: Adapted from the Baldrige National Quality Program Health Care Criteria for Performance Excellence Framework, 2007.

As senior leadership starts to manage this organizational change, it should share a road map for change. Kotter suggested a practical and useful change process that can serve as a useful guide for the leadership team starting the quality improvement journey. The following eight-stage change process, modified from Kotter's seminal work *Leading Change* (1996), serves as a realistic and viable framework to guide leaders who are managing a change to quality:

1. Unfreezing the old culture
2. Forming a powerful guiding coalition
3. Developing a vision and strategy
4. Communicating a vision and strategy
5. Empowering employees to act on the vision and strategy
6. Generating short-term wins
7. Consolidating gains and producing more change
8. Refreezing new approaches in the culture

Implementing Quality in Healthcare Organizations

Unfreezing the Old Culture

The time to repair the roof is when the sun is shining.

—John F. Kennedy

The essential trait of leadership is the courage to set a direction. Leadership establishes the vision. The transition to a high-performance healthcare organization requires a leader to define a culture that has quality at its core and to establish clear and specific expectations for employees involved in the quality journey.

This step is the most difficult because of culture's influence on employee behavior and some employees' desire to resist change and impede progress. Organizational culture comprises values, underlying assumptions, behaviors, ceremonies, symbols, language, and activities that a group learns and shares. Culture is like an iceberg. Some elements of culture are more visible (i.e., above the waterline), such as management information systems, organizational structure, and behaviors that employees are encouraged to follow. However, like an iceberg, the less visible and more significant elements of culture are those below the waterline—elements like shared values and behaviors that influence employees and persist over time (Kotter and Heskett 1992). Culture contributes significantly to employees' identification and contributes to the success or failure of strategy execution. Leadership often overlooks or minimizes the role of culture and tends to focus on highly visible changes such as improved financial performance, new service lines, and employee layoffs. The real changes in behavior that will hold the new culture in place long term are the elements of culture below the waterline that take years to change.

Before this process can begin, leaders must motivate employees to change. To transform behaviors, leaders must "encourage both personal and organizational transformation" and deal with employees' resistance to change (Rooke and Torbert 2005). The first step is for leadership to define and communicate the idea that the status quo is no longer acceptable. This step is not an easy task, especially if the organization is not in a financial crisis. Although numerous conflicts occur in the typical healthcare organization, this movement toward quality should be easier when conflict is minimal and the financial strength of the organization is sound. This movement seldom happens because most organizations prefer to stand pat when times are good or at best make only superficial changes to appear as though they are making improvements.

Leaders who can communicate the sense of urgency about an opportunity or a potential crisis effectively without creating a sense of fear or resistance among employees are rare. More often than not, weakening financial performance, employee discontent, or a declining dominance in the marketplace brings about urgency for change. Schein (2002) suggests that "the essence of an effective unfreezing process is a balancing of enough disconfirmation to arouse an optimal level of anxiety or guilt, without arousing so much learning anxiety as to cause denial, repression, projection, or some other defense mechanism." Unfreezing the cultural iceberg and transforming the organization must start with education: making employees understand that changing the organization to embrace quality is required for growth and survival.

High-performing organizations spend time on what is important. If quality is the desired focus, leadership must create a sense of urgency that will move people from the comfort of the status quo to a new culture that reflects the values of quality. Culture can be changed without a sense of urgency, but change occurs more readily if leadership recognizes or perceives a sense of urgency. As an example, the leadership of Baptist Health Care recognized that the organization could not compete in the marketplace by outspending its competitors and that it had to change because its flagship hospital was losing market share. In its search for ways to regain market dominance, it examined many options but eventually embraced quality, which started it on its successful journey to winning the coveted Malcolm Baldrige National Quality Award and regaining its competitive advantage (Stubblefield 2005).

Creating a Guiding Coalition

You can accomplish anything in life, provided you do not mind who gets the credit.

—Harry S. Truman

"Leaders get the right people on the bus (and the wrong people off the bus) and set the direction," says Jim Collins, author of *Good to Great* (2001). Creating a strategy for quality improvement requires a team; no single leader can drive a sustainable change without the rest of the leadership on the bus and in the correct seat. The organization's change effort will determine the skills it needs in specific leadership positions. Senior leaders must coach, promote, and hire people who clearly understand the urgency, see the need to change, and have the set of skills essential to guide and support the change. At this stage of the journey, a few key leaders may be asked to get off the bus or change seats because they are unwilling to embrace the shift to the new culture or do not have the required skills. For example, if a CEO realizes that lower reimbursements are challenging the hospital's market position, all the senior leaders on the bus must accept the strategy to address this threat or risk losing their jobs.

Leadership that is responsible for communicating this challenge in a troubled organization must recognize the feelings and perspectives of employees. Atchison and Bujak (2001) provide the following insight about this situation.

Individuals go through three stages: egocentric, rolecentric, and missioncentric. Egocentric behavior is distinguished by self-interest. An employee faced with change will often respond to this new situation by asking: how does this affect me? Rolecentric focuses on issues related to the job. A common question that is asked by an employee in this stage is: how will this change affect my work? The third stage, missioncentric, is characterized by employees who understand and share the vision and mission of the organization. Employees at this stage begin to ask questions like: what can I do help the organization achieve their strategy?

The first step is moving senior leadership to a mission-centric position. The leadership team must understand its job and expected objectives as the journey to quality improvement begins. Thus, the CEO must ensure that team members clearly understand expectations for their performance and then must provide effective and timely feedback on their behavior. Senior leaders, including the board, must be held accountable for their performance, which requires the tenacity, focus, and skills of what George (2003) calls *authentic leadership*. This common understanding about expectations and accountability helps to create what Kotter (1995) labels the *guiding coalition*, which is responsible for leading the change effort. Team members must have the desire, knowledge, and skills to support the vision, to direct change, and to deal with resistance, and they must be passionate about quality. The role of the guiding coalition is to help the organization develop a shared understanding of the vision and the goal to move toward a new organizational culture based on quality.

Executives must include key clinical leaders and staff in the guiding coalition. Executives can prod and support change, but the real drivers of clinical care improvement are physicians, nurses, and other clinical staff. Executives may attempt to inspire a shared vision through effective communication and common ground; however, key clinical leaders must lead improvement initiatives in patient care areas.

Team members' most critical asset is trust in each other. Without trust, they cannot achieve true teamwork and the strategy will fall short of its goals.

Developing a Vision and a Strategy

A great hockey player skates to where the puck is going to be.
—Wayne Gretzky

Establishing a vision and creating a new strategic direction are exercises that allow everyone in the organization to understand what the future will look like and what they will have to do to achieve the future state. Most for-profit organizations create visions and strategies that focus on improving profits, which is only one necessary element of the Balanced Scorecard. Historically, most not-for-profit organizations have focused on the opportunity to pursue a more mission-oriented existence without great concern for fiscal stability and strength. In the increasingly competitive healthcare market, most nonprofit organizations now recognize that if there is no margin, there is no mission. This view reflects a more balanced perspective of what organizations need to achieve success. As organizations experience financial challenges, the focus is necessarily fiscal, not quality. This phenomenon is similar to that illustrated by Maslow's hierarchy of needs, which suggests that survival requirements take priority over higher-level needs until the survival needs are met (Maslow 1943).

In a world where many healthcare organizations continually face financial pressures, the trade-off between bottom line and quality has a predictable result. The organization in financial straits does not focus on quality and emphasizes a positive bottom line, which may compromise improvement and lead to a less-competitive organization.

The critical step that will remove the organization from this downward spiral starts with a leader who creates a succinct and inspiring vision that will transform the organization to one that will be attractive to employees, have achievable goals, and allow for individual interest. A simple and effective way to think of vision is in terms of one question: what do we want to be? The vision statement that answers this question should motivate employees to move in a common direction and give them a clear sense of the future. For a vision to have this level of influence, it also must reflect the essence of the mission and values of the organization. Vision, values, and mission are the bedrock of any strategy and must be aligned with and totally integrated into the organization's culture. Employees should understand that they are engaged in an effort to build a cathedral rather than to lay stones.

Bower and Gilbert (2007) suggest that a "reasonable definition of strategy in the real world" is "which opportunities a company will pursue and which it will pass by." An effective strategy must be built on the organization's vision, values, and mission and describe activities needed to implement the strategy. These activities can be referred to as goals, which should answer another question: what do we expect to achieve? Tactical initiatives clarify how the organization will accomplish the goals. They answer a third question: how will we accomplish our goals? An organization must excel at these activities to implement its strategy successfully. Porter (1996) supports the critical importance of these activities in arguing that "the essence of strategy is in activities—choosing to perform activities differently or to perform different activities than rivals."

The final elements of an effective strategy are the metrics that answer this question: how do we know we are there? As the adage suggests, "what gets measured is what gets done." The failure to develop key metrics that will drive the change and to measure the organization's performance consistently on those metrics contributes significantly to the break between strategies and performance. Metrics are critical to strategy adjustment and reinforce new behaviors and processes. Healthcare can drown in metrics, but knowing which areas to measure will drive the strategy directly and motivate employee behavior. Fewer metrics are usually better.

Key stakeholders need to be fully involved in selecting the metrics and determining how they will measure them. Although this process is more time consuming, it will ensure their ownership of the strategy and the efforts to measure progress. Clinical staff's engagement in this step is imperative. Physicians and other providers will support efforts to measure quality if there is real commitment and involvement from the beginning. If physicians and other providers are involved from the beginning, they will be better translators to other providers.

In particular, physicians need to understand how the proposed quality improvement initiatives will affect their practice style and behavior. Physicians will support change but, as most employees, are often skeptical at first. As suggested earlier, change will occur when they understand the inadequacy of the current behavior or process.

Physicians often have divergent views based on past personal experience. Physicians who have participated in similar but unsuccessful quality improvement programs will be reluctant to spend time or lend support to measuring some aspects of clinical care and may see the initiative as a waste of time.

Physicians often have financial conflicts of interest in working on these projects as well. These conflicts can be direct. For example, the internist who is paid for every day the patient is admitted will have a financial conflict with the hospital that is paid on a diagnosis-related group fixed payment basis. Senior leaders must understand that the private practice physician is an independent businessperson and sees the hospital only as a place to admit patients. Hospital committee work and time spent on improvement initiatives infringe on time the physician can use to see patients and earn money for the private practice. The leadership team must understand these conflicts when targeting physicians' participation in improvement and change programs.

In addition to strategy, a strategic management system includes three other processes: resource allocation to support the strategic initiatives, action plans, and a communication plan. These elements must be aligned for the strategy to be successful. The biggest challenge for organizations that do not have a strategy focus is distinguishing strategic planning from other types of planning, such as operational. "Improving operational effectiveness is a necessary part of management, but it is not strategy" (Porter 1996). Strategy has more of an external focus. As Porter (1985) advocates, "competitive strategy is the search for a favorable competitive position in an industry, the fundamental arena in which competition occurs."

The strategic planning process involves deciding what to do rather than how to do it and therefore must look beyond organizational boundaries. Understanding opportunities in the external environment that match internal strengths is the starting point of a solid strategy.

Communicating a Vision and a Strategy

Think like a wise man but communicate in the language of the people.
                                                        —William Butler Yeats

A vision and a strategic plan are the cornerstones of transformation, but they will not drive change successfully if only a few employees understand and hear the message. Senior leadership must manage the communication of the vision and strategy. It must repeat the message continuously by word and action. Personal meetings with credible messengers have the best chance of building rapport and credibility with key individuals. Committee discussions can be effective; however, key leaders must be enthusiastic supporters of the change before the meeting begins. The process of effective change implementation can be time consuming. Presentation of new initiatives to a group may seem to be more time efficient; however, unless key people have seen and support the information before the group meeting, the initiative is unlikely to move forward. Similarly, letters, phone calls, newsletters, bulletin board messages, and e-mail tend to be ineffective in moving projects forward. These impersonal methods of communication can benefit employees as sources of information, but leadership must do the real work through a series of one-on-one and small-group discussions to explain the initiative to supervisors who will move the change forward with the employees who report to them.

To communicate the change effectively, leaders must eliminate the "we versus them" mentality and work toward expanding the guiding coalition. Medical staff is not a homogenous group; one common voice cannot generally represent it. Elected leaders often assume that physicians agree with both vision and strategic direction. In reality, they must test their support through direct and open discussions with individuals on the medical staff. The chief of staff may have clout, but other practicing physicians may not recognize this individual as their representative.

Effective communication depends on a clear understanding of terminology and language. Healthcare has become increasingly specialized. This specialization can impair effective communication about quality improvement efforts. Physicians use a clinical and patient-specific lexicon, whereas administrators speak the language of teams, systems, and populations (Ransom, Tropman, and Pinsky 2001). Frequently, words used by an administrator to communicate quality improvement may not convey the intended message to the physician. For example, a large healthcare system, including more than 40 hospitals nationwide, conducted an experiment with its leadership team. This leadership team consisted of all site CEOs and chief medical officers. The team members were asked individually to write ten words that describe or support the term *quality healthcare*. Less than 25 percent of the group wrote three or more of the same terms. In fact, only 60 percent of the group wrote just one of the same terms. Although everyone in the room was an expert in hospital leadership, the group had inconsistent definitions of healthcare quality. This simple experiment shows the difficulty with effective communication of even basic concepts to healthcare workers.

"CEOs who fail to define success and communicate their vision of it, and fail to make their expectations clear to employees, produce meaningless cultures" (Hamm 2006). There is no substitute for communicating this change toward a new vision clearly, simply, and using multiple forums to do so (Kotter 1996). Leadership by example is the most powerful communication tool, and senior leadership and all members of the guiding coalition must serve consistently as role models.

Empowering Employees to Act on the Vision and Strategy

One does not "manage" people. The task is to lead people. And the goal is to make productive the specific strengths and knowledge of each individual.
—Peter F. Drucker

The ultimate measure of a strategy's success is how well it is executed. The research of Mankins and Steele (2005) suggests that "companies on average deliver only 63 percent of the financial performance their strategies promise." Leaders often look first to areas like poor planning or lack of clear priorities as hindrances to the successful execution of their strategies. These barriers may play a significant role in strategy implementation, but they are not the most basic factors in the execution of a new strategy. George and Sims (2007), in their book *True North*, say, "Individuals usually have their own passions that drive them." They go on to suggest that "results achieved by empowering people throughout their organizations with passion and purpose are far superior to what can be accomplished by getting them to be loyal followers." Leaders often overlook this factor. They can use a crisis to empower people, but building a culture that supports these values takes time, and an organization usually does not have this time during a crisis.

Senior leaders have failed to execute many excellent strategies because they did not trust employees and give them the responsibility and authority to make decisions on a day-to-day basis. In implementing a new strategy, leadership often makes the critical mistake of acting like the implementation process is centrally controlled—a level of control seldom found in an organization (Bower and Gilbert 2007). This lack of appreciation for the important role other employees play in implementing the new strategy may result from a lack of trust and respect for anyone who is not in the executive suite. No leadership team can transform an organization to a culture of quality without empowering employees. George and Sims (2007) suggest that effective leaders use the following six approaches at different times and in different ways to empower employees:

1. Show up—take the time to be there for these people
2. Engage a wide range of people—share with these people work, family, personal, and career concerns
3. Help teammates—offer suggestions or assist them with their concerns
4. Challenge leaders—ask people why they made particular decisions and engage them in a discussion to help them become better leaders
5. Stretch people—assess people and give them assignments that will help them develop and grow
6. Align everyone with a mission—show people how the organization's mission can fulfill their existing passion and drive

The ability to create a new culture of quality and implement a strategy to reinforce this culture requires sensitivity to organization history, the resistance of employees to change, and the need to empower people through passionate leadership that clearly and repeatedly communicates the new vision.

Generating Short-Term Wins

Victorious warriors win first and then go to war, while defeated warriors go to war first and then seek to win.

—Sun-Tzu

The commitment to establishing a culture that will focus on quality as its core objective is a process that takes time. As with any change that occurs slowly, people need to see their efforts are contributing to the change and making a difference. "Not all wins are equal. In general, the more visible victories are, the more they help the change process" (Kotter and Cohen 2002). If people do not identify and share wins, the risk that the change effort will lose momentum increases. Consider golf. If we didn't go to the course until we shot par, few people would ever play golf. Rather, we celebrate every small victory along the way, from a longer drive off the tee to an improved putt.

Does the need for positive reinforcement apply to people involved in a transformational effort? Employees need feedback and recognition to know that their efforts are paying a dividend and that leadership cares about their efforts. As successes are noted, the benefit of the effort becomes widespread and the desire to accelerate the change grows. A spotlight on these wins reinforces the success of the transformation effort to the guiding coalition and demonstrates to doubters that the change efforts are working.

Celebrated wins must be central to change efforts and appear genuine to employees. A critical challenge for leadership is to keep the sense of importance high in the organization. Short-term wins play a critical role in keeping the urgency level high and building momentum. Kotter (1995) takes the position that "in a successful transformation, managers actively look for ways to obtain clear performance improvements, establish goals in the yearly planning system, achieve the objectives, and reward the people involved with recognition, promotions, and even money." One argument against this approach is that some may see this added pressure as unnecessary and even harmful to the overall acceptance of the drive toward quality because many systems are not yet in place to measure the quality effort. This argument may be true, but the Japanese proverb that "pressure makes diamonds" is a reminder that urgency is useful during a transformational effort. If leadership does not maintain a sense of urgency, employees easily can stop short of executing the change to quality.

Consolidating Gains and Producing More Change

This is the power of the flywheel. Success breeds support and commitment, which breeds even greater success, which breeds more support and commitment—round and round the flywheel goes. People like to support success!
—Jim Collins

The process of effective change implementation takes years and is a time-consuming task for leadership and the guiding coalition. As mentioned earlier, people have an instinctive resistance to change, and doubters will continue to exist in the organization for months into the change process. These doubters will vocalize their concerns that leadership is "going too fast" or complain about having to focus on learning new skills with everything else they already have to do. If leadership lets these voices muffle the change effort, they can reverse gains quickly; the new behaviors that will create a culture of quality have yet to materialize.

This stage relies more on the employee empowerment efforts discussed earlier, which will expand the guiding coalition to a larger group of employees. The training and process efforts that contributed to the short-term wins should be leveraged and focused on larger projects that affect the organization more widely. The celebration of continued successes will help change employee behaviors, solidify the change, and minimize resistance. Leadership must ensure that performance expectations are realistic and fulfilled. Mankins and Steele (2005) contend that "unrealistic plans create the expectations throughout the organization that plans simply will not be fulfilled. Then, as the expectations become experience, it becomes the norm that performance commitments won't be kept." They describe this backward slide as an "insidious shift in culture" and attest that "once it takes root it is very hard to reverse."

Refreezing New Approaches in the Culture

The biggest impediment to creating change in a group is culture.
—John P. Kotter

One vital purpose of the process up to this point is to unfreeze the old culture and refreeze the new culture that has new behaviors that support quality at its core. Refreezing new behaviors and approaches in the new culture is necessary because culture drives employees who are responsible for strategy execution. The keys to solidifying the new culture are to measure the success of the strategic goals and share these data throughout the organization. Sharing data in a transparent way will help to drive the change to quality and reinforce the new behaviors that have brought about the positive results.

The challenge for the leadership team and the guiding coalition is to decide how detailed and precise the information has to be to support the change and anchor the new culture. Information paralysis is a common problem in healthcare organizations. Despite the promise of data from powerful management systems, the effective leader must act on trends rather than wait for statistical significance. Statistical significance for critical management decisions may take years to achieve. An executive who waits for perfect information may impede the change process and damage the organization's competitive position.

The powerful data systems in most hospitals churn out reams of data, but only a few pieces of information are useful in implementing improvement. Michael Lewis (2003), in his book *Moneyball*, presents the story of how the Oakland Athletics created championship baseball seasons despite having one of the lowest-salaried teams in the major league. The team's manager found that the traditional measures of batting average and home runs were not the most important in determining winning team strategy. He understood that on-base percentage was far more important than these other measures. From this new way of thinking, the Athletics were able to recruit less-expensive players with consistently high on-base percentages, who helped the team win games. This simple story demonstrates the importance of knowing the critical few measures that will drive change. Healthcare leaders can learn from this story by looking at their data in a different way. By identifying the right measures to achieve the organizational vision, executives can lead the organization to success.

Although risk does exist in making decisions without full information, top leaders use available information combined with their instincts to make decisions. Sutcliffe and Weber (2003) suggest that "the returns on accurate knowledge are initially positive, taper off, and then turn negative....The way executives interpret their business environment is more important for performance than how accurately they know their environment." The concept of leading with "good-enough information" is a challenge for executives and contradicts several research principles. However, just as a physician sees a patient and makes a reasonably accurate, but not precise, judgment on the patient's condition and offers treatment, the executive must make decisions in a timely way given the information available at the time, without procrastination.

The executive must consider the effect of decisions from all perspectives. A decision to improve financial performance may have a downstream effect on clinical quality or patient satisfaction. Similarly, a program to improve patient satisfaction may have a negative effect on the bottom line. The effective executive must quickly understand the implications of these decisions and act accordingly. Waiting for statistically significant information is not operationally feasible in the highly competitive healthcare environment. As executives ponder options and conduct further studies to make the best decisions, a competitor may have acted already and eliminated the window of opportunity.

Case Study: An Academic Medical Center's Quality Journey

This case study describes a journey that began less than 18 months ago. Because cultural changes take a long time, only a few steps in the journey have been implemented, and they have yet to affect the organization. Remember that the journey is incomplete and that the road is long, tricky, and treacherous. The final effect of the change process on the culture is still three or more years down the road. However, the story does illustrate the value of applying the change model described earlier to unfreeze a culture and the critical role of leadership in managing change.

The University of North Texas Health Science Center at Fort Worth (UNTHSC) is one of nine public health-related institutions in Texas. The initial school was chartered as the Texas College of Osteopathic Medicine (TCOM), which accepted its first students in 1970. In addition to TCOM, UNTHSC includes a physician assistant studies program; UNT Health, the entity responsible for the practice plan; the Graduate School of Biomedical Sciences; the School of Public Health; and the School of Health Professions. UNTHSC became part of the UNT system in 1999. Currently there are over 1,200 students, over 300 faculty members, and approximately 1,100 staff members.

The Health Science Center (HSC) has cultivated a successful research culture that has brought about a steady growth in research funding. In 2007, it received approximately $30 million in extramural research support. UNT Health has approximately 200 physicians who see patients in 31 clinics throughout the county as well as in the patient care center located on campus. Over

385,000 clinic visits occurred in 2007. Revenues in 2007 for UNT Health were in the region of $50 million. The HSC has long-standing ties to the community and is actively engaged in supporting annual events such as the Cowtown Marathon and delivering educational outreach programs to children in local school districts. These programs are designed to encourage young adults' interest in health and science. As a result of its research activity, the HSC has gained state and national stature and recognition in the area of medical education; TCOM has been ranked in *U.S. News and World Report*'s Top 50 Medical Schools in primary care education for seven consecutive years.

The other side of this coin is a state institution that has had its difficulties over the past decade. It has dealt with the vicissitudes of state funding and a physician practice plan that, over this same period, struggled with declining reimbursements, increased competition, and the closing of its primary teaching hospital. In addition, within the past 18 months, UNT Health has added approximately 100 physicians who had been practicing at the local county hospital. These clinicians joined UNT Health as a result of a contract dispute at the local county hospital. Many of these physicians had not been part of an academic medical center and found themselves dealing with a new and, in some instances, conflicting set of clinical, teaching, and research expectations. Finally, the School of Public Health, which had experienced tremendous growth since it became a school in 1999, started to experience declines in enrollment.

Unfreezing the Old Culture

Against this backdrop, UNTHSC charged its search committee with identifying a transformational leader who could leverage the strengths of the HSC and address the challenges the institution was facing. It hired this new president in the summer of 2006. As required by state law, the new president was an osteopathic physician but, in contrast with all previous presidents, had two additional degrees: a Master of Public Health (MPH) and a Master of Business Administration (MBA).

He arrived at the campus in July 2006, and the leadership team presented him with a strategic plan that it had completed over the past ten months. Before assuming the presidency, he had acquired an understanding of the HSC, but once on campus was able to learn firsthand and in greater depth about the overall operation of the HSC. The urgency to learn more about the academic, clinical, research, and community missions of the HSC was a function of the upcoming legislative session that was to start in January 2007 and the search committee's mandate to lead the HSC in a new direction. During this biannual legislative session, the school's budget would be determined for the next two years. The recently completed strategic plan and the rapidly approaching legislative session created a perfect stage for the president to launch his change effort.

As a result of his discussions with key HSC leaders, faculty, and staff; the chancellor of the UNT system; Board of Regents members; and community leaders, and extensive review of the academic, research, clinical, and financial picture, he determined why business as usual was not working and which areas had to change. Enrollment concerns facing the School of Public Health, the continued challenges of declining reimbursements for healthcare, increasing competitive pressures in the healthcare marketplace, increased demands for accountability, growing concerns about declining federal funding for research, and new research models that were driving funding agencies such as the National Institutes of Health all suggested that a new strategy was necessary to be successful in the future. The Board members and chancellor had recognized many of these issues and hired the new president to guide the change process. Convincing HSC senior leadership, faculty, and staff of this view was the first challenge of many that he would face over the months ahead.

The change effort required more candid discussion than in the past regarding realities such as enrollment trends, challenges facing UNT Health, and the need to measure performance and hold leadership accountable. Addressing these and other opportunities required a new focus. A commitment to four areas anchored this new focus:

1. Excellence in everything the HSC does
2. Goals determined and executed by a strategic map
3. Budgets dedicated to plan priorities
4. Accountability through measurement of results

Holding people accountable through measurement of results had not been common practice at the HSC. To support this commitment with reliable, timely, and accurate data, the Office of Strategy and Measurement (OSM), which had been called Institutional Planning and Performance Improvement, was established. The OSM was responsible for collecting, analyzing, and reporting internal and external data in support of the newly refined strategy map, metrics, and required external reporting.

At five weeks into the change process, as anticipated, many stakeholders still did not fully appreciate the sense of urgency and need for change, and the pace of change caught many administrators, faculty, and staff off guard. The Board of Regents approved the strategy map in early September, which solidified the reasons for change and the sense of urgency. The process passed the first road sign in the journey.

Forming a Powerful Guiding Coalition

Recognizing that some of his direct reports (the executive team), other key leaders (e.g., department chairs and heads), and most faculty and staff had not yet embraced the sense of urgency and the need for change, the president took a number of significant actions. First, he completely restructured his office by moving a number of staff members to different positions on the campus, hired a new executive director with an MBA, and consolidated some responsibilities among senior leaders, which caused a senior administrator to retire. This reorganization of the administration on the "eighth floor" was both symbolic and practical.

Next, he established strategic thinking councils (STCs). Each council represented one of the five mission-centric areas of the strategic map: administrative, academic, research, clinical, and community engagement. Each STC comprised key stakeholders from all levels of the organization and from across the campus. The STCs also included the president, the president's executive director, and the vice president for strategy and measurement. The STCs met monthly and were charged with examining issues that affected their area of the strategic plan, as well as obtaining input from and providing feedback to other interested persons on campus. The president's involvement in each STC communicated a consistent message about the sense of urgency and need for change.

During the fall of 2006, the STCs addressed a number of concerns and listened carefully to long-standing issues that fit under the rubric "we have always done things that way." Empowered to act by the president, one by one the STCs challenged the status quo and examined approaches and solutions that reflected the drive toward excellence. As team members saw their ideas change the way things were being done, they began to appreciate how they were affecting the existing bureaucracy directly. This process created a culture of increased participation in the change effort. When suggestions brought about significant change, team members sensed their ideas were being put into action. Welch and Byrne (2001) referred to these types of efforts as "true bureaucracy busters" because of the impact they have on the existing culture. These efforts not only challenged the status quo but also helped many members of the STCs understand the president's message regarding the need to change and the slowly evolving shared vision of the future.

An additional activity that enlarged the guiding coalition was the establishment of the leadership team, which comprised the executive team and all academic and nonacademic department heads. The purpose of this group was to communicate the vision and message of change correctly and to provide a direct line of communication about concerns and issues between the leadership team and the president. This group's first meeting was a one-day program held off campus. An outside facilitator ran the meeting, and the agenda was designed to clarify the reasons for the sense of urgency, pace of change, vision, strategic direction, and critical role the group must play in executing the new strategy. The most significant event during this meeting was a video presentation that showed the chancellor's formal introduction of the president to the public as a transformational leader. This video reinforced the president's vision of the university as a top 10 HSC and his sense of urgency. Few members of the leadership team left the meeting without a clearer sense of the importance and need to change and a better sense of how the vision would act as the lighthouse for the journey.

Along with these efforts, the president's executive team had been meeting monthly to discuss operational and strategic issues as well as the upcoming legislative session. Although the importance of change became clearer with each meeting, the executive team still needed a greater understanding of the need to change and move toward a culture of excellence. Working with each team member, the president developed a written set of performance expectations with stretch targets. These performance expectations also included appropriate team goals that reinforced the dependency among team members. Having written performance expectations was a new experience for most team members and initially met with some skepticism; they doubted the value of the approach and whether the targets were attainable. These performance expectations wove accountability into every activity of the executive team. As a result of this effort to set expectations, and other activities that required the executive team to address changes required to move forward, a member of the executive team announced his resignation from the HSC. This announcement demonstrated to the campus community that the president was serious about change. It caused many senior leaders and faculty members to examine whether they were on the right bus.

Next, accountability had to extend beyond the executive team to the entire campus community. Transparency beyond the "eighth floor" demonstrated a significant shift in culture and contributed to stakeholders' belief that business was being done in a very different way. Accountability moved beyond the eighth floor when the evaluation process for faculty and staff was reenergized. Each faculty and staff member was required to be evaluated through standardized forms developed by either a committee of faculty members or the human resources department. Faculty and staff members reacted to this evaluation with varying levels of resistance, but the requirement sent a clear message that accountability extended to every employee at the HSC and business as usual was not acceptable.

As the legislative session approached, the executive team built an agenda around what was called the Health Institutes of Texas (HIT). The idea behind HIT was that chances for funding would be increased if a unique bench-to-bedside program could be developed that would address the unmet healthcare needs of Texans. The second purpose behind HIT was to create a new organizational structure that would have at its core research programs built around interdisciplinary research teams. This model would leverage the strengths of faculty from different schools, breaking down the traditional culture of doing research encouraged by the National Institutes of Health.

Some members of the leadership team and most faculty and staff members perceived the pace of change to be rapid. In spite of this pace, few members of the executive team could argue with the fact that the efforts to date had expanded the guiding coalition, built trust, and sent the message that senior leadership accepted and encouraged new ways of doing business. Overcoming the resistance of some faculty and staff members remained a challenge, but the good news was that more senior leaders, faculty, and staff were getting on the bus.

Developing a Vision and Strategy

While the president was focusing his efforts on sharing his sense of urgency with the executive and leadership teams, a process was under way to refine the newly developed strategic plan that ultimately would drive the change process. Leadership, faculty, and staff polished the strategy map and brought about a new vision, which was "to become a top 10 health science center." This vision was consistent with the president's transformation direction and influenced the goals and tactical initiatives of the revised strategy map. In addition to the focused vision, the process clarified the mission statement and values so that they supported and aligned with the vision.

The strategy map had five central areas crucial to the mission of the HSC. One major difference in the strategic plan was that for the first time, each mission-centric area had specific and focused goals, tactical initiatives, and metrics. The metrics were developed with input from the appropriate stakeholders and the executive team. This process ensured that managers, who would be held accountable for the metrics, had ownership of the targets. Measurement with accountability meant that for the first time, the strategic plan was not a document that a senior leader would dust off once a year and use as a prop to support a presentation. Senior leaders, deans, and vice presidents clearly recognized that performance now mattered. Senior leaders understood that they would be responsible for the success or failure of their respective schools and units. To convey the importance of the change and accountability, each senior leader was responsible for creating a strategy map and action plans that would be in alignment with the HSC strategy map for their areas of responsibility. All academic and nonacademic schools and departments also were responsible for creating strategy maps and action plans. The development of strategy maps for each area of the institution required all stakeholders to think about not just what they wanted to do but how they would accomplish the activity and how they would measure their success. Strategy maps were developed within the context of a new strategic management system (SMS) built around the president's new focus. It paid particular attention to programs that would be determined and executed on the basis of strategies and budgets dedicated to planned priorities. This new SMS also focused on action and communication plans.

Communicating the Vision and Strategy

Communicating the vision and strategy relied heavily on the efforts of the president, the executive team, and the newly formed leadership team. In addition to the meetings with these groups, the president and other members of senior leadership held numerous meetings with key individuals to explain the vision and strategy. Some of these meetings were formal, whereas others were spontaneous, occurring in the hallway or elevator. They overlooked no opportunity to beat the drum of change.

They used a number of approaches to engage faculty and staff. Starting in early January, they scheduled town hall meetings with all employees. These meetings were held after each Board of Regents meeting, giving the president the opportunity to share what was presented at the most recent meeting and to answer questions that faculty and staff had about campus activities. Normally, they scheduled three meetings during the day to accommodate the various staff schedules. They paid particular attention to the schedules of clinical faculty and staff. These meetings always included a presentation on quarterly metrics, progress on the new strategy, and the rapidly evolving master plan for the campus. Although attendance was limited, questions were often provocative and reflected a growing interest in the president's change efforts. These meetings communicated the new vision and strategy and addressed the latest rumors concerning the change.

Another communication effort revolved around the revision of the *Campus Connection*, which was the campus's main communication vehicle. This online publication focused on a number of critical issues affecting the campus community (e.g., the campus master plan) and always included a column by the president. Key leaders selectively highlighted vision and strategy in many of the issues, and with each issue, a growing number of faculty and staff became regular readers.

Effective leaders in change communication must eliminate the "we versus them" mentality and work toward expanding the guiding coalition. This tactic is particularly useful when dealing with medical staff. HSC physicians were not a homogenous group and could not be represented by one common voice. The president was careful not to assume that the physicians would agree with both the vision and strategic direction. He engaged physicians and their key leaders in direct and open discussion about the new direction and vision for the HSC and the expectations he had about their clinical, educational, and research roles.

Recognizing the importance of changing the culture, the executive team decided in early spring to assess the HSC culture with the use of the Denison Organizational Culture Survey (Denison and Mishra 1995). TCOM and the School of Public Health had used this survey in the past, but the rest of the faculty and staff had never completed it. This survey examines four elements of culture, with three indices for each area. The cultural elements are:

1. mission, which includes vision, goals and objectives, and strategic direction;
2. involvement, which examines empowerment, team orientation, and capability development;
3. adaptability, which includes questions about creating change, customer focus, and organizational learning; and
4. consistency, which includes core values, agreement, coordination, and integration.

Not surprisingly, the overall result left room for improvement, but the area that had the highest results was mission, with vision having the highest score. The area of consistency followed, with core values having the highest score. All faculty and staff received the results of the Denison survey, and departments were challenged to examine the opportunities the results presented in their areas. These data demonstrated that the message of vision was taking hold but that much work remained in creating the new culture.

Another effort was to brand UNT Health. This branding effort was designed to create an identity in the community for the clinical services provided by UNT Health physicians. This campaign included UNT's first billboards and new marketing collaterals, including a physician directory. This marketing campaign coincided with a focus on improving patient satisfaction and access to care through patient satisfaction surveys and creation of a call center, which were central elements to becoming a provider of choice. These quality improvement efforts linked directly to the vision of becoming excellent in all areas of performance and one of the top 10. This branding effort also benefited the clinicians who were central to driving change in clinical care.

The newly expanded and reenergized marketing and communications department coordinated a number of other efforts, including an annual HSC golf tournament, the Campus Pride Campaign, the restructuring of the UNTHSC Foundation Board, and revision of the faculty bylaws, which it carried out in a very deliberate way, engaging stakeholders and ensuring effective communication of the new vision and direction. Before the president's arrival, this department had minimal staff and budget support. As the marketing and communication team gained momentum, the message of change was becoming clearer and more people, both inside and outside the organization, were starting to hear and understand the message.

Although the change was moving forward, a small number of faculty members chose to leave the institution. Reasons for their departure varied. Comments by those who still doubted the need for change—that the departure of faculty was a direct result of the change to a culture of higher standards and quality—were hard to overcome. The departures affected the medical school faculty the most, who, more than other faculty, was feeling added pressure to increase its clinical revenues. In most cases, individuals who left the faculty either were advancing their careers by assuming administrative positions (e.g., dean) or recognized that the emerging culture was not a good fit for their behaviors and career expectations.

Empowering Employees to Act on the Vision and Strategy

Strategy execution was completely dependent on faculty and staff empowerment to act on the vision and strategy. The previous culture had relied heavily on centralized control, specifically in the areas of finance and budgets. Most faculty members are highly motivated and productive individuals who enjoy working in higher education because this environment allows them to exercise a level of professional freedom found in few other work situations.

All the efforts to date were designed to align everyone with the vision and strategy map, but one critical element was missing. Traditionally, the deans and vice presidents controlled departmental budgets. Department chairs and unit heads, who had the greatest impact on implementation, had no real control over or accountability for their budgets. The president, with the support of the executive team and the budget office, decided to expand budget management and accountability from the deans and vice presidents to the chairs and unit heads of each department. This process required a significant number of changes in how the budget accounts were set up and reported. During this shift in responsibility, the president and executive team decided to eliminate deficit spending in all accounts. This decision required account holders to alter a long-standing practice of the old culture that deflected accountability. This change challenged many senior leaders to learn new financial skills and cemented transparency and accountability, values central to the new culture. This change paved the way for additional financial accountability and responsibility, which was assigned to senior leaders during the fiscal year 2008 budgetary process that occurred in the summer of 2007. These additional change efforts converted many chairs and department heads, but a number of doubters remained in the organization.

Generating Short-Term Wins

The wave of change was evident across the campus, and the time had come to celebrate some of the successes. Because the change was less than eight months old, identifying specific improvements was difficult, although many activities were under way that had broad-based support. The Denison results dealing with vision and values were encouraging, but the effects of the changes on the everyday lives of faculty, staff, and students were not yet fully evident.

The president and the executive team planned the HSC's first employee appreciation lunch. On the day of the lunch, the president delivered onetime bonus checks to eligible staff members. Although the lunch did not celebrate a specific win, it championed the most important asset of the HSC—its faculty and staff and their efforts over the past eight months to create a new culture and become a top 10 HSC. The lunch, served by the executive team, was a success and demonstrated the value that leadership placed on faculty and staff. The other significance of the lunch was the number of people who attended. The members of the expanded guiding coalition could see that more faculty and staff were beginning to appreciate their efforts in bringing about a new culture that valued transparency, accountability, and excellence. During the lunch and for weeks afterward, faculty and staff expressed their appreciation to the president and many senior leaders and endorsed the efforts to improve the HSC. As successful as this appreciation lunch was, the real work of solidifying the new culture and executing the strategic direction still had a long way to go.

Consolidating Gains and Producing More Change

A discipline was established to collect, analyze, and share information about the strategy map and metrics. Early in the process, it recognized that reliable, transparent data were essential to refreeze the new culture, drive the change process, and support new behaviors. It limited the metrics for each mission-centric area to three or fewer critical measures. It saw these metrics as being measurable and understandable to all stakeholders, and the executive team accepted them as credible indicators of the success or failure of the strategy. The metrics were imperfect but represented a good balance of what was obtainable, measurable, and "good enough" to drive the change process.

When the foundation established the metrics, some members of the team felt there should have been more. This view was prevalent in the development of strategy maps at the levels of schools and departments. Because the entire strategic management process was new to so many people, the foundation decided not to let perfect be the enemy of good during the development of the strategy maps and corresponding metrics. Wherever possible, it took great pains to ensure alignment of the strategy maps and metrics. It set realistic stretch targets for all the metrics, and the executive team, which was responsible for ensuring that these targets were met, generally felt comfortable with them. The foundation collected and reported the metrics on a quarterly basis and shared them with the Board of Regents and all faculty and staff during the quarterly town hall meetings. It posted the results on the HSC website and on a quality wall maintained on the campus. Everyone saw the impact of setting targets, holding people accountable for achieving results, and sharing information in a transparent way as positive. This effort contributed to the establishment of new behavioral patterns that will drive the change process toward the goal of becoming a top 10 HSC.

Refreezing New Approaches in the Culture

In summary, the HSC has started down a new path and is in the process of creating a new culture. It has laid a solid foundation for this new culture, but status as a top 10 HSC is far from certain. Refreezing these new behaviors and processes will depend on successful execution by the leadership team and an increasing number of employees. As the HSC addresses new and larger change projects, it must continue to share results to enforce the desired new behaviors. As it begins its next leg of the journey, it is paying particular attention to expansion of the leadership team, the skills that team members need to understand their leadership styles, the importance of teamwork, and the management of data-driven change. One thing is certain—hard work and many surprises lie ahead.

Conclusion

Changing the culture of a healthcare organization to one that has quality improvement at its core is a demanding, time-consuming, challenging task for senior leadership. This journey of change requires a road map that recognizes the significant role of leadership and the influence culture has on employee behavior and performance. This chapter provided a practical road map for change and an example of how one health science center applied this road map.

Many lessons are still to be learned from this journey, which will unfold over the next few years. Implementing a culture of excellence has many different stories, each with a different starting point (Kotter and Cohen 2002; Stubblefield 2005). These stories share a comment element: the importance of courageous, principled, effective leadership. Anyone starting a journey or already on the road to quality must remember that there is no substitute for the guidance of experienced leadership. Faced with the state of healthcare organizations today and the approaching demographic tidal wave, we must start creating organizations that have quality at their core and do a better job of balancing cash and care. Good luck on your journey.

Study Questions

1. Did the new president of UNTHSC take the necessary steps to unfreeze the old culture?
2. How should the leadership team build a sense of trust that will support the vision of becoming a top 10 HSC?
3. What activities could the executive team initiate that would empower more faculty and staff to act on the strategy?

4. What are the most critical steps in refreezing the new culture, and who should be responsible for these steps?

Notes

1. See IOM's website at www.iom.edu.
2. See the group's website at www.leapfroggroup.org.
3. See IHI's website at www.ihi.org.
4. See NQF's website at www.qualityforum.org.
5. For more information, see www.qualitylongtermcarecommission.org.
6. See the Brookings Institution's website at www.Brookings.edu.
7. See the Commonwealth Fund's website at www.commonwealthfund.org.
8. See www.rwjf.org for more information.
9. See RAND Corporation's website at www.rand.org.
10. For more information, see www.healthtransformation.net.

References

Andrews, R. M., and A. Elixhauser. 2007. "The National Hospital Bill: Growth Trends and 2005 Update on the Most Expensive Conditions by Payer." *Healthcare Cost and Utilization Project*, December. [Online information; retrieved 4/11/08.] http://ahrq.hhs.gov/data/hcup/.

Atchison, T. A., and J. S. Bujak. 2001. *Leading Transformational Change: The Physician-Executive Partnership*. Chicago: Health Administration Press.

Baldrige National Quality Program. 2007. "Health Care Criteria for Performance Excellence." [Online information; retrieved 4/11/08.] www.quality.nist.gov/HealthCare_Criteria.htm.

Bower, J. L., and C. G. Gilbert. 2007. "How Managers' Everyday Decisions Create—or Destroy—Your Company's Strategy." *Harvard Business Review* 85 (2): 72–79, 154.

Collins, J. 2001. *Good to Great: Why Some Companies Make the Leap...and Others Don't*. New York: Harper Collins.

Denison, D. R., and A. K. Mishra. 1995. "Toward a Theory of Organizational Culture and Effectiveness." *Organization Science* 6 (2): 204–23.

George, B. 2003. *Authentic Leadership: Rediscovering the Secrets to Creating Lasting Value*. New York: Wiley.

George, B., and P. Sims. 2007. *True North: Discover Your Authentic Leadership*. New York: Wiley.

Hamm, J. 2006. "The Five Messages Leaders Must Manage." *Harvard Business Review* 84 (5): 114–23, 158.

Herzlinger, R. 2007. *Who Killed Health Care?* New York: McGraw-Hill.

Kaplan, R. S., and D. P. Norton. 2001. *The Strategy Focused Organization*. Cambridge, MA: Harvard Business School Press.

Kotter, J. P. 1995. "Leading Change: Why Transformation Efforts Fail." *Harvard Business Review* (March): 58–67.

———. 1996. *Leading Change*. Cambridge, MA: Harvard Business School Press.

Kotter, J. P., and D. S. Cohen. 2002. *The Heart of Change*. Cambridge, MA: Harvard Business School Press.

Kotter, J. P., and J. L. Heskett. 1992. *Corporate Culture and Performance*. New York: Free Press.

Lewis, M. 2003. *Moneyball*. New York: W. W. Norton.

Mankins, M. C., and R. Steele. 2005. "Turning Great Strategy into Great Performance." *Harvard Business Review* 83 (7): 64–72, 191.

Maslow, A. H. 1943. "A Theory of Human Motivation." *Psychological Review* (July): 370–96.

Porter, M. E. 1985. *Competitive Advantage: Creating and Sustaining Superior Performance*. New York: Free Press.

———. 1996. "What Is Strategy?" *Harvard Business Review* 74 (6): 61–78.

Porter, M. E., and E. O. Teisberg. 2004. "Redefining Competition in Health Care." *Harvard Business Review* 82 (6): 64–76, 136.

Ransom, S. B., J. Tropman, and W. W. Pinsky. 2001. *Enhancing Physician Performance*. Tampa, FL: American College of Physician Executives Press.

Rooke, D., and W. R. Torbert. 2005. "Seven Transformations of Leadership." *Harvard Business Review* 83 (4): 66–76, 133.

Schein, E. H. 2002. "Models and Tools for Stability and Change in Human Systems." *Reflections* 4 (2): 34–46.

Schoen, C., R. Osborn, M. M. Doty, M. Bishop, J. Peugh, and N. Murukutla. 2007. "Toward Higher-Performance Health Systems: Adults' Health Care Experiences in Seven Countries." *Health Affairs* 26 (6): w717–w734.

Stubblefield, A. 2005. *The Baptist Health Care Journey to Excellence: Creating a Culture That WOWs!* New York: Wiley.

Sutcliffe, K. M., and K. Weber. 2003. "The High Cost of Accurate Knowledge." *Harvard Business Review* 81 (5): 74–82.

Welch, J., and J. A. Byrne. 2001. *Jack: Straight from the Gut*. New York: Warner Books.

IMPLEMENTING HEALTHCARE QUALITY IMPROVEMENT: CHANGING CLINICIAN BEHAVIOR

Valerie Weber and John Bulger

Mastery of change implementation skills is essential for current and future healthcare leaders. Without a solid knowledge of change management, healthcare leaders will not be able to improve the quality of healthcare in their organizations at the rate needed to bring about substantial improvement. In the field of healthcare quality, often the lack of both leadership for change management and focus on implementation, not weak initiatives, has slowed progress.

Another important aspect of healthcare change management is understanding how physicians behave with respect to quality improvement initiatives and the adoption of best practices. This knowledge is necessary to implement strategies effectively and to prevent repeated failure of new initiatives.

Understanding Change Management in Healthcare

Healthcare has undergone a more dramatic technological explosion in the past few decades than perhaps any other industry, yet our healthcare organizations have not reacted with the same speed and agility to improve quality processes and decrease error as have other industries, such as airlines or manufacturing. Motorola, Allied Signal, and other manufacturers have made great strides in Six Sigma quality programs. In contrast, many healthcare organizations are still approaching patient care using the same outmoded paradigms they have used for decades, despite their tendency to be inefficient and error prone. The ability to embrace change will be the distinguishing feature of the successful healthcare organization—and the successful healthcare leader—in the twenty-first century.

No matter how well a system or solution is conceived, designed, and executed, if people do not like it, it will fail. Conversely, no matter how poorly a system or solution is conceived, designed, and executed, if people want it to work, it will succeed (Shays 2003). The goal of the change leader is to create well-designed solutions that will gain wide acceptance.

Diffusion of Innovations and Other Change Theories

How do some new ideas in healthcare, such as a new drug or treatment, gain broad acceptance, whereas other ideas that present an equally strong—or even stronger—case for change never catch on? An often-cited example in healthcare is the use of laparoscopic surgery. Within a few years of its invention, it became widely used and is now considered the standard approach for most routine surgery. However, simpler innovations, such as the use of beta-blockers and aspirin after myocardial infarction, for which strong evidence of their value has been available for years, are still not widely used.

The science of innovation diffusion focuses on the rate at which change spreads and can help to explain these differences. These theories center on three basic themes: the perception of the innovation; characteristics of the people who choose to adopt or not adopt an innovation; and context, that is, how the change is communicated and led (Berwick 2003).

How an innovation is perceived is an important predictor of the rate at which the variation will spread. Why do certain innovations spread more quickly than others? The characteristics that determine an innovation's rate of adoption are relative advantage, compatibility, complexity, trial-ability, and observability.

- *Relative advantage* is the degree to which the innovation is seen as better than the convention it replaces. The greater the perceived relative advantage of an innovation, the more rapid its rate of adoption will be. In medicine, the decision to adopt a new idea usually results from a risk-benefit calculation made by the individual physician. For example, most physicians will make the decision to try a new medication by weighing its efficacy against the need for monitoring, potential side effects, and cost. A physician will prescribe a new medication if it is cheaper, is easier for the patient to take (e.g., once a day as opposed to multiple doses), is safer, or requires less monitoring.
- *Compatibility* is the degree to which potential adopters perceive the innovation as being consistent with their values, past experiences, and needs. It is less risky to try a new drug that is similar to one a physician has tried with success in the past. There is a plethora of drugs on the market that are similar to other drugs. These drugs are easy to introduce successfully into the market because of the compatibility factor.
- *Complexity* is the perception of the ease of the innovation's application. The simpler the change is, the more likely it is to take root. Again, using a medication example, physicians are unlikely to try a new drug if they must write a letter to a health maintenance organization (HMO) for approval because the drug is not on that HMO's formulary. This

requirement would make trying the new drug more complex and make its use unlikely.

- *Trial-ability* implies that the innovation can be used on a trial basis before deciding to adopt it and enhances the perception that trying the innovation is low risk. Availability of a medication to physicians in a trial form (pharmaceutical sampling) increases the likelihood that the physician will adopt it.
- *Observability* is the ease with which a potential adopter can view others trying the change first. Pharmaceutical companies, in marketing new drugs to physicians and patients, use the observability and trial-ability concepts extensively. The use of in-office pharmaceutical samples decreases complexity, increases trial-ability and observability, and allows for compatibility once the physician experiences success with the new drug.

Social science helps us understand how individual characteristics of the members of a social group aid the spread of an innovation. Everett Rogers's (1995) theory of innovation diffusion explains that any innovation within a social group is adopted over time by a process he terms *natural diffusion*. These processes were first described by a group of Iowa farmers adopting a new form of hybrid seed corn. Over time, this theory has become recognized as applicable to any institution, societal fad, or organization, including healthcare.

A few adopters, whom Rogers terms *innovators*, who are excited by change and cope well with uncertainty, generally initiate the change process. They often perform a gatekeeping role for the introduction of new ideas into a system. Although this role is important, the rest of the group generally regards innovators as somewhat radical; innovators do not help the majority of the group to enact an innovation but rather are the first to introduce it.

The next, and most important, group of individuals to adopt an innovation is the *early adopters*. This group includes the opinion leaders. Others look to these individuals for guidance about the innovation. They often are the informal leaders and decrease uncertainty about the innovation by networking with their peers.

Innovations generally begin to spread when members of the early majority, hearing from satisfied adopters of the new idea, begin to create a critical mass for change. The late majority eventually will follow the lead of others after increasing pressure from their peers. The laggards, the last group of individuals in a system to adopt, remain suspicious of change agents and innovations. They tend to be socially isolated and resist change efforts. These groups tend to be represented in a social group over a normal distribution (see Figure 16.1).

The rate of diffusion of innovations has much to do with organizational context, that is, the characteristics of an organization's culture that

FIGURE 16.1

Rogers's
Adopter
Categories
Based on
Degree of
Innovativeness

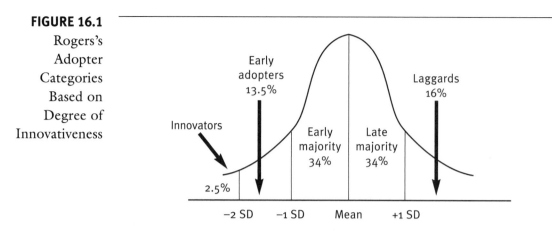

Time to Adoption (Standard Deviations [SD] from Mean)

tend to support (or discourage) innovation and spread. Clear goal setting; strong support from physicians, nurses, and administrative staff; and the use of high-quality feedback data are important factors contributing to success (Bradley et al. 2001).

In his book *The Tipping Point*, Malcolm Gladwell (2000) makes several observations regarding change that organization leaders may find useful. Some ideas, behaviors, and products start epidemics, whereas others do not. The tipping point is that moment of critical mass, a threshold or boiling point for change with three identified agents, including the law of the few, the stickiness factor, and the power of context.

The *law of the few* describes three types of people critical to spreading epidemics—connectors, mavens, and salesmen. *Connectors* are important for both the numbers and kinds of people they know. They maintain this high connectedness by spanning many different worlds. The connectors use the power of weak ties (i.e., word of mouth) to spread ideas that impress them. Other key individuals, called *mavens,* have a talent for accumulating and passing on knowledge. *Salesmen* help create epidemics through their power to persuade others. Acting in concert, these individuals can spread an innovation rapidly. The implication is that the identification of these individuals in an organization enables them to be enlisted as champions of the change process.

The *stickiness factor* relates to the innovation or characteristics of the message itself that determine the rapidity with which an innovation or change "tips" (Gladwell 2000). Anything a change agent can do to enhance the "stickiness" of the message will increase the rate at which the change will tip.

The power of context again addresses the framework for delivery of the message. Gladwell (2000) discusses what he calls the *broken-window theory*: "If a window is broken and left unrepaired, people walking by will conclude that no one cares . . . soon more windows will be broken and the sense of anarchy will spread from the building to the street on which it faces." His statement implies that quality initiatives will be received more effectively in a healthcare organization that has a pervasive background of quality.

Physician-Specific Research

To implement changes in healthcare quality successfully, we must understand how and why physicians change. A behavioral study targeted at general practitioners in London showed that rarely did a single trigger for behavior change exist, but rather an accumulation of evidence that change was possible, desirable, and worthwhile. These cues came from educational interactions in some cases, but more often from contact with professional colleagues, particularly those who were especially influential or respected (Armstrong, Reyburn, and Jones 1996). When enough of these cues accumulated, the behavior would change (accumulation model). Furthermore, only a limited number of changes could be made over a fixed amount of time—on average three to four changes over a six-month period.

At other times, though, changes occurred abruptly when an immediate challenge arose; the authors term this phenomenon the *challenge model of change*. One particularly strong source of influence was the practitioner's personal experience of a drug or an illness. Another was a clinical disaster, or a negative outcome that tended to change the practitioner's prescribing behavior abruptly. A patient's experience with a particularly serious or life-threatening side effect could cause a physician to discontinue a medication's use.

The *continuity model of change* describes how sometimes practitioners change readily on the basis of a level of preparedness for a particular change (e.g., the provider was waiting for a more acceptable treatment because of the current treatment's difficulty of use or cost). The strongest reinforcer of continuing change is patients' feedback. A patient's positive report reinforces the behavior change; conversely, a negative result, such as a major side effect, is often enough to stop the experiment. In the initial stages of the change, high risk of reverting to the original prescribing pattern exists.

Although many clinicians espouse evidence-based medicine—which emphasizes the importance of proving effectiveness in large numbers of patients—in this study, most physicians seemed to base prescription changes on the results of a few initial experiments with a small number of patients (Armstrong, Reyburn, and Jones 1996). Most changes required a period of preparation through education and contact with opinion leaders. Educational efforts were necessary, but by no means sufficient, to produce the needed change.

Physicians often fail to comply with best practices. One study analyzed self-reports by physicians explaining why in particular instances, after chart review, they did not follow best practices for diabetes, such as screening for microalbuminuria, hyperlipidemia, and retinopathy. Reasons included inadequate oversight (it slipped through the cracks), system issues, and patient nonadherence, but in a surprising number of cases, physicians made a conscious decision not to comply with the recommendation (Mottur-Pilson, Snow, and Bartlett 2001). Individual physicians often balk at the idea of practice guidelines as "cookbook medicine." Many physicians view themselves as craftsmen or artists and consider individual variation as acceptable or even desirable. Scrutiny of physicians' practices by the government, third-party payers, and consumers has increased. From this perspective, lack of championing by the medical profession, although improved in recent years, has clearly slowed the pace of change in the quality improvement movement.

Leading Change

Change within organizations cannot occur in the absence of skilled leadership. Among its many definitions, leadership has been described as "a set of processes that creates organizations . . . or adapts them to significantly changing circumstances. Leadership defines what the future should look like, aligns people with that vision, and inspires them to make it happen, despite the obstacles" (Kotter 1996). Many feel that leadership is entirely about creating change. Managers create order and predictability, whereas leaders establish direction and motivate and inspire people. Although both management and leadership are necessary, change depends on skilled leadership.

Reinertsen (1998) describes leaders as "initiators" who "define reality, often with data . . . they develop and test changes, persuade others, are not daunted by the loud, negative voices, and are not afraid to think and work outside their immediate areas of responsibility." Similarly, Kotter (1996) has proposed a road map to create change that includes establishment of a sense of urgency, creation of a guiding coalition, creation of a vision, effective communication of the vision, and creation of short-term wins to show success can be achieved (see Figure 16.2).

Leaders of change find it necessary to remove structural barriers to ensure that the needed changes are possible. For example, if time resources are an issue, it may be necessary to dedicate a percentage of time to key employees to direct quality initiatives or to restructure reward and incentive systems to promote quality improvement. Increasingly, physicians are taking on leadership roles; these roles are important in serving as boundary spanners to champion quality initiatives in healthcare (Zuckerman et al. 1998). Developing this leadership within healthcare organizations is key to maximizing cooperative leadership between physicians and administration.

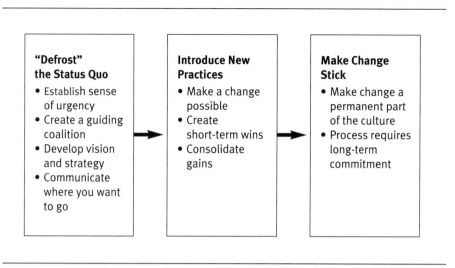

SOURCE: © Joint Commission Resources: "Effecting and Leading Change in Health Care Organizations." *Joint Commission Journal on Quality Improvement* Volume 26(7): 388–399, 2000. Reprinted with permission.

FIGURE 16.2
Kotter's Stages of Creating Major Change

Reducing Variation: The Example of Clinical Practice Guidelines

Large variations in standards of care exist for many healthcare conditions. Studies (Jencks, Huff, and Cuerdon 2003) have demonstrated that higher healthcare expenditures in Medicare populations have not resulted in better quality, increased access to services, improved satisfaction, or better health outcomes. Underuse, overuse, and misuse abound in U.S. medicine (Chassin 1998).

Industry, however, has achieved quality by reducing variation. The clinical practice guideline movement was born from this concept in the last decades of the twentieth century.

Since the 1980s, the knowledge base required to practice high-quality medicine has increased dramatically. Each month, thousands of articles in medical literature can result in practice changes. The clinical practice guideline movement aims to translate the medical literature into concise statements meant to change practice. This translation is especially important when one considers that 50 percent of the knowledge physicians learn becomes obsolete within five to ten years after their training.

By 1995, more than 60 organizations in at least ten countries were producing clinical practice guidelines (Rogers 1995). Although this movement continues, observations show that its basic mission has been unsuccessful. Clinical guidelines are gathering dust on every clinician's bookshelf because of a lack of attention to implementation.

During the development of most guidelines, data are synthesized from the literature by the sponsoring body, often a national specialty organization. Experts review the quality of the evidence and then collate the information as guidelines. Although these guidelines are widely available, most practitioners are not using them in everyday practice. Why not? A number of possible reasons have been proposed.

First, some qualities of the guidelines themselves may influence their adoption by clinicians. In the implementation of disease management strategies, clinicians insist that they (1) be simple, (2) be practical, and (3) not increase their or their staff's workload. The less complicated the guideline is, the more compatible the recommendation will be with existing beliefs or values; the easier the guideline is to use, the more likely it is to be adopted. Other variables, such as the characteristics of the healthcare professional (age and country of training in particular), characteristics of the practice setting, and use of incentives and imposed regulations, also can influence a guideline's adoption. A review by Cabana et al. (1999) discussed other barriers to guideline implementation, including physician knowledge (e.g., lack of awareness and familiarity), attitudes (e.g., lack of agreement, self-efficacy, and outcome expectancy; inertia of previous practice), and behavior (e.g., external barriers) (see Figure 16.3).

One report studied the use of a pneumonia practice guideline in an emergency department. The authors report influence of a variety of patient factors, including age greater than 65, comorbidities, and social factors. Physician factors also affected adherence to guidelines; most notably, the more experience the physician had in treating pneumonia, the less likely the physician was to follow the guideline (Halm et al. 2000).

Active Implementation Strategies

Greco and Eisenberg (1993) note that, at times, changes in medical practice are rapid and dramatic, as with the replacement of many open surgical procedures with laparoscopic procedures in the span of just a few years, and, at other times, slow to proceed, as with the use of beta-blockers for patients after myocardial infarction. Continuing medical education (CME) is most often used to attempt to improve the dissemination of new medical knowledge, yet this approach has consistently been shown to have little effect on performance or health outcomes (Davis 1998). In particular, most studies that used only printed materials failed to demonstrate changes in performance or health outcomes, a finding that also has been associated with the distribution of guidelines (Oxman et al. 1995). Similarly, conferences, particularly those during which no explicit effort was made to facilitate practice change, failed to demonstrate change in performance or health outcomes. More interactive workshops have demonstrated some positive, but overall mixed, results. One publication demonstrated that the exposure of Canadian family practice physicians to a 90-minute workshop on the ordering of preventive tests

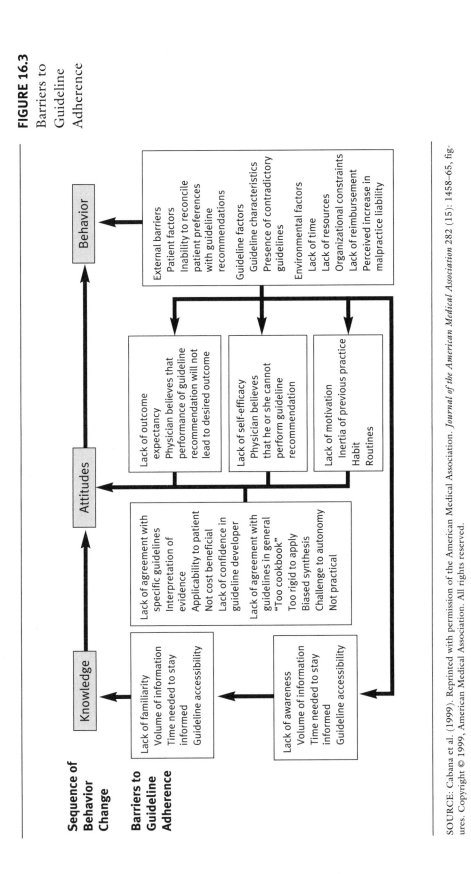

FIGURE 16.3
Barriers to
Guideline
Adherence

**Sequence of
Behavior
Change**

Knowledge → Attitudes → Behavior

**Barriers to
Guideline
Adherence**

Lack of familiarity
Volume of information
Time needed to stay
informed
Guideline accessibility

Lack of awareness
Volume of information
Time needed to stay
informed
Guideline accessibility

Lack of agreement with
specific guidelines
Interpretation of
evidence
Applicability to patient
Not cost beneficial
Lack of confidence in
guideline developer
Lack of agreement with
guidelines in general
"Too cookbook"
Too rigid to apply
Biased synthesis
Challenge to autonomy
Not practical

Lack of outcome
expectancy
Physician believes that
performance of guideline
recommendation will not
lead to desired outcome

Lack of self-efficacy
Physician believes
that he or she cannot
perform guideline
recommendation

Lack of motivation
Inertia of previous practice
Habit
Routines

External barriers
Patient factors
Inability to reconcile
patient preferences
with guideline
recommendations

Guideline factors
Guideline characteristics
Presence of contradictory
guidelines

Environmental factors
Lack of time
Lack of resources
Organizational constraints
Lack of reimbursement
Perceived increase in
malpractice liability

SOURCE: Cabana et al. (1999). Reprinted with permission of the American Medical Association. *Journal of the American Medical Association* 282 (15): 1458–65, figures. Copyright © 1999, American Medical Association. All rights reserved.

did not increase the ordering of items recommended for inclusion but did decrease unnecessary test ordering (Beaulieu et al. 2002).

Other, more active strategies of diffusing medical knowledge have shown more promise. The use of opinion leaders, locally influential physicians whose opinions hold sway with their peers, has been shown to be effective in improving outcomes (Davis 1998). Other studies have shown that the recruitment of these leaders to disseminate information via local implementation of clinical practice guidelines can change prescribing patterns and health outcomes effectively (Davis 1998).

A strategy termed *academic detailing*, which involves outreach visits to a practice site by opinion leaders, has been found to be effective in accelerating the dissemination of best practices. This strategy was modeled on the methods of pharmaceutical sales representatives, who have trained physicians or pharmacists to deliver one-on-one education or feedback sessions. Evidence from controlled trials shows that academic detailing alters prescribing, affects blood pressure product transfusion practices, and improves hypertension control (Goldberg et al. 1998). These studies suggest that, although the content of the guidelines is indeed important, the presentation of the guidelines is critical to their acceptance. Guidelines distributed in a poor format—such as mass mailings, didacticism, and CME—were not accepted as well as guidelines distributed through proven methods such as academic detailing and the use of opinion leaders.

The use of reminders involves interventions (manual or computerized) that prompt the healthcare provider to perform a clinical action. Examples include concurrent or intervisit reminders to professionals regarding follow-up appointments or enhanced laboratory reports, or administrative systems that can prompt these reminders. These methods are moderately effective in some settings (Oxman et al. 1995).

Audit and feedback systems provide clinicians with information comparing their practices and outcomes with those of other physicians in their group or an external benchmark. The use of these methods has resulted in decreased laboratory ordering (Ramoska 1998), increased compliance with preventive care and cancer-screening guidelines (Mandelblatt and Kanetsky 1995), and more appropriate drug-prescribing behavior (Schectman et al. 1995).

Administrative interventions that control test ordering have been shown to be effective in various settings. For example, evidence shows that simple modifications to laboratory order forms or changes to funding policy decrease the use of certain laboratory studies (Van Walraven, Goel, and Chan 1998).

The use of continuous quality improvement teams also has been described. Practice sites are trained in quality improvement techniques, including the Plan-Do-Study-Act (PDSA) methodology. Although healthcare has shown a great deal of enthusiasm for the adoption of Six Sigma methodology, which details initiatives for quality improvement in industry, the success of such strategies in healthcare has a limited track record. One report using local team-based quality improvement practices found variable success in improving guideline conformity but increased effectiveness when used in conjunction with other techniques such as academic detailing (Goldberg et al. 1998).

The use of multifaceted interventions, including combinations of audit and feedback, reminders, academic detailing, and opinion leaders, has demonstrated changes in professional performance and, less consistently, changes in health outcomes. A systematic review of interventions intended to change clinician behavior found that 62 percent of interventions aimed at one behavioral factor were successful in changing behavior, whereas 86 percent of interventions targeted at two or more behavioral factors reported success (Solomon et al. 1998). Healthcare leaders must combine strategies to produce effects that are cumulative and significant (see Figure 16.4).

The 100,000 Lives Campaign, sponsored and implemented in a variety of hospital systems by the Institute for Healthcare Improvement from 2004 through 2006, provides a robust example of how combined implementation strategies can improve performance. The campaign led efforts focused on improving patient safety in hospitals, including the prevention of ventilator-associated pneumonia, catheter-associated sepsis, and other initiatives. In this program, an interdisciplinary team, led by physician opinion leaders with multidisciplinary representation, first obtained data on performance and communicated the shortfalls within the organization. Using PDSA cycles and other well-established implementation strategies, the team then worked to create sustained changes. This program was successful at many organizations, and many U.S. hospitals have adopted its interventions as expected standards of care (Gosfield and Reinertsen 2005).

Decision Support/Informatics

The use of reminder systems has long been suggested as a method of increasing clinicians' adherence to guidelines. Many early studies used manual chart review strategies that provided reminders to physicians during their office visits. Such strategies included chart stickers or tags, medical record checklists, flowsheets, and nurse-initiated reminders. Patient-directed reminders also have been used, including letters, telephone calls, and questionnaires. Proven efficacy exists for many of these interventions (McPhee et al. 1991). Limitations of these efforts center on the labor-intensive nature of these processes and the inability to sustain them over time.

Information technology and electronic medical records (EMRs) promise to streamline this process. Beginning in the early 1990s, computerized reminder systems began to appear. Early trials showed significant performance differences in cancer prevention (McPhee et al. 1991).

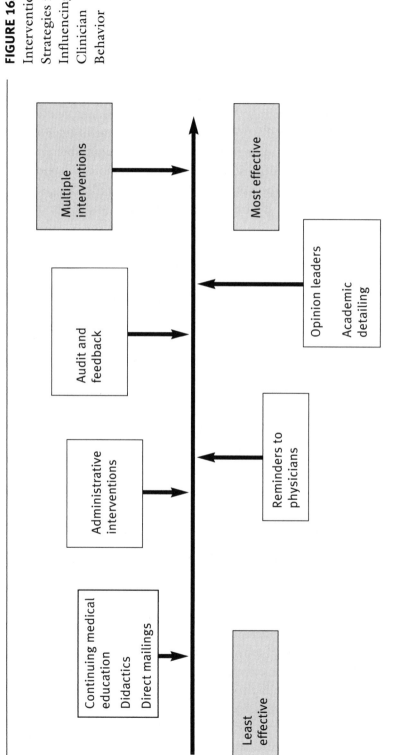

FIGURE 16.4
Intervention Strategies for Influencing Clinician Behavior

Subsequent trials demonstrated that computerized reminders can increase the performance of preventive care activities in hospitalized patients (Dexter et al. 2001) and improve adherence to guidelines for the prophylaxis of deep venous thrombosis (Durieux et al. 2000). More recent work has shown that the use of informatics-based interventions can improve the use of statin drugs for the secondary prevention of coronary disease (Lester et al. 2006) and reduce polypharmacy and falls in the elderly (Weber, White, and McIlvried 2008). Most computer-based interventions in the literature are either computer-prompted reminders to physicians that usually occur during visits or online guidelines available to physicians on the EMR.

For EMRs to live up to this early promise, however, much work will need to be done to understand which uses of the EMR improve care the most, taking into account issues such as the preservation of work flows and physician autonomy (Lester et al. 2006). For example, busy physicians usually ignore reminders occurring at the wrong time during a clinical encounter.

Recent work on the interface of chronic disease management and information technology focuses on the use of computerized chronic disease registries, which shifts the attention from what is occurring in individualized patient visits to strategies that allow for enhanced management of populations. For example, many EMRs identify patients with important conditions, such as diabetes, hypertension, asthma, or congestive heart failure. Patients whose care does not conform to best practice guidelines then can be pulled in for various interventions by other members of the healthcare team (with physician consent), or, alternatively, the registry information can be fed back to the physicians for action (Hunt et al. 2001). Such approaches have demonstrated improvements in chronic disease management (Weber et al. 2008).

EMRs also can influence physician behavior through more advanced decision support systems. Thus far, computerized test ordering systems with embedded clinical practice guidelines have demonstrated the ability to reduce laboratory test ordering by primary care physicians (Van Wijk et al. 2001) and increase the use of aspirin in patients with coronary artery disease in the outpatient setting (Walker 2003). Preliminary work in this area shows that alerts for aspects of preventive medicine vary in effectiveness depending on where in the course of the encounter such prompts appear. As mentioned earlier, if physicians are reminded during the wrong portion of the encounter, they generally ignore the prompts. Alerts are also more effective when supported by other enabling strategies, such as audit and feedback (Walker 2003).

Disease Management

Disease management has been instrumental in motivating physicians to conform to best practices. *Disease management* can be defined as any program devoted to the care of populations characterized by the presence of a chronic disease. Most of these programs have been designed by third parties, such as managed care organizations, to reduce costs through increased conformity. The underlying strategy of disease management is to improve health outcomes while lowering use and costs.

Many believe that the most effective method of changing physician behavior is to make "doing the right thing" the path of least resistance by taking responsibility for the guideline from the physician and sharing the management of chronic diseases with an expanded healthcare team. Such programs have proven effective in improving outcomes and reducing costs of diabetes care (Sidorov et al. 2002), asthma (Bolton et al. 1991), and congestive heart failure (CHF) (Rich et al. 1995). Characteristics of such programs include population disease management (a method of identifying the population of patients with a symptom management plan), education and case management, and health promotion/disease prevention activities. Barriers to the use of such programs include lack of financial and staffing resources as well as cultural issues that emerge when physicians evolve to a more team-based method of disease management. As with any implementation, adequate attention to physician buy-in as well as administrative support and involvement are crucial (Waters et al. 2001).

Financial Incentives

In the aftermath of the Institute of Medicine's *Crossing the Quality Chasm* (2001) publication, the government and large employers, responsible for paying the nation's healthcare bill, have wanted to accelerate the pace of change in healthcare. Financial incentives are being introduced to reward physicians and healthcare organizations for delivering high-quality medical care. Yet, until very recently, few empirical studies of the effect of direct quality incentives on physician performance have been conducted (Conrad et al. 2006; Petersen et al. 2006). However, the use of pay-for-performance schemes has quickly outstripped the evidence, and such programs are now in use at over half of private-sector health management organizations (Rosenthal et al. 2006). In addition, Centers for Medicare & Medicaid Services (CMS) is piloting pay for performance in various demonstration projects and will be including performance indicators as means for providers to obtain additional reimbursement for fulfilling these criteria.[1] In the largest report published to date, Lindenauer et al. (2007) measured changes in 14 quality measures over two years during a CMS pay-for-performance demonstration project. Although pay-for-performance hospitals outperformed control hospitals, improvements after adjusting for baseline performance and hospital characteristics were modest, ranging from 2.6 to 4.1 percent.

Concerns about such programs include whether they would deter physicians from caring for sicker or economically disadvantaged populations. For example, "cherry picking" healthier patients would improve a provider's overall performance; similarly, caring for patients with multiple health problems or psychiatric diagnoses would put providers at a disadvantage. These groups may challenge adherence to guidelines and therefore disproportionately affect our country's "safety net" hospitals and healthcare providers. Whether pay for performance will have enough of an effect on quality to justify its costs remains to be seen.

Addressing the Cost of Implementation

Many guidelines do not include information about how implementation will affect health resources. As a result, one barrier to implementation may be the misperception that the value gained is not worth the cost. Efforts to change physicians' clinical behavior should be in accord with administrative and reimbursement policies. For example, if an organization asks physicians to spend more time identifying and treating depression and at the same time pressures them to see more patients, depression care is unlikely to improve. If the structure of the healthcare system, in particular its reimbursement structure, runs counter to medical guidelines, even the best guidelines will not be implemented successfully (Brook 1995).

It is necessary to distinguish between treatment cost-effectiveness (i.e., the incremental costs and benefits of a treatment) and policy cost-effectiveness (the cost in relation to treatment cost-effectiveness and the cost and magnitude of the implementation method needed to enact the change). Having to invest resources to change physician behavior imposes an additional cost on treatment cost-effectiveness.

Policy cost-effectiveness will remain attractive only when effective but inexpensive implementation methods exist or if large health gains per patient exist for a high-prevalence disease. For example, the use of angiotensin converting enzyme inhibitors for heart failure is considered cost-effective at $2,602 per life year gained. Estimates of successful implementation based on academic detailing programs used in the United Kingdom by the National Health Service, which had a significant effect at a small cost per patient ($446 per life year gained), allow the intervention to retain its cost-effectiveness. However, the cost of academic outreach to promote a reduction in newer classes of antidepressants in favor of less-expensive tricyclic antidepressants is not economical because the outreach cost per patient exceeds the cost saved from behavioral change. Thus, the cost and efficacy of the implementation method must be added to the cost-effectiveness of the treatment to make a policy decision (Mason et al. 2001) (see Figure 16.5).

Furthermore, whether quality improvement initiatives make financial sense for an organization is a complex problem. A healthcare organization

FIGURE 16.5
Evaluating
Cost-
Effectiveness

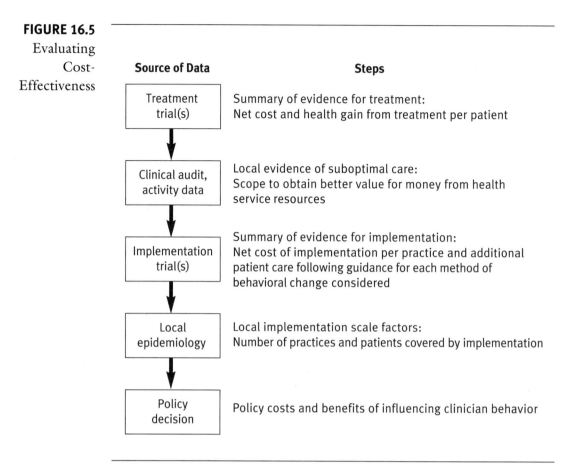

Source of Data

Steps

Treatment trial(s) — Summary of evidence for treatment:
Net cost and health gain from treatment per patient

Clinical audit, activity data — Local evidence of suboptimal care:
Scope to obtain better value for money from health service resources

Implementation trial(s) — Summary of evidence for implementation:
Net cost of implementation per practice and additional patient care following guidance for each method of behavioral change considered

Local epidemiology — Local implementation scale factors:
Number of practices and patients covered by implementation

Policy decision — Policy costs and benefits of influencing clinician behavior

operating under capitated payment structures is likely to benefit from a strategy that reduces utilization or hospital admissions. A health system that is reimbursed under fee-for-service plans or relies on diagnosis-related group payments from Medicare would lose money from a program that reduced hospital admissions. Successful chronic care programs have been discontinued because financial incentives did not exist to support the expense of such programs (Rich et al. 1995). In the ambulatory setting, increased utilization of ambulatory resources for unreimbursed chronic disease management results in decreased revenue per visit in a capitated managed care setting.

Thus, to create a favorable business case for quality improvement initiatives, the savings or increased revenue from improved care must accrue to the organization paying for the improvements. External incentives are likely to become increasingly important in driving quality improvement and the use of clinical guidelines/chronic disease models.

Keys to Successful Implementation and Lessons Learned

From the preceding discussion, you should have gained knowledge of specific tools that improve dissemination of healthcare quality initiatives. This section summarizes key steps to the successful implementation of such initiatives.

1. *Focus on high-impact interventions.* What disease processes are most prevalent in your population? For most adult populations, the three major processes are diabetes, hypertension, and CHF. What is your goal? A goal to reduce hospitalizations for patients with CHF is attainable in the short term, whereas a goal to reduce the number of amputations in diabetes patients will take longer to realize.

2. *How are you performing now?* To know what to focus on, you need to know your current performance relative to benchmarks. Initially, the things furthest from benchmarks are easiest to correct. Keep in mind the Pareto principle, or 80/20 rule, recognizing that you will expend the greatest amount of effort trying to accomplish that final 20 percent.

3. *For every hour spent discussing the content of the initiative, spend four hours planning its implementation.* Your practice guideline will do no good in your organization unless it is used. Emphasizing the structural or developmental phase without adequate attention to implementation is a sure recipe for failure. Use proven implementation methods, not merely passive education and dissemination, and use multiple interventions simultaneously.

4. *Who needs to change?* Analyze which individuals in the organization must respond to the proposed change and what barriers exist. Invest in the innovators and early adopters. Know who your opinion leaders are, and enlist them as your champions. Spend little time with the laggards, recognizing that in an era of constrained resources, change leaders must direct efforts at those who are on board or coming aboard.

5. *Do a cost-benefit analysis.* Weigh the costs of implementation, taking into account the implementation method, against both the costs of inaction and the gains of a successful result. Too often, leaders fail to factor in the cost of a change early enough in the process. As a result, a great deal of work is done in an area that will not be sustainable long term. As described previously, the party expending the resources generally must be the same party reaping the financial benefits of the change.

6. *Enlist multidisciplinary teams.* Teams should consist of individuals who actually do the work, not the formal leadership. For example, an office redesign project should include representation from the front desk personnel, secretaries, nursing staff, and operational leadership, not just physicians.

7. *Think big, but start small.* The old saying "Rome wasn't built in a day" applies here. Projects that are too ambitious may cause an early failure—you need to achieve an early short-term gain to keep the bosses on board and silence the naysayers. Is your real goal to convert your

practice from a traditional scheduling scheme to an open-access scheduling system? Start with a small project—either piloting this idea with one physician or working on a smaller, related project—before redesigning the entire system.

8. *Once you have defined your goal, construct a timeline and publicize it.* Teams sometimes spin their wheels forever without accomplishing anything. This timeline will give the team accountability to keep moving along in the process. You can change milestones midstream—flexibility is important—but procrastination cannot be an excuse.

9. *Change must be well communicated.* Many initiatives have failed because the changes were poorly communicated. Make use of multiple and informal forums, everything from meetings to e-mail to water cooler conversations. Make sure your vision can be clearly articulated in 30 to 60 seconds—if the new way is transparent, seems simple, and makes sense, it will be easier to spread.

10. *Leaders should back up their talk with actions.* Leaders should not be exempt from following the new path, and they also must be perfect role models of the new process. Do you want to implement open access in your practice? Do it yourself first. Have you reconstructed a new patient identification process to reduce the chance of wrong-site surgery? Do it yourself, 100 percent of the time.

11. *Is your change working?* Celebrate its success. Hold systemwide meetings highlighting how your new medication error reduction system is reducing errors. Ensuring that everyone in your organization is aware of the successes makes change less threatening the next time around. Moreover, publishing and speaking outside your organization about your successes can spread successful techniques externally. In exchange, from others, you may learn successful approaches to apply in your organization.

12. *Create a culture of continual change within your organization.* Successful organizations and industries understand that their survival is dependent on a continual reinvention of themselves—continuous quality improvement. Many experiencing the ongoing change will ask, "Are we almost there yet?" The answer is *no.* Our organizations should strive continuously for a state of perfection, which we may approach but likely will never reach. Figure 16.6 summarizes common pitfalls encountered in the change process.

Case Studies

Case 1: A Good Strategy at the Wrong Time

A large East Coast healthcare organization rooted in an academic medical center was located in a highly competitive market. A rising number

FIGURE 16.6

Common
Implementation
Pitfalls

- Lack of attention to implementation
  - Overemphasis on guideline development
  - No knowledge of effective implementation strategies

- Involvement of the wrong people
  - Lack of recognition of informal leadership
  - Failure to enlist opinion leaders

- Failure to commit adequate resources to the implementation process
  - Lack of commitment of time and staffing
  - Lack of visible leadership support

- Inadequate communication
  - Message too complex
  - Lack of establishing a sense of urgency

- Implementation too costly/failure to assess cost-effectiveness
  - Program too expensive or incentives misaligned

- Competing crises or uncontrollable factors in the external environment

of managed care organizations in the marketplace were approaching the organization to negotiate full-risk contracts. An early experiment showed this business to be very costly to the organization.

To prepare for this wave of risk contracting, the CEO and chief quality officer embarked on a major endeavor to make quality the driving force of the organization. The belief was that a strategy of providing the best care with assistance from disease management programs throughout the organization's practice network would allow the organization to engage in full-risk capitation, earn the organization a competitive advantage of offering the best quality, and thus help the organization negotiate favorable contracts in the healthcare marketplace.

The program addressed deviations from best practice in the care of high-volume chronic conditions such as CHF, diabetes, and asthma. Clinical champions—well-known physicians respected by their peers—led teams in designing outpatient clinical guidelines according to evidence-based best practices. The multipronged effort included educational strategies, academic detailing to individual physician practices, clinical decision support with prompts and reminder systems, and office-based coordinators to disseminate the guidelines.

At its peak, the department contained three medical directors, employed 70 persons, and enrolled more than 14,000 patients in 28 programs. It was successful in demonstrating improved outcomes in asthma care, including reduced hospitalizations and emergency room visits, as well as improved compliance with best practices in CHF and asthma care. The program was successful because of its intense focus on implementation. Particularly effective was the focus on the use of opinion leaders and clinical champions, as well as the use of multiple interventions to increase physician enrollment and buy-in. In addition, the system's leadership communicated a strong mandate for quality improvement and disease management, and strong physician leadership for the programs existed. Initial programs in high-impact areas were able to demonstrate short-term wins.

However, the organization began suffering financial losses, and the entire program was abruptly dismantled during a round of consultant-driven expense reduction. The expected rush to full-risk capitation never occurred, and the organization's emphasis on quality did not seem to garner it a special place in the crowded marketplace. In reality, the party incurring the cost was not the party obtaining the financial benefit. The insurers and managed care organizations benefited financially from the program, but the health system paid the expense. Thus, the cost of the program was not sustainable over time.

Case 2: A Novel Approach

An integrated healthcare delivery system implemented a disease management effort that emphasized both short- and long-term goals. The system included two acute care hospitals, a large academic physician group practice, and an HMO. The leadership of the disease management effort established goals to drive the process; these goals included improving the quality of patient care (appealing to the providers in the group practice), decreasing the variation in care (appealing to health system leadership, who realized that decreased variation means increased cost efficiency), and decreasing long- and short-term utilization by health plan members (appealing to the HMO by decreasing medical loss ratios). These goals formed a viable financial model, and each stakeholder gained ownership in the success of the endeavor.

Physicians actively engaged in the group practice led the disease management program, although it was centered in the HMO. These leaders were respected clinicians and continued to practice at the grassroots level, helping to sell the program to peers and creating instant credibility for the program.

The model began with the target population and sought to find strategies to affect this group. The chosen populations were high-prevalence, high-impact areas including tobacco cessation, asthma, diabetes, CHF, hypertension, and osteoporosis. Each condition was rolled out individually in steps. Strategies for this mix of conditions offered both short-term (decreased hospitalizations for asthma and CHF) and long-term (decreased lung disease from smoking and decreased complications from diabetes) gains. The implementation team included physicians, case management nurses, information systems, triage systems, physician office staff (e.g., nurses, medical records personnel, and scheduling coordinators), and patients themselves.

The implementation plan included the following strategies:

- Place health plan–employed care coordination nurses in local physician offices to coordinate care and assist primary care physicians and their staffs
- Establish evidence-based guidelines by employing nationally recognized basic guidelines and engaging opinion leaders from the academic group practice to review and disseminate the data
- Enroll all members of a population in the program and allow them to opt out if they choose
- Stratify patients according to risk and target the highest-risk members of the population first, thereby achieving early successes
- Use regional case managers to help oversee management of difficult or high-acuity cases
- Use timely electronic decision support to allow providers a greater opportunity to follow guidelines (Providers were given up-front input on the content, and each new intervention was pilot tested on a small group.)
- Promote member self-management, allowing the patient, the true consumer of the service, to become a stakeholder
- Provide frequent member and provider education in multiple media and forums, including regional group sessions, face-to-face contact, and print and electronic active and passive communication
- Maintain an active data acquisition and processing department to measure progress, fine tune procedures, and recognize successes

The health plan had approximately 250,000 members in more than 1,200 primary care providers' offices. These physicians included those employed by the health system and those contracted by the health plan. The disease management program employed more than 70 full-time equivalent professionals, with more than two-thirds in direct patient care at the point of service. The health plan received "excellent" accreditation status from the National Committee for Quality Assurance (NCQA), and NCQA and the American Diabetes Association recognized the disease management program for excellence and innovation. The program realized tangible positive results, including increased quality of care, decreased variation in practice, decreased cost to the system, and decreased utilization for the health plan.

Why did this disease management system succeed? First, it used a stepwise approach (think big, but start small), and pilot projects were launched before large-scale rollouts. Attainable goals were set using high-impact diseases, outcomes were measured, and successes were celebrated.

Second, all constituencies were stakeholders in the change process. The program took a global, multifaceted approach to implementation, involving as many different resources and tools as possible. It enlisted thought leaders from each affected area and used innovative approaches to implement, maintain, publicize, and remediate processes. Most importantly, the downstream cost savings produced by the program accrued directly to the health system that financed the programs, which allows for sustainability over the long term (i.e., the party bearing the cost of the program directly benefited).

Case 3: System Implementation of Clinical Office Redesign

One mid-Atlantic region integrated health system, heeding complaints from referring physicians and patients regarding access issues, joined a collaborative initiated by the Institute for Healthcare Improvement called the Idealized Design of Clinical Office Practices. This initiative centered on multiple facets of office practice, including access (the ability to get into the system), interaction (the experience of the patient in the system), reliability (practicing state-of-the-art medicine), and vitality (financial sustainability). This healthcare system chose to focus its early efforts on redefining access as a means of gaining market share, increasing patient satisfaction, and enhancing clinical and financial performance. The system began with implementation in two practice sites, with rapid-spread methods for implementing successful processes across multiple sites. Lessons learned from these early sites were then used to spread the process to the entire system and medical center specialties.

The deployment model included a team of dedicated, trained staff to support the rollout. The staff was trained in change management and quality improvement and taught local leadership how to lead the practice through these changes. Local teams took ownership of the process and tailored it to fit their needs. The support team worked with the sites for eight to ten weeks to assist with team formation, facilitate team leadership, introduce data collection tools, and encourage change. The team also provided periodic follow-up support and review. Positive early prototype results incited interest throughout the system practices. Rolling, scheduled spread then occurred across community practice sites, followed by sites at the medical center. These sites were able to markedly improve access, demonstrate improved patient satisfaction, and increase market share.

This model included the following key components of a successful rollout:

- Visible support from leadership
- Demonstration of short-term successes with early results from the prototype sites
- Use of multidisciplinary, local teams

- Structural support for the teams
- Active communication of the process through multiple forums
- Development of a structured timeline for the rollout
- Accountability at the local leadership level
- Celebration of successes both locally and nationally

The success of this initiative has been a model for other quality improvement initiatives within the organization.

Conclusion

This chapter has reviewed practical methods of leading healthcare organizations through change. American healthcare needs substantial improvement in care delivery; for healthcare leaders, mastery of skills that will contribute to effective quality improvement is critical. We must conduct further research on the use of informatics, pay for performance, and other strategies to expand our knowledge and discover additional methods of inducing change in the healthcare system.

Study Questions

1. You are the medical director for a practice network. You would like to improve diabetes care for the patients in your network. You have an EMR that allows you to send feedback to each physician outlining his or her performance relative to a benchmark. Outline your implementation plan.

2. Your organization is participating in a CMS demonstration project. The goal of this project is to improve preventive measures in the Medicare population (cancer screening and immunizations) as well as to reduce overall healthcare costs in the Medicare population. You are in charge of this three-year project. Outline a strategy for implementing the changes needed to carry out such a large project.

3. You are the lead cardiac surgeon in a large group. The hospital's chief medical officer calls and informs you that the outcome data for coronary artery bypass surgery is going to be made public on a state website. You obtain the data for wound infection rates and discover that it is double the state average. What steps would you take to correct this problem?

Note

1. See www.cms.hhs.gov/DemoProjectsEvalRpts/MD.

References

Armstrong, D., H. Reyburn, and R. Jones. 1996. "A Study of General Practitioners' Reasons for Changing Their Prescribing Behaviour." *British Medical Journal* 312: 949–52.

Beaulieu, M. D., M. Rivard, E. Hudon, C. Beaudoin, D. Saucier, and M. Remondin. 2002. "Comparative Trial of a Short Workshop Designed to Enhance Appropriate Use of Screening Tests by Family Physicians." *Canadian Medical Association Journal* 167 (11): 1241–46.

Berwick, D. M. 2003. "Disseminating Innovations in Health Care." *Journal of the American Medical Association* 289: 1969–75.

Bolton, M. B., B. C. Tilley, J. Kuder, T. Reeves, and L. R. Schultz. 1991. "The Cost and Effectiveness of an Education Program for Adults Who Have Asthma." *Journal of General Internal Medicine* 6: 401–7.

Bradley, E. H., E. S. Holmboe, J. A. Mattera, S. A. Roumanis, M. J. Radford, and H. M. Krumholz. 2001. "A Quality Study of Increasing Beta-Blocker Use After Myocardial Infarction: Why Do Some Hospitals Succeed?" *Journal of the American Medical Association* 285 (20): 2604–11.

Brook, R. H. 1995. "Implementing Medical Guidelines." *Lancet* 346 (8968): 132.

Cabana, M. D., C. S. Rand, N. R. Powe, A. W. Wu, M. H. Wilson, P. A. Abboud, and H. R. Rubin. 1999. "Why Don't Physicians Follow Clinical Practice Guidelines? A Framework for Improvement." *Journal of the American Medical Association* 282 (15): 1458–65.

Chassin, M. R. 1998. "Is Health Care Ready for Six Sigma Quality?" *Milbank Quarterly* 76: 565–91.

Conrad, D. A., B. G. Saver, B. Court, and S. Heath. 2006. "Paying Physicians for Quality: Evidence and Themes from the Field." *Joint Commission Journal on Quality and Patient Safety* 32 (8): 443–51.

Davis, D. 1998. "Does CME Work? An Analysis of the Effect of Educational Activities on Physician Performance or Health Care Outcomes." *Journal of Psychiatry in Medicine* 28 (1): 21–39.

Dexter, P. R., S. Perkins, J. M. Overhage, K. Maharry, R. B. Kohler, and C. J. McDonald. 2001. "A Computerized Reminder System to Increase the Use of Preventive Care for Hospitalized Patients." *New England Journal of Medicine* 345 (13): 965–70.

Durieux, P., R. Nizard, N. Ravaud, and E. Lepage. 2000. "A Clinical Decision Support System for Prevention of Venous Thromboembolism: Effect on Physician Behavior." *Journal of the American Medical Association* 283 (21): 2816–21.

Gladwell, M. 2000. *The Tipping Point: How Little Things Make a Big Difference.* New York: Little, Brown.

Goldberg, H. I., E. H. Wagner, S. D. Fihn, D. P. Martin, C. R. Horowitz, D. B. Christensen, A. D. Cheadle, P. Diehr, and G. Simon. 1998. "A Randomized Controlled Trial of CQI Teams and Academic Detailing: Can They Alter Compliance with Guidelines?" *Joint Commission Journal of Quality Improvement* 24 (3): 130–42.

Gosfield, A. G., and J. L. Reinertsen. 2005. "The 100,000 Lives Campaign: Crystallizing Standards of Care for Hospitals." *Health Affairs* 24 (6): 1560–70.

Greco, P., and J. Eisenberg. 1993. "Changing Physician Practices." *New England Journal of Medicine* 329: 1271–73.

Halm, E. A., S. J. Atlas, L. H. Borowsky, T. I. Benzer, J. P. Metlay, Y. C. Change, and D. E. Singer. 2000. "Understanding Physician Adherence with a Pneumonia Practice Guideline: Effects of Patient, System and Physician Factors." *Archives of Internal Medicine* 160: 98–104.

Hunt, J., J. Siemienczuk, P. Erstgaard, J. Slater, and B. Middleton. 2001. "Use of an Electronic Medical Record in Disease Management Programs: A Case Study in Hyperlipidemia." In *MedInfo 2001: Proceedings of the 10th World Congress on Medical Informatics,* edited by V. L. Patel, R. Rogers, and R. Haux. Amsterdam: IOS Press.

Institute of Medicine. 2001. *Crossing the Quality Chasm.* [Online information; retrieved 04/07.] www.iom.edu/cms/8089/5432.aspx.

Jencks, S. F., E. D. Huff, and T. Cuerdon. 2003. "Change in the Quality of Care Delivered to Medicare Beneficiaries, 1998–1999 to 2000–2001." *Journal of the American Medical Association* 289 (3): 305–12.

Kotter, J. P. 1996. *Leading Change.* Cambridge, MA: Harvard Business School Press.

Lester, W. T., R. W. Grant, G. O. Barnett, and H. C. Chueh. 2006. "Randomized Controlled Trial of an Informatics-Based Intervention to Increase Statin Prescription for Secondary Prevention of Coronary Disease." *Journal of General Internal Medicine* 21: 22–29.

Lindenauer, P. K., D. Remus, S. Roman, M. B. Rothberg, E. M. Benjamin, A. Ma, and D. W. Bratzler. 2007. "Public Reporting and Pay for Performance in Hospital Quality Improvement." *New England Journal of Medicine* 356: 486–96.

Mandelblatt, J., and P. A. Kanetsky. 1995. "Effectiveness of Interventions to Enhance Physician Screening for Breast Cancer." *Journal of Family Practice* 40: 162–67.

Mason, J. M., N. Freemantle, I. Nazareth, M. Eccles, A. Haines, and M. Drummond. 2001. "When Is It Cost-Effective to Change the Behavior of Health Professionals?" *Journal of the American Medical Association* 286 (23): 2988–92.

McPhee, S. J., J. A. Bird, D. Fordham, J. E. Rodnick, and E. H. Osborn. 1991. "Promoting Cancer Prevention Activities by Primary Care

Physicians: Results of a Randomized, Controlled Trial." *Journal of the American Medical Association* 266: 538–44.

Mottur-Pilson, C., V. Snow, and K. Bartlett. 2001. "Physician Explanations for Failing to Comply with 'Best Practices'." *Effective Clinical Practice* 4: 207–13.

Oxman, A. D., M. A. Thomson, D. A. Davis, and R. B. Haynes. 1995. "No Magic Bullets: A Systematic Review of 102 Trials of Interventions to Improve Professional Practice." *Canadian Medical Association Journal* 153 (10): 1423–27.

Petersen, L. A., L. D. Woodard, T. Urech, C. Daw, and S. Sookanan. 2006. "Does Pay for Performance Improve the Quality of Health Care?" *Annals of Internal Medicine* 145: 265–72.

Ramoska, E. A. 1998. "Information Sharing Can Reduce Laboratory Use by Emergency Physicians." *American Journal of Emergency Medicine* 16: 34–36.

Reinertsen, J. L. 1998. "Physicians as Leaders in the Improvement of Health Care Systems." *Annals of Internal Medicine* 128: 833–38.

Rich, M. W., V. Beckham, C. Wittenberg, C. L. Leven, K. E. Freedland, and R. M. Carney. 1995. "A Multidisciplinary Intervention to Prevent Readmission of Elderly Patients with Congestive Heart Failure." *New England Journal of Medicine* 333: 1190–95.

Rogers, E. M. 1995. "Lessons for Guidelines from the Diffusion of Innovations." *Joint Commission Journal of Quality Improvement* 21: 324–28.

Rosenthal, M. B., A. B. E. Landon, S. L. Normand, R. G. Frank, and A. M. Epstein. 2006. "Pay for Performance in Commercial HMOs." *New England Journal of Medicine* 355: 1895–902.

Schectman, J. M., N. K. Kanwal, W. S. Schroth, and E. G. Elinsky. 1995. "The Effect of an Education and Feedback Intervention on Group-Model and Network-Model Health Maintenance Organization Physician Prescribing Behavior." *Medical Care* 33 (2): 139–44.

Shays, M. 2003. "Helping Clients to Control Their Future." *Consulting to Management* 14 (2): 1.

Sidorov, J., R. Shull, J. Tomcavage, S. Girolami, N. Lawton, and R. Harris. 2002. "Does Disease Management Save Money and Improve Outcomes? A Report of Simultaneous Short-Term Savings and Quality Improvement Associated with a Health Maintenance Organization–Sponsored Disease Management Program Among Patients Fulfilling Health Employer Data and Information Set Criteria." *Diabetes Care* 25 (4): 684–89.

Solomon, D. H., H. Hashimoto, L. Daltroy, and M. H. Liang. 1998. "Techniques to Improve Physicians' Use of Diagnostic Tests: A New Conceptual Framework." *Journal of the American Medical Association* 280 (23): 2020–27.

Van Walraven, C., V. Goel, and B. Chan. 1998. "Effect of Population-Based Interventions on Laboratory Utilization: A Time Series Analysis." *Journal of the American Medical Association* 280: 2028–33.

Van Wijk, M. A. M., J. van der Lei, M. Mosseveld, A. M. Bohnen, and J. H. van Bemmel. 2001. "Assessment of Decision Support for Blood Test Ordering in Primary Care: A Randomized Trial." *Annals of Internal Medicine* 134: 274–81.

Walker, J. 2003. Personal communication, May 13.

Waters, T. M., P. P. Budett, K. S. Reynolds, R. R. Gillies, H. S. Zuckerman, J. A. Alexander, L. R. Burns, and S. M. Shortell. 2001. "Factors Associated with Physician Involvement in Care Management." *Medical Care* 39 (7, Suppl.): I19–I91.

Weber, V., F. Bloom, S. Pierdon, and C. Bloom. 2008. "Employing the Electronic Health Record to Improve Diabetes Care: A Multifaceted Intervention in an Integrated Delivery System." *Journal of General Internal Medicine* 23 (4): 379–82.

Weber, V., A. White, and R. McIlvried. 2008. "A Multifaceted Intervention to Reduce Polypharmacy and Falls in an Ambulatory Rural Elderly Population." *Journal of General Internal Medicine* 23 (4): 399–404.

Zuckerman, H. S., D. W. Hilberman, R. M. Andersen, L. R. Burns, J. A. Alexander, and P. Torrens. 1998. "Physicians and Organizations: Strange Bedfellows or a Marriage Made in Heaven?" *Frontiers of Health Services Management* 14 (3): 3–34.

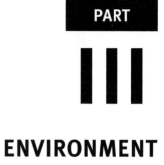

PART

III

ENVIRONMENT

THE QUALITY IMPROVEMENT LANDSCAPE

Jean Johnson, Ellen Dawson, and Kimberly Acquaviva

The quality improvement landscape in the United States is in a dynamic state of development; both established and new organizations are fostering change. Understanding the roles of these organizations is foundational to understanding the decisions underlying current quality improvement initiatives and anticipating the future direction of quality improvement nationwide. A complex network of public and private entities plays a major role in shaping quality improvement efforts, and many of these organizations' efforts overlap. The ways in which organizations influence quality vary. Some influence quality through the accreditation process, others develop measures of quality, and others advocate the integration of quality improvement into our health system.

Organizations approach quality improvement from different perspectives, depending on their mission as well as key stakeholders' needs and desires. Purchasers and insurers strive to link quality and cost containment to create more value for each dollar spent on healthcare. Healthcare providers work to improve patient care through internal quality improvement and the use of measures. The ultimate stakeholder of all these organizations—patients—expect (and in many cases, demand) to know more about the quality of care their healthcare providers deliver. Policymakers require data to drive rational policy decisions related to healthcare. This chapter examines the organizations that play major roles in shaping the quality improvement landscape, details important trends in quality improvement, and provides an overview of quality initiatives in specific health settings.

Quality Improvement Organizations

The interactions between organizations in the complex quality improvement landscape may be collegial or contentious depending on the issue under discussion, but almost without exception, the interactions are dynamic. Figure 17.1 illustrates the roles of organizations and notes that consumers currently are involved in quality improvement and are likely to become even more involved in the future. The illustration includes organizations that create incentives to quality through payment; organizations that are involved in the measurement process, including development, review, endorsement, and approval of measures; and organizations that use these measures.

Table 17.1 describes the roles of the major organizations. Many organizations are involved in quality improvement, but this chapter focuses on organizations whose main missions center on quality improvement.

Drivers of Quality

Several forces push the national quality agenda. These forces (payers, purchasers, certifiers, regulators, accrediting bodies, professional organizations, and advocates/technical support) directly or indirectly shape and advance the national quality agenda.

FIGURE 17.1
Roles of Organizations in the Quality Improvement Process

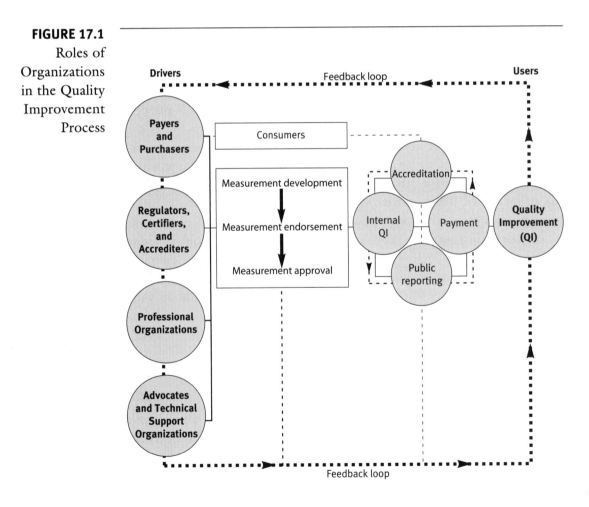

Payers and Purchasers

The main entities that influence quality improvement are those who pay for care. One of the largest and most powerful of these entities is the Centers for Medicare & Medicaid Services (CMS). With healthcare costs exceeding $1.4 billion (Poisal, Truffer, and Smith 2007) and public dollars accounting for approximately 45 percent of total costs, CMS is deeply vested in ensuring that Medicare and Medicaid enrollees receive the best care for each dollar they spend. CMS has driven the accreditation process in all settings and recently has emerged as a major influence in linking financial incentives to improving quality. Because of its role as the largest single

TABLE 17.1

Organizations by Type with Major Role in Quality

Type	Name of Organization	Mission	Website
Business Groups	National Business Group on Health	•National voice of *Fortune* 500 employers concerned about cost and quality; seeks solutions to important health issues	*www.business grouphealth.org*
	National Business Coalition on Health	•Organization of employer-based healthcare coalitions; seeks to improve quality through value-based purchasing	*www.nbch.org/ about/index.cfm*
	Pacific Business Group on Health (50 businesses)	•Regional coalition; seeks to improve the quality and availability of healthcare, moderate costs through value-based purchasing, use quality measurement and improvement, and engage consumers	*www.pbgh.org*
	Leapfrog Group	•Seeks to mobilize employer purchasing power to improve care through access to health information and by rewarding good care	*www.leapfrog group.org/home*
Federal Agencies	Centers for Medicare & Medicaid Services	•Major governmental agency that is a purchaser and payer of care and regulator of care through certification and licensure processes for providers receiving Medicare and Medicaid funds; provides consumer information and conducts demonstration projects	*www.cms.hhs. gov*
	Agency for Healthcare Research and Quality	•Seeks to improve the quality, safety, efficiency, and effectiveness of healthcare through research and provision of guidelines and other tools to educate and support providers and consumers	*www.ahrq.gov*
Accrediting Organizations	The Joint Commission	•Supports performance improvement in healthcare organizations	*www.joint commission.org*
	National Committee for Quality Assurance	•Accredits health plans and other organizations, develops measures, and engages in education of policymakers related to quality issues	*http://web.ncqa.org*

(continued)

TABLE 17.1
(continued)

Type	Name of Organization	Mission	Website
Alliances	Ambulatory Quality Alliance	•Reviews and approves measures for use in ambulatory care; supports public reporting of measures	*www.aqa alliance.org/ default.htm*
	Hospital Quality Alliance	•Reviews and approves measures of quality, cost, and value of hospital care; shares useful hospital performance information with the public	*www.hospital qualityalliance.org/ hospitalquality alliance/index.html*
	Physician Consortium for Performance Indicators	•AMA sponsored, over 100 groups; reviews and approves use of measures	*www.ama-assn.org/ama/pub/ category/2946.html*
Public/ Private	National Quality Forum	•Sets national priorities and goals for performance improvement, endorses national consensus standards for measuring and publicly reporting on performance, and promotes the attainment of national goals through education and outreach programs	*www.quality forum.org*
Technical Assistance/Advocate	Institute for Healthcare Improvement	•Reduces needless deaths, pain, and waiting; accelerates the measurable and continual progress of healthcare systems throughout the world using IOM's six aims	*www.ihi.org*
	National Patient Safety Foundation	•Awards small grants; resource for knowledge and public awareness; enhances culture of patient safety	*www.npsf. org*
Foundations	Robert Wood Johnson Foundation	•Supports regional initiatives in quality; continues to support measure development; communication strategies targeted to communities	*www.rwjf. org*
	California HealthCare Foundation	•Improves the care of chronically ill individuals; creates incentives to improve care	*www.chcf. org/aboutchcf*
	Commonwealth Fund	•Promotes a high-performing healthcare system with better access, improved quality, and greater efficiency, particularly for society's most vulnerable, including low-income individuals, the uninsured, minority Americans, children, and elderly adults	*www. commonwealth fund.org*

Note: The professional organizations noted in Figure 17.1 are not listed individually in Table 17.1 because their missions are broader than quality improvement.

health payer in the United States, CMS has the power to catalyze quality improvement through financial incentives such as the voluntary reporting programs that provide incentive Medicare payments. CMS is pushing several quality initiatives, many of which can be expected to have a significant impact on the quality improvement landscape in the United States for years to come. Examples of CMS projects include Doctor's Office Quality, which focuses on improving ambulatory care, and Premier Hospital Quality, which intends to improve hospital care. These projects are discussed later in the chapter (CMS 2006a; Premier 2006).

Businesses (purchasers) and health plans have been able to leverage quality through financial incentives similar to those of CMS. As health costs continue to rise, purchasers and health plans are looking to quality improvement to help control costs and maximize return on investment. The business groups on health—coalitions of businesses that provide health insurance benefits to employees—also have provided leverage to improve quality through the development of measures and system changes. Many states, regions, and even cities have business groups on health. Notable among the business groups are the National Business Group on Health, which brings the perspective of large employers to quality issues, and the National Business Coalition on Health, an organization of employer-based healthcare coalitions working to enhance value-based purchasing of healthcare services. At the regional level, business coalitions such as the Pacific Business Group on Health, which is very active in influencing policy to improve health and control costs, play a significant role in quality improvement. The Leapfrog Group is an offshoot of the business sector's concern about the quality and cost of hospital care. It was officially chartered in 2000 and gained considerable attention when it identified four practices that would create a "leap" in quality and patient safety. These practices are (1) computer physician order entry in hospitals, (2) evidence-based hospital referral, (3) intensive care unit (ICU) staffing by physicians experienced in critical care medicine, and (4) the Leapfrog Safe Practices Score (Leapfrog Group 2007). As hospitals improve their quality, Leapfrog Group members provide financial rewards.

Regulators, Certifiers, and Accrediting Bodies

CMS is the agency within the executive branch that has regulatory control over much of the healthcare system, particularly hospitals, nursing homes, home care, and some aspects of outpatient care. Regulations are a powerful influence on quality and serve to put legislation into operation. CMS also influences quality through the development of standards, survey instruments, and interpretation guidelines (guides to interpreting regulation). An example of CMS regulatory influence is the federally mandated requirements of nursing home surveys conducted by state survey agencies. In addition, through "deemed status," CMS recognizes The Joint Commission as the accrediting body of hospitals.

Entities that certify providers as safe and competent practitioners have a significant impact on quality. Several certifying boards now are integrating questions about quality improvement in their exams to highlight the importance of being knowledgeable about and engaged in quality improvement.

Professional Organizations

Healthcare professional organizations representing the entire spectrum of disciplines are embracing quality improvement through the development of educational initiatives, tools for providers to use in practice, and certification programs that recognize competence in specific areas. Through seminars, workshops, webinars, and other means, professional organizations have worked to make their members more aware of the need to improve quality. They also have developed measures, such as the American Nurses Association's (ANA) National Database for Nursing Quality indicators, in which over 1,000 hospitals report nursing-sensitive measures (ANA 2007), and the American Medical Association's (AMA) measures for ambulatory care, part of the Physician Consortium for Performance Improvement (AMA 2006). Professional organizations have been key partners in consortia that include a wide array of stakeholders who are involved in reviewing, endorsing, and approving the use of measures for different settings. Boards of medicine, nursing, and allied health professionals play a major role in quality improvement through certification and licensure programs and the establishment of standards for entry into practice as well as for continued competence.

Advocates/Technical Support

The Institute for Healthcare Improvement (IHI) has worked to engage healthcare providers, as well as stakeholders and the public, to improve the quality of care and reduce the number of needless deaths and errors. IHI has promoted the Plan-Do-Study-Act method of quality improvement and has created a number of collaboratives to bring providers together to work on projects related to a specific area. (See case study titled "IHI Campaigns" later in this chapter).

Quality improvement organizations (QIOs) evolved from the Medicare Utilization and Quality Control Peer Review Program created by statute in 1982. CMS has contracts with 53 QIOs covering all 50 states, Washington, DC, Puerto Rico, and the Virgin Islands. Although QIOs continue to have a role in ensuring that Medicare pays only for necessary and reasonable services, a recent Institute of Medicine (IOM 2006) report has recommended that the scope of work of QIOs be restructured to promote quality-of-care initiatives more actively by providing technical assistance to accomplish national goals.

The National Patient Safety Foundation's (2007) mission is to improve patient safety. It identifies and creates core bodies of knowledge;

identifies pathways to which it can apply the knowledge; and develops and enhances the culture of receptivity to, raises public awareness of, and fosters communications about patient safety.

Another group of supporting organizations comprises foundations that have served as catalysts in innovative quality program creation. For instance, the Robert Wood Johnson Foundation has a team that focuses on developing and funding programs to improve quality. It has supported quality improvement initiatives such as Transforming Care at the Bedside, an initiative to reengineer nursing care on medical-surgical units in hospitals. It also funded Rewarding Results, which supported programs providing incentives to improve care and now is investing in regional projects to improve care through Aligning Forces for Quality. The California HealthCare Foundation has funded a number of projects to improve care, such as pay-for-performance initiatives, and explores ways to improve the quality of chronic illness care. The Commonwealth Fund develops measurements and improves systems of care through its Improve Health Care Quality and Efficiency projects as well as through its work on patient-centered medical homes.

Measurement Development Process

Measure Development

The major developers of measures are the National Committee for Quality Assurance (NCQA), Agency for Healthcare Research and Quality (AHRQ), AMA, ANA, and Joint Commission. NCQA (2006) continues to add and delete measures from the Healthcare Effectiveness Data Information Set (HEDIS) database, and it develops measures for other programs such as the Diabetes Physician Recognition Program. AHRQ (2006) developed the Consumer Assessment of Healthcare Providers and Systems (CAHPS) for hospital, outpatient, nursing home, and home health settings. AMA (2006) has developed a number of measures as part of the Physician Consortium for Performance Indicators. ANA (2007) developed the National Database of Nursing Quality Indicators, which comprises nursing-sensitive measures of hospital care. In 1997, The Joint Commission (2007) developed the ORYX measures, which integrate patient outcome measures into the accreditation process.

Measure Endorsement

In 1998, a recommendation by the President's Advisory Commission on Consumer Protection and Quality in the Health Care Industry (1998) gave birth to the National Quality Forum (NQF). NQF was chartered in 1999 and has been developing the roles of scientific review provider and endorser of measures for public reporting purposes. CMS recognizes NQF as a voluntary, national consensus, standards-setting organization that adheres to the guidelines established by the National Technology Transfer and Advancement Act of 1995 and Office of Management and Budget Circular A-119, which allows CMS to use the standards rather than create an internal entity with similar function. NQF is a membership organization with a broad array of stakeholders who participate in the review and endorsement of measures. NQF works to create a coherent approach to measurement and reporting at the national level.

Measure Approval

A relatively new phenomenon is the emergence of consortia that bring together a wide group of stakeholders to review performance measures to ensure they are science-based, important measures of quality. The first consortium was the Hospital Quality Alliance (HQA). Founded in 2002 by the Association of American Medical Colleges (AAMC), the American Hospital Association (AHA), and the Federation of American Hospitals (FAH), HQA worked closely with CMS to review and approve measures for hospital reporting. HQA has numerous other participating organizations and a broad array of stakeholders, including consumers, purchasers, health plans, and providers. Another important consortium is the Ambulatory Quality Alliance (AQA), formally known as the Ambulatory Care Quality Alliance. Initiated in 2004 by the American Academy of Family Physicians (AAFP), the American College of Physicians (ACP), America's Health Insurance Plans (AHIP), and AHRQ to work collaboratively on performance measurement and reporting issues in ambulatory care, this consortium now has a broad-based collaborative of physicians, consumers, purchasers, health insurance plans, and others representing nearly 150 organizations. AQA works closely with CMS to adopt appropriate measures for ambulatory care.

Measure Use

There are four primary uses of quality measures: (1) internal quality monitoring, (2) accreditation, (3) payment incentives to improve care, and (4) public reporting. The first use is for health professions to improve care; the other three uses are related to holding providers accountable.

The first use of quality measures—internal monitoring and improvement—helps providers and institutions track specific measures to improve care. It is related to professional and personal commitments to care as well as expectations of institutions. Although they long have used quality measures for internal monitoring and reporting, providers have had difficulty comparing themselves to others because institutions collect different data, or similar data using different specifications. By collecting and reporting the same data using the same specifications, organizations and providers understand how they perform in comparison with others and can identify opportunities for focused quality improvement efforts.

The second use—accreditation—is carried out by organizations such as The Joint Commission (for hospitals) and NCQA (for health plans). The Joint Commission accredits nearly all of the hospitals in the United States and has an international accrediting arm, The Joint Commission International. The Joint Commission developed the ORYX system, which is composed of a core set of measures used in the hospital accreditation process. NCQA uses the HEDIS measures for accreditation of health plans. Accreditation began in the early 1990s with the initial set of HEDIS measures. HEDIS now includes 71 measures representing eight different areas (domains of care) (NCQA 2006). Currently 95 percent of health plans are accredited, but fewer PPOs are accredited (NCQA 2006).

The third use of quality measures—payment incentives to improve care—is carried out by payers. CMS projects in pay for performance, as well as health plans' use of measures to reward the provision of high-quality care, depend on having valid and reliable measures on which to base payment decisions.

The fourth use of quality measures—public reporting—entails reporting of the same data by all similar institutions, such as all hospitals, which allows consumers to compare institutions on the basis of the same data. Organizations such as CMS, The Joint Commission, and NCQA provide the public with information obtained from the quality measures. The Hospital Compare and Nursing Home Compare sites sponsored by CMS are examples. NCQA's health plan report card is another example. Findings from The Joint Commission accreditation results are also available to the public online.

Trends in Quality Improvement

Consumer Information

Consumers are being charged with increased responsibility for making rational decisions about healthcare. Because consumers may not have a comprehensive understanding of the interrelatedness of consumer behavior and healthcare costs, mainly because of the effect of health insurance, they may behave in ways that drive up healthcare costs unnecessarily. One could argue that coverage insulates consumers from bearing the full cost of care, thus leading them to conclude that healthcare costs equal whatever their co-payment amount is. Hence, consumers may perceive that a visit to the doctor "costs" $10 and that a visit to the emergency room "costs" $50. A landmark study supports the contention that consumer sensitivity to costs reduces use of healthcare services with few adverse effects (Brook et al. 1984). The emergence of consumer-driven health plans—plans that make consumers more vulnerable to the costs of healthcare—is changing the dynamic of consumer involvement in quality and cost issues. Consumer-driven health plans attempt to make consumers more sensitive to costs by requiring them to pay a higher share of the costs through higher premiums, deductibles, and co-pays. Some plans, such as health savings accounts, allow consumers to roll over unspent funds to the next year, providing an incentive for consumers to spend their healthcare dollars carefully. However, to make informed decisions, consumers must know about both cost and quality. If consumers have a greater financial stake in the healthcare they receive, they likely will choose the greatest value for the lowest cost. This economic concept is reasonably straightforward, but the level of information consumers need to make an informed decision based on cost and quality of care has been difficult to provide.

To support efforts to make information about quality of care available to consumers, CMS has created consumer information websites that inform people about the quality of care in nursing homes, home care, and hospitals (CMS 2005b, 2007a, 2007b). Many people visit these comparison sites, but how useful these sites actually are in helping consumers select care on the basis of quality is not clear. For instance, the Nursing Home Compare site provides facility-level information on 19 measures of quality as well as information about staffing and the number of deficiencies in the last survey. Although public availability of this information may be useful, concerns continue about the accuracy of the data and how people make informed decisions based on these data. To date, there is no composite scoring system providing consumers with an indication of overall quality. The Home Health Compare and the Hospital Compare websites have similar issues related to accuracy of data and interpretation, and whether information provided on these websites is useful to consumers in making healthcare decisions is not yet clear.

Despite these challenges and limitations, consumers are beginning to access information relevant to decision making. Evidence suggests that consumer information does make a difference in choosing healthcare on the basis of quality (Turnbull and Hembree 1996; Marquis et al. 2005; Hoy, Wicks, and Forland 1996). In addition to the current information on the websites, CMS will be adding the results from CAHPS for each of the settings. The Hospital CAHPS has been completed, and initial data collection is being done. Full implementation of the CAHPS surveys will allow comparison of hospitals based on consumer experience in addition to technical measures of care. The Hospital CAHPS asks consumers whether nurses and physicians treated them with respect and courtesy and informed them about what to expect. It also includes questions about specific aspects of care, such as pain management.

Pay for Performance/Value-Based Purchasing

Pay for performance is a major force moving the quality agenda forward. This movement has caught the attention of providers by directly linking payment incentives to quality improvement. Pay for performance also is referred to as *value-based purchasing* because payers are looking not only at quality but also at cost. Defining *value* as high-quality healthcare at the lowest cost assumes that the appropriate care is delivered in an efficient and effective manner.

Both private payers and CMS are embracing pay for performance. Payers have a keen interest in ensuring that patients receive the most appropriate and efficient care possible, and CMS is moving ahead with several pay-for-performance initiatives geared toward achieving this goal. As healthcare costs continue to rise at a rate greater than that of inflation in the general economy, prevention of the overuse, underuse, and inappropriate use of healthcare is seen as critical to both quality and cost. In the United States, more than 50 percent of commercial health plans representing 81.3 percent of enrollees use pay-for-performance programs (Rosenthal et al. 2006). More than one-half of the health plans include pay for performance in contracts, and almost all specify quality measures. Health plans more commonly have pay for performance for physicians than for hospitals. About a third of the plans reward the top-rated physicians but not the physicians who improved the most (Rosenthal et al. 2006). AHRQ has developed and disseminated a report to help public and private purchasers who are considering implementation of a pay-for-performance program (Dudley and Rosenthal 2006).

The Medicare Prescription Drug, Improvement, and Modernization Act of 2003 directed IOM to report on the best methods of aligning financial incentives to achieve the best outcomes for Medicare patients. IOM stated that the purpose of pay for performance is not to reward the best hospitals or providers but to align incentives so that there will be ongoing improvement in quality by all providers. IOM (2007) determined that the objectives for aligning incentives with quality improvement will:

- encourage the most rapid, feasible performance improvement by all providers;
- support innovation and constructive change throughout the healthcare system; and
- promote better outcomes of care, especially through coordination of care across provider settings and time.

In *Crossing the Quality Chasm*, IOM (2001) recommended consolidating the six aims (patient safety, patient centeredness, efficiency, effectiveness, timeliness, and equity) into three domains for developing performance measures and incentives: high clinical quality, patient-centered care, and efficiency.

Pay for performance has strong advocates, but some people are less enthusiastic about its cost/effectiveness. The question of whether pay for performance actually produces better care at reduced costs is only beginning to be answered. A comprehensive study on pay for performance conducted in the United Kingdom yielded promising results. On the basis of performance on 146 measures related to select chronic illnesses, organization of care, and patient experiences, the National Health Service provided incentive payments of nearly 25 percent of the usual general practitioner income. The initial findings suggested that the incentive payment produced higher-than-expected quality scores, and on average, physicians earned an additional $40,000 per year (Doran et al. 2006). Although these early results suggest that incentive payments produce better quality, critical questions remain. Were the expectations for improved quality set too low? Were incentive payments set too high? Can the system continue to afford the incentive payments? Further study is needed if definitive answers to these questions are to be found. Another study conducted in the United Kingdom examined pay for performance on smoking cessation among people with diabetes and found that increased support from providers to stop smoking coincided with an actual reduction in smoking (Millett et al. 2007). However, a recent study examining pay for performance on hospital care for acute myocardial infarction found no significant improvement in patient outcomes (Felt-Lisk, Gimm, and Peterson 2007). Overall data on pay for performance suggest mixed short-term results, and no long-term data are available (Chassin 2002; Dudley 2004; Hibbard, Stockard, and Tusler 2005; Rosenthal 2005).

Concerns remain regarding pay for performance. First, use of measures is meaningful only if it produces desired behavioral changes in providers; otherwise, the measures are merely informative and do not improve quality. Another concern is that some providers, hospitals, and other healthcare organizations that care for underserved minority populations and treat very ill patients may score lower on reported measures (Casalino 2006). Possible adverse impacts include reduced payment to physicians working in areas serving a large minority population, health plan avoidance of patients who may cause lower-quality scores, and poorer public outcome reports (Casalino et al. 2007). Risk adjustment in reported measures is needed. In addition, some practices may see more patients with multiple chronic diseases, and as of today, there are no good measures of care related to multiple diseases. Another concern is that practices and health organizations may focus their attention on the diseases being measured, to the exclusion of other important aspects of healthcare.

Questions remain regarding the ideal way to structure and level payments. This challenge is complex because different payment levels may be effective for different settings and different populations within those settings. In addition, sustaining long-term change may be difficult and costly. Practices may become accustomed to receiving incentive payments, and if benchmarks are raised at some point and these practices no longer receive incentive payments, there may be a negative effect on the program.

One clear result of the recent nationwide quality improvement efforts is the increasing number of measures that healthcare organizations are required to report or asked to report voluntarily. Organizations currently focused on quality improvement are working to ensure the validity and reliability of measures as well as advocating the inclusion of useful measures only. All organizations, whether accrediting bodies or payers, should use the same measures and specifications to reduce the onerous task of collecting vast amounts of information to fulfill accreditation, payment, or recognition programs' requirements.

Trends and Initiatives in Specific Healthcare Sectors

Ambulatory Care

Significant quality improvement efforts have only recently begun to focus on ambulatory care. Outpatient quality improvement programs have been difficult to develop because of the diffuse nature of outpatient settings as well as the lack of electronic health records, the presence of which would facilitate data collection and reporting. On December 20, 2006, President Bush signed the Tax Relief and Health Care Act of 2006. Section 101 under Title I authorizes the establishment of a physician quality reporting system by CMS. CMS has titled the statutory program the Physician Quality Reporting Initiative (PQRI).

PQRI establishes a financial incentive for eligible professionals to participate in a voluntary quality-reporting program. Eligible professionals who successfully report a designated set of quality measures codified on claims for dates of service from July 1 to December 31, 2007, may earn a bonus payment, subject to a cap of 1.5 percent of total allowed charges for covered Medicare physician fee schedule services (CMS 2005a).

The Patient Centered Medical Home (PCMH) is a new movement within healthcare spurred on by ACP, AAFP, the American Academy of Pediatrics (AAP), the American Osteopathic Association (AOA), and NCQA. The PCMH concept builds on the foundation of primary care as described in IOM's (1996) report on the future of primary care, as well as the work done by AAP in developing a medical concept for the care of children with chronic illnesses. Two important aspects of the PCMH concept are that it incorporates quality and safety as hallmarks and emphasizes recognition of the non-face-to-face costs of providing an effective, high-quality medical home. These costs include those associated with coordinating care, managing e-mail communication with patients, and adopting health information technology into practice. This concept is gaining traction with legislatures, and several organizations are advocating for a patient-centered medical home demonstration project (Arvantes 2007).

Supporters of the PCMH concept offer evidence of the success of several models in increasing quality while decreasing costs. North Carolina Medicaid created 15 medical home networks providing 24-hour access to providers, disease management, and hospital care through a program started in 1998 by Community Care of North Carolina. Medicaid paid each participating physician $2.50 per Medicaid enrollee per month in addition to payment for face-to-face visits. Although the cost of providing primary care physicians with this additional payment totaled $10.2 million, the return on investment was significant; the program saved the State of North Carolina an estimated $120 million in 2004 (Wilson 2005). The State of North Carolina accrued similar savings from the program in 2005 and 2006. Although there are data that support elements of the PCMH model, additional rigorous investigation of the costs and benefits needs to be undertaken.

Hospitals

During the past several years, quality improvement initiatives in healthcare have focused primarily on hospital-provided care. In one such initiative, CMS sought to improve the quality of inpatient care for Medicare patients by creating an incentive program that monetarily rewards hospitals for providing high-quality care. The Premier Hospital Quality Incentive Demonstration, which began in 2003, used quality measures based on the work of QIOs, The Joint Commission, AHRQ, and NQF, as well as on the work of other healthcare organizations that partner with CMS. There are 34 reportable quality measures (see Table 17.2) that demonstrate evidence-based clinical treatment for five clinical conditions: acute myocardial infarction, coronary artery bypass graft, heart failure, community-acquired pneumonia, and hip and knee replacement. This demonstration project sought to assess the impact of pay for performance on the quality of healthcare delivery and involved the voluntary participation of more than 250 hospitals in the Premier Perspective data system. Hospitals received scores on quality measures for each of the five clinical conditions. Hospitals scoring in the top 20 percent received a financial payment in recognition of their high-quality care. Conversely, those that did not perform well were financially penalized through the diagnosis-related group (DRG) payment scale (CMS 2005b).

HQA serves as another example of recent quality improvement initiatives focused on hospital-based healthcare. HQA was a collaborative endeavor launched in 2002 by partners including CMS, AHA, FAH, and AAMC, among others. HQA sought to create a set of publicly reportable quality measures that would be understood and recognized by accrediting bodies, purchasers, payers, providers, and consumers. Thanks to the overwhelming support HQA has received from organizations including AARP,

AFL-CIO, AHRQ, AMA, ANA, The Joint Commission, and NQF, among others, the results of this initiative have been impressive. As of July 2007, 4,059 hospitals were participating and reporting on HQA's hospital quality measures for heart attack, heart failure, pneumonia, surgical infection prevention, and patient experience of care (Premier 2006).

TABLE 17.2

The Premier Hospital Quality Incentive Demonstration: Clinical Conditions and Measures for Reporting

The CMS/Premier quality measures are based on clinical evidence and industry-recognized metrics. For example, they include:

- all 10 indicators from the starter set of "The National Voluntary Hospital Reporting Initiative: A Public Resource on Hospital Performance" (AHA initiative);
- 27 NQF indicators;
- 24 CMS 7th Scope of Work indicators;
- 15 Joint Commission core measures indicators;
- 3 indicators proposed by the Leapfrog Group; and
- 4 AHRQ patient safety indicators.

Clinical Conditions	Measures
Acute Myocardial Infarction (AMI)	1. Aspirin at arrival [1,2,3,4,P]
	2. Aspirin prescribed at discharge [1,2,3,4,P]
	3. ACEI for LVSD [1,2,3,4,P]
	4. Smoking cessation advice/counseling [1,2,3,P]
	5. Beta-blocker prescribed at discharge [1,2,3,4,P]
	6. Beta-blocker at arrival [1,2,3,4,P]
	7. Thrombolytic received within 30 minutes of hospital arrival [1,2,10,P]
	8. PCI received within 120 minutes of hospital arrival [1,5,10,P]
	9. Inpatient mortality rate [1,3,6,O]
Coronary Artery Bypass Graft (CABG)	10. Aspirin prescribed at discharge [5,P]
	11. CABG using internal mammary artery [1,5,P]
	12. Prophylactic antibiotic received within 1 hour prior to surgical incision [1,2,10,P]
	13. Prophylactic selection for surgical patients [1,2,10,P]
	14. Prophylactic antibiotics discontinued within 24 hours after surgery end time [1,2,10,P]
	15. Inpatient mortality rate [7,O]
	16. Postoperative hemorrhage or hematoma [8,O]
	17. Postoperative physiologic and metabolic derangement [8,O]
Heart Failure (HF)	18. Left ventricular function (LVF) assessment [1,2,3,4,P]
	19. Detailed discharge instructions [1,2,3,P]
	20. ACEI for LVSD [1,2,3,4,P]
	21. Smoking cessation advice/counseling [1,2,3,P]
Community-Acquired Pneumonia (CAP)	22. Percentage of patients who received an oxygenation assessment within 24 hours prior to or after hospital arrival [1,2,3,4,P]
	23. Initial antibiotic consistent with current recommendations [1,2,10,P]
	24. Blood culture collected prior to first antibiotic administration [1,2,3,P]
	25. Influenza screening/vaccination [1,2,10,P]
	26. Pneumococcal screening/vaccination [1,2,3,4,P]
	27. Antibiotic timing, percentage of pneumonia patients who received first dose of antibiotics within four hours after hospital arrival [1,2,4,10,P]
	28. Smoking cessation advice/counseling [1,2,3,P]
Hip and Knee Replacement [9]	29. Prophylactic antibiotic received within 1 hour prior to surgical incision [1,2,9,10,P]
	30. Prophylactic antibiotics selection for surgical patients [1,2,9,10,P]
	31. Prophylactic antibiotics discontinued within 24 hours after surgery end time [1,2,9,10,P]
	32. Postoperative hemorrhage or hematoma [8,9,O]
	33. Postoperative physiologic and metabolic derangement [8,9,O]
	34. Readmissions 30 days post-discharge [9,O]

1 National Quality Forum measure
2 CMS 7th Scope of Work measure
3 Joint Commission Core Measure
4 The National Voluntary Hospital Reporting Initiative (AHA initiative)
5 The Leapfrog Group proposed measure
6 Risk adjusted using Joint Commission methodology
7 Risk adjusted using 3M™ All Patient Refined DRG methodology
8 AHRQ Patient Safety Indicators and risk adjusted using AHRQ methodology
9 Medicare beneficiaries only
10 CMS and/or Joint Commission was to align with this measure in 2004
O Outcomes measure
P Process measure

Launched in 1995, CAHPS is a collaboratively developed AHRQ survey of patients' experiences with ambulatory facility care. Building on this foundation, CMS and AHRQ developed an instrument designed for hospital use in 2005 called Hospital Consumer Assessment of Healthcare Providers and Systems (HCAHPS). This nationally standardized survey was designed to generate publicly reported data on patients' perception of their hospital care, increase hospitals' motivation to improve the quality of care they provide, and increase public accountability and investment in healthcare. The 27-item survey, endorsed by NQF, solicits information regarding communication with nurses, doctors, and staff; communications about medications and discharge plans; cleanliness and quietness of the hospital; and pain control. Other questions elicit the patient's perceptions of the overall quality of the hospital as well as whether the patient would recommend this hospital to others. HCAHPS was launched in 2006 as a voluntary, incentive-free program under the sponsorship of HQA. CMS encourages hospitals to survey patients and submit results monthly.

AHA and The Joint Commission currently are developing and implementing other examples of hospital-focused quality improvement initiatives. AHA's quality program is based on the six aims of IOM's 2001 report *Crossing the Quality Chasm*. AHA and other state and federal healthcare organizations are focusing their quality improvement efforts on integrating these aims into the healthcare system and using them to create public awareness regarding quality performance. As the accrediting body for hospitals, The Joint Commission's purpose is to ensure patient safety through review of hospital performance and distribution of information. In partial fulfillment of this purpose, The Joint Commission provides each hospital with a selection of ORYX performance sets from which to choose, according to the hospital's mission. Included in the survey are items pertaining to heart attack care, pneumonia care, and surgical infection interventions. Quarterly reporting on these core measures gives The Joint Commission insight into its on-site hospital visits.

Nursing Homes

Quality monitoring and improvement in the nursing home industry have been deeply rooted in the regulatory process. Because of the frailty of the population served as well as historical issues related to quality of care, nursing homes have been the target of many sustained efforts to monitor and improve care. In the early 1980s, the nursing home industry developed quality improvement programs such as the Quest for Quality program offered by state nursing home organizations. At the same time, the industry established and used more defined standards for care as the basis for

TABLE 17.3

Nursing Home
Quality
Measures

Long-Term Measures

- Percentage of long-stay residents given influenza vaccinations during the flu season
- Percentage of long-stay residents who were assessed and given pneumococcal vaccinations
- Percentage of residents whose need for help with daily activities has increased
- Percentage of residents who have moderate to severe pain
- Percentage of high-risk residents who have pressure sores
- Percentage of low-risk residents who have pressure sores
- Percentage of residents who were physically restrained
- Percentage of residents who are more depressed or anxious
- Percentage of low-risk residents who lose control of their bowels or bladder
- Percentage of residents who have/had a catheter inserted and left in their bladder
- Percentage of residents who spent most of their time in bed or in a chair
- Percentage of residents whose ability to move about in and around their room got worse
- Percentage of residents with a urinary tract infection
- Percentage of residents who lose too much weight

Short-Stay Measures

- Percentage of short-stay residents given influenza vaccinations during the flu season
- Percentage of short-stay residents who were assessed and given pneumococcal vaccinations
- Percentage of short-stay residents with delirium
- Percentage of short-stay residents who had moderate to severe pain
- Percentage of short-stay residents with pressure sores

SOURCE: CMS (2007b).

the survey process. It has developed specified measures of quality for both long-term and short-stay patients and currently reports these measures to the public on the Nursing Home Compare website. See Table 17.3 for a listing of the measures.

Nursing homes are also unique in having a standardized, federally required assessment for every resident in a Medicare- and Medicaid-certified facility. The Minimum Data Set (MDS) is an instrument that includes information about resident function and major health problems and risks and generates a plan of care based on the assessment. The same assessment is performed on every resident in every certified facility, thus providing patient-level data that are useful in monitoring quality of care.

A new quality indicator survey is being tested. It is based on a two-step process. In the first phase, surveyors will collect data from a variety of sources—including the MDS; interviews of staff, residents, and family members; and observations—that will generate 162 quality-of-care and quality-of-life indicators. These indicators will be benchmarked against national averages. The second phase will include a more in-depth review of nursing facilities that have indicators suggesting a quality-of-care problem when compared to other facilities. Six states—Connecticut, Kansas, Ohio, California, Louisiana, and Florida—are testing this survey approach. Consumers can find information about nursing home staffing survey results and specific quality measures on the Nursing Home Compare website (CMS 2007b).

Home Healthcare

CMS began the Home Care Quality Initiative (HCQI) in 2003. HCQI centers on the collection of information from the 8,100 Medicare-certified home health agencies in the United States. In 2000, as part of a broad quality improvement initiative, the federal government began requiring each Medicare-certified home health agency to complete and submit health assessment information for its clients using a data collection instrument called the Outcome and Assessment Information Set (OASIS). This nationally mandated instrument consists of 54 items based on functional measures. A technical expert group engaged by AHRQ to review 41 of the OASIS measures recommended public reporting of 10 measures, deemed important to consumers, in which home health agencies have substantial impact. All of the measures are risk adjusted, except for the Improvement in Pain Interfering with Activity, and were reviewed and endorsed by NQF. These measures are part of the report on the Home Health Compare website. Table 17.4 provides a summary of the measures.

Since fall 2003, CMS has posted a subset of OASIS-based quality performance information at www.medicare.gov that shows how well home health agencies assist their patients in regaining or maintaining

TABLE 17.4 Home Healthcare Measures of Quality (Collected from OASIS)	Improvement in ambulation/locomotion Improvement in bathing Improvement in transferring Improvement in management of oral medication Improvement in pain interfering with activity Acute care hospitalization Emergent care Discharge to community Improvement in dyspnea (shortness of breath) Improvement in urinary incontinence

SOURCE: CMS (2007a).

their ability to function. Core measures of how well people can perform activities of daily living in their homes are supplemented with questions about physical status and two use-of-service measures (hospitalization and emergent care).

Case Studies

Premier Hospital Demonstration

The CMS/Premier Health Quality Incentive Demonstration (HQID) project began in early 2003 and tracks process and outcome measures for healthcare delivery in five clinical areas using 33 nationally standardized quality indicators. Hospitals are graded and receive a composite quality score (CQS) for each clinical area. Hospitals participating in the HQID project receive financial incentives depending on their performance in each clinical area. For CQS performance in the top decile of any of the five clinical areas, they receive a 2 percent bonus on their Medicare DRG payments. Performance in the second decile results in a 1 percent bonus. At the end of the third year of the demonstration project, low-performing hospitals can receive a financial disincentive. For example, hospitals that do not achieve a CQS above the ninth decile (based on the threshold established in the first year of the project) have their Medicare DRG payments reduced by 1 percent. Similarly, hospitals whose CQS does not exceed the tenth decile have their Medicare DRG payments reduced by 2 percent.

Cleveland Regional Medical Center (CRMC) implemented a quality improvement program to enhance the value of its healthcare offerings. Among many initiatives, it chose to explore the impact of pay for performance on the quality of healthcare by participating in the Premier/CMS HQID project.

The results from the first two years of the HQID project for CRMC indicated that among congestive heart failure patients, there was a 37 percent decrease in readmission rates. Mortality related to acute myocardial infarctions decreased by 25 percent. Knee infections decreased by 70 percent, and hip infections decreased by 36 percent. During these two years, CRMC demonstrated a marked improvement from negative to positive quality performance.

Hospital Public Reporting

In 2002, the U.S. Department of Health and Human Services recognized the leadership in the hospital industry (specifically AHA, FAH, and AAMC) for supporting voluntary reporting by hospitals as part of the CMS effort to provide public information about hospital quality of care. At the urging of CMS, these organizations joined together initially as the National Voluntary Hospital Reporting Initiative, now known as HQA. The initial set of voluntary measures included ten measures related to three disease areas: acute myocardial infarction, heart failure, and pneumonia. These measures were part of a database that was to be put on a Hospital Compare website available to consumers. However, relatively few hospitals (fewer than 500) reported data in 2003. The 2003 Medicare Prescription Drug, Improvement, and Modernization Act introduced an incentive to report data. It stipulated that hospitals failing to report data would receive 0.4 percent less in their Medicare Annual Payment Update (APU) for fiscal year 2005. To receive the full APU, hospitals had to sign up with the QIOs' data warehouse. As part of their contract with CMS, the QIOs were charged with providing technical assistance to hospitals for the data reporting. By 2004, nearly all of the 3,906 inpatient acute care hospitals eligible to report data did so (CMS 2005b).

Beginning in 2007, the measure set expanded to 21 measures, including 5 measures of surgical care. Hospitals that fail to report data will receive a reduction of 2 percent of the APU. CMS will require the reporting of 24 measures in 2008, including the HCAHPS data of patient experiences.

HQA has worked closely with CMS to review and approve measures for hospital reporting. This relationship has been vital to creating a public-private partnership that involves the representatives of providers affected by reporting requirements. HQA's participation in the measure approval process provides a mechanism for bringing hospitals to the table as decision makers and working with CMS to get the public reporting projects under way. The push by CMS for the public reporting of data has been balanced by HQA's efforts to ensure that the product of the reporting is an honest appraisal of the quality of hospital care related to specific health problems.

IHI Campaigns

IHI initiated a campaign in 2004 to save 100,000 lives. In response to an IOM report estimating that more than 100,000 lives are lost annually in hospitals from medical errors, IHI partnered with ANA, the Centers for Disease Control and Prevention, the National Business Group on Health, AMA, the Leapfrog Group, and The Joint Commission, among others, to launch the 100,000 Lives Campaign (IHI 2007).

Funded by Blue Cross and Blue Shield Massachusetts, the Cardinal Health Foundation, the Colorado Trust, the Gordon and Betty Moore Foundation, Baxter International, Inc., the Blue Shield of California Foundation, and the Robert Wood Johnson Foundation, IHI's 100,000 Lives Campaign yielded impressive results. After 18 months, an estimated 122,000 lives had been saved. One health system alone—the Henry Ford Health System—estimated that it saved 165 lives between January and August of 2005 (Henry Ford Health System 2005). The 100,000 Lives Campaign united hospitals and health systems in a collective commitment to improving quality and generated considerable excitement among providers as well as the media.

Several key elements were instrumental in the success of the 100,000 Lives Campaign, the most significant of which was having a credible organization with committed, highly visible, highly respected people in healthcare promoting the campaign. Another key element was IHI's development of the structure and process by which participants could learn from one another and reinforce change. As part of the promise to create change, participating hospitals were required to provide data as evidence of outcomes achieved, thus further strengthening (and exemplifying) the organizational commitment of participants in this groundbreaking initiative.

The 100,000 Lives Campaign laid the groundwork for a campaign with a slightly different focus. The 5 Million Lives Campaign focuses on reducing the number of incidents of medical harm to hospitalized patients, a number currently estimated to be 15 million each year. With the powerful slogan "Do No Harm," this two-year campaign (scheduled to end in December 2008) builds on lessons learned from the 100,000 Lives Campaign, particularly lessons related to rapid response teams, evidenced-based care for acute myocardial infraction, adverse drug events, central line infections, surgical site infections, and ventilator-associated pneumonia. In addition, six areas are targeted for harm prevention/reduction, including high-alert medications, surgical complications, pressure ulcers, methicillin-resistant *Staphylococcus aureus*, and congestive heart failure. Along with the ambitious goal of preventing 5 million instances of medical harm, the 5 Million Lives Campaign seeks to increase the number of quality improvement-committed providers appointed to the boards of hospitals and health systems.

The campaigns launched by IHI exemplify quality improvement efforts that use evidence to identify high-priority areas on which to focus, change individual provider behavior, and mobilize public action for policy change. The IHI campaigns demonstrated a great deal of campaign sophistication with clear objectives and documented results. For a campaign to be deemed a success, success needs to be defined operationally at the outset so that there are clear relationships among goals, activities, and measurable outcomes. To create this definition, the target audience must be understood, desired actions must be identified, and clear strategies for implementation must be provided. IHI defined the goal—saving 5 million lives from medical harm—and defined the 12 target areas. Experience gained during the first campaign provided insight into which implementation strategies would be most effective. Part of the success of the campaigns hinges on its simple message—a message that echoes and builds on the "do no harm" charge given to physicians since the time of Hippocrates. The slogan engages both providers and media and is a clear message to consumers that participating provider hospitals are committed to protecting their patients from medical harm.

Chronic Care Initiative

The economic burden of chronic illness in the United States is expected to increase significantly as the population ages (Centers for Disease Control and Prevention 2005). Certain chronic illnesses account for a high proportion of Medicare expenditure. For instance, an estimated 14 percent of Medicare beneficiaries have heart failure, accounting for 43 percent of Medicare costs (CMS 2006b). In addition, care for chronically ill individuals often is fragmented, resulting in poor health outcomes (McGlynn et al. 2003). To begin addressing this issue, the Medicare Prescription Drug, Improvement, and Modernization Act of 2003 authorized a demonstration project to evaluate chronic care improvement programs. This program first was known as the Voluntary Chronic Care Improvement Program and was renamed the Medicare Health Support Program in 2007. The program seeks to improve the quality of care provided to Medicare enrollees with chronic illness, improve enrollee satisfaction with care, and hit savings targets. Payment to participating organizations is based on a pay-for-performance model through which monthly fees are paid, but organizations must meet specified standards to keep the funds. If a participating organization fails to meet the agreed-upon standards, the organization is required to pay back a portion of the Medicare payments.

The first phase of the program was initiated in 2005 with the selection of eight chronic care improvement organizations. Each organization is required to have a designated contact person to facilitate communication with the enrollee and the other healthcare providers, provide self-care education to the enrollee, educate healthcare providers about relevant clinical information, and educate the enrollee to use monitoring technologies effectively to provide relevant information to healthcare providers. Participating organizations are required to report specific data to CMS to facilitate the comparison of enrollees in the intervention program to a control program. In Phase I, CMS identified beneficiaries using claim data in the geographic areas of the participating organization. It assigned each enrollee randomly to an intervention or control group, and enrollees assigned to the intervention group were given the option to refuse to participate. Phase II is an expansion phase in which participating programs can increase the number of enrollees or expand parts of the program that were particularly effective. Initial results of Phase I are due to Congress in 2008.

Conclusion

Spurred on by IOM's reports, the quality improvement environment has been active over the past decade. The context is complex; many different organizations are exerting forces in different ways, yet they all share the goal of improving patient care. The commitment to improving quality by purchasers, providers, regulators, patients, and others is creating a significant culture change in healthcare. The challenge for the future will be to ensure that quality measures and processes can be integrated into systems efficiently and that there are common measures that payers, insurers, and health systems use to measure care. In addition, more work needs to be done to understand what information is important and useful to consumers in making decisions and how they use the information.

Study Questions

1. What are the driving forces of quality improvement?
2. What are the roles of various organizations working on quality issues? How do these organizations relate to each other?
3. Discuss the uses of quality improvement information and the benefits and costs of each.
4. What are the dominant trends in quality improvement, and what is their impact on quality of patient care?
5. Compare and contrast the quality improvement activities that are under way in several healthcare settings.

References

Agency for Healthcare Research and Quality. 2006. "CAHPS." [Online information; retrieved 7/15/06.] www.cahps.ahrq.gov/content /cahpsOverview/Over_AboutUN.asp?p=101&s=14.

American Medical Association (AMA). 2006. "Physician Consortium for Performance Improvement." [Online information; retrieved 7/25/06.] www.ama-assn.org/ama/pub/category/2946.html.

American Nurses Association (ANA). 2007. "National Database for Nursing Quality Indicators: Transforming Data into Quality Care." [Online information; retrieved 7/20/07.] www.nursingworld.org/quality /ndnqi.pdf.

Arvantes, J. 2007. "State Legislators Champion Patient-Centered Medical Home." [Online information; retrieved 7/20/07.] www.aafp.org/ online/en/home/publications/news/news-now/government-medi-cine/20060702statelegislators.html.

Brook, H. R., J. E. Ware, W. H. Rogers, E. B. Keeler, A. R. Davies, C. A. Sherbourne, G. A. Goldberg, K. N. Lohr, P. Camp, and J. P. Newhouse. 1984. *The Effect of Coinsurance on the Health of Adults: Results from the RAND Health Insurance Experiment.* No. R-3055-HHS. Santa Monica, CA: RAND.

Casalino, L. P. 2006. "Medicare, the National Quality Infrastructure, and Health Disparities." *Medicare Brief* 14 (October): 1–7.

Casalino, L. P., A. Elster, A. Eisenberg, E. Lewis, J. Montgomery, and D. Ramos. 2007. "Will Pay-for-Performance and Quality Reporting Affect Health Care Disparities?" *Health Affairs Web Exclusives* 26 (3): w405–w414.

Centers for Disease Control and Prevention. 2005. "Chronic Disease Overview." [Online information; retrieved 7/23/07.] www.cdc.gov/nccdphp/overview.htm.

Centers for Medicare & Medicaid Services. 2005a. "Ambulatory Measures Owned and Maintained by the Ambulatory Consortium." [Online information; retrieved 6/5/07.] www.cms.hhs.gov/PhysicianFocused QualInits/Downloads/PFQIAMA.pdf.

———. 2005b. "Hospital Quality Initiative." [Online information; retrieved 4/7/08.] www.cms.hhs.gov/HospitalQualityInits.

———. 2006a. "Doctors Office Quality Project." [Online information; retrieved 1/8/07.] http://www.cms.hhs.gov/PhysicianFocused QualInits/05_PFQIDOQ.asp#TopOfPage.

———. 2006b. "Medicare Health Support." [Online information; retrieved 7/15/07.] www.cms.hhs.gov/CCIP/downloads/Overview_ ketchum_71006.pdf.

———. 2007a. "Home Health Compare." [Online information; retrieved 3/14/07.] www.medicare.gov/HHCompare/Home.asp? version=default&browser=IE%7C6%7CWinXP&language=English&defa ultstatus=0&pagelist=Home&CookiesEnabledStatus=True.

———. 2007b. "Nursing Home Compare." [Online information; retrieved 3/7/07.] www.medicare.gov/NHCompare/Home.asp?version =alter- nate&browser=IE%7C6%7CWinXP&language=English&defaultstatus=0 &pagelist=Home&CookiesEnabledStatus=True.

Chassin, M. R. 2002. "Achieving and Sustaining Improved Quality: Lessons from New York State and Cardiac Surgery." *Health Affairs* 4: 40–51.

Doran, T., C. Fullwood, H. Gravelle, C. Reeves, E. Kontopantelis, U. Hiroeh, and M. Roland. 2006. "Pay-for-Performance Programs in Family Practices in the United Kingdom." *New England Journal of Medicine* 355 (4): 375–84.

Dudley, R. A. 2004. *Strategies to Support Quality-Based Purchasing: A Review of the Evidence.* AHRQ Publication No. 04-P024. [Online information; retrieved 4/7/08.] www.ahrq.gov/clinic/tp/qpurchtp.htm.

Dudley, R. A., and M. B. Rosenthal. 2006. *Pay for Performance: A Decision Guide for Purchasers.* AHRQ Publication No. 06-0047. [Online infor- mation; retrieved 4/7/08.] www.ahrq.gov/qual/p4pguide.htm.

Felt-Lisk, S., G. Gimm, and S. Peterson. 2007. "Making Pay-for-Performance Work in Medicaid." *Health Affairs Web Exclusives* 26 (4): w516–w527.

Henry Ford Health System. 2005. "Progress Report on 100,000K Lives Campaign." [Online information; retrieved 7/20/07.] www.ihi.org/ NR/rdonlyres/CADB66C8-81ED-45F8-B5CF-8A1E0AFA980A/ 2457/ProgressReporton100K.pdf.

Hibbard, J. H., J. Stockard, and M. Tusler. 2005. "Hospital Performance Reports: Impact on Quality, Market Share, and Reputation." *Health Affairs* 24 (4): 1150–60.

Hoy, E. W., E. K. Wicks, and R. A. Forland. 1996. "A Guide to Facilitating Consumer Choice." *Health Affairs* 15 (4): 9–30.

Institute for Healthcare Improvement (IHI). 2007. "The 100,000 Lives Campaign: An Initiative of the Institute for Healthcare Improvement." [Online information; retrieved 7/20/07.] www.ihi.org/NR/rdonlyres/ 65F20C8A-5DCC-4178-98F3-A571F71E1151/0/100kLivesCampaign CaseStatement.pdf.

Institute of Medicine (IOM). 1996. *Primary Care: America's Health in a New Era.* Washington, DC: National Academies Press.

———. 2001. *Crossing the Quality Chasm: A New Health System for the 21st Century.* Washington, DC: National Academies Press.

———. 2006. *Medicare's Quality Improvement Organization Program: Maximizing Potential.* Washington, DC: National Academies Press.

———. 2007. *Rewarding Provider Performance: Aligning Incentives in Medicare.* Washington, DC: National Academies Press.

The Joint Commission. 2007. "Facts About ORYX for Hospitals, Core Measures and Hospital Core Measures." [Online information; retrieved 5/25/07.] www.jointcommission.org/AccreditationPrograms /Hospitals/ORYX/oryx_facts.htm.

Leapfrog Group. 2007. "Fact Sheet." [Online information; retrieved 7/19/07.] www.leapfroggroup.org/media/file/leapfrog_ factsheet.pdf.

Marquis, M. S., M. B. Buntin, K. Kapur, and J. M. Yegian. 2005. "Using Contingent Choice Methods to Assess Consumer Preferences About Health Plan Design." *Applied Health Economics and Health Policy* 4 (2): 77–86.

McGlynn, E. A., S. M. Asch, J. Adams, J. Keesey, J. Hicks, A. DeCristofaro, and E. A. Kerr. 2003. "The Quality of Health Care Delivered to Adults in the United States." *New England Journal of Medicine* 348 (26): 2635–45.

Millett, C., J. Gray, S. Saxena, G. Netuveli, and A. Majeed. 2007. "Impact of a Pay-for-Performance Incentive on Support for Smoking Cessation and on Smoking Prevalence Among People with Diabetes." *Canadian Medical Association Journal* 176 (12): 1705–10.

National Committee for Quality Assurance (NCQA). 2006. "HEDIS Program." [Online information; retrieved 7/25/06.] www.ncqa.org/ Programs/HEDIS/index.htm.

National Patient Safety Foundation. 2007. "NPSF Research Projects and Principal Investigators 2005–2007." [Online information; retrieved 7/19/07.] www.npsf.org/r/ga/.

Poisal, J., S. Truffer, and A. Smith. 2007. "Health Spending Projections Through 2016." *Health Affairs* 26 (2): w242–w253.

Premier. 2006. *Centers for Medicare and Medicaid Services (CMS)/Premier Hospital Quality Incentive Demonstration Project: Findings from Year One.* Charlotte, NC: Premier, Inc.

President's Advisory Commission on Consumer Protection and Quality in the Health Care Industry. 1998. *Quality First: Better Health Care for All Americans.* Derby, PA: Diane Publishing.

Rosenthal, M. B. 2005. "Early Experience with Pay-for-Performance: From Concept to Practice." *Journal of the American Medical Association* 294 (14): 1788–93.

Rosenthal, M. B., B. E. Landon, S. L. Normand, R. G. Frank, and A. M. Epstein. 2006. "Pay for Performance in Commercial HMOs." *New England Journal of Medicine* 355 (18): 1895–902.

Turnbull, J. E., and W. E. Hembree. 1996. "Consumer Information, Patient Satisfaction Surveys, and Public Reports." *American Journal of Medical Quality* 11 (1): S42–S45.

Wilson, C. F. 2005. "Community Care of North Carolina: Saving State Money and Improving Patient Care." *North Carolina Medical Journal* 66 (3): 229–33.

ACCREDITATION: ITS ROLE IN DRIVING ACCOUNTABILITY IN HEALTHCARE

Greg Pawlson and Paul Schyve

There is a large, growing body of evidence that today's level of quality and safety in healthcare is substantially lower than what is possible with currently available treatments and technology. This evidence was summarized in the Institute of Medicine's (IOM 2001) report *Crossing the Quality Chasm*. Recognition of this gap and growing purchaser and consumer demand for information about healthcare quality and safety have incited demand for more accountability in the healthcare system. More recently, the Presidential Executive Orders in August 2006 and the subsequent effort of the secretary of Health and Human Services, Michael Leavitt, have given additional impetus to transparency and performance reports, including accreditation reports, at all levels of the healthcare system. This chapter examines the role of accreditation in both its past and prospective roles in driving accountability in the healthcare system.

Background and Terminology

Accountability is defined as "the procedure and process by which one party provides a justification and is held responsible for its actions by another party who has an interest in the action" (Emanuel and Emanuel 1996; Emanuel 1996). Accountability in healthcare has been driven by three major forces: the marketplace, regulation, and professionalism. In healthcare, the parties that may seek accountability include those directly affected by health services (patients) and those who directly or indirectly pay for the services (insurers, employers, employees, or taxpayers). This chapter refers collectively to this group of interested parties as *the public*.

Accountability can be achieved by informal, subjective means or through the exchange of information using a formal set of metrics. One mechanism that has been used to create accountability is accreditation. *Accreditation* is a process by which an entity external to the organization providing goods or services evaluates that organization against a set of predetermined requirements or desirable attributes and publicly attests to the results.

The term *certification* often is used to denote a similar process, except that certification more often is used in reference either to the determination of an individual's (rather than an organization's) competency or to the government's determination of an organization's eligibility to participate in a government program. Although organizational accreditation or certification—as contrasted with licensure—is usually thought of as voluntary, the decision to seek accreditation can be truly optional, linked to participation in an insurance program,[1] or required for licensure by government at the federal or state level.[2] Throughout the world, either private-sector bodies or government agencies provide organizational accreditation and certification; in the United States, private-sector bodies provide organizational accreditation, and either private-sector or government agencies provide certification. In contrast, *licensure* is always the domain of government, is nearly always mandatory, and requires that organizations meet certain legally defined requirements to practice or exercise a certain activity.

Regulation and Accreditation

Trade associations or professional societies within the field usually create and govern the bodies that provide accreditation. Thus, a major genesis of accreditation or private-sector certification is professionals' desire to define adherence to professional norms and standards in the delivery of services at both individual and organizational levels. However, regulatory and market forces also have a strong influence on the presence of accreditation. Regulatory forces, including licensure and federal or state regulations or mandates, and the justice system, including malpractice litigation, urge professional groups to offer accreditation—both to encourage adherence to standards of performance beyond those required by licensure and as an alternative to additional regulatory control. Some see the implicit delegation of a portion of accountability to accreditation as a manifestation of the self-monitoring that society has historically granted—and expected—through implicit and explicit contracts it establishes with professionals. Market forces play a role in some forms of accreditation, as in the case of health maintenance organizations (HMOs); some private purchasers either encourage or require HMO accreditation as a prerequisite to inclusion in the insurance programs they offer to employees. Thus, in most situations, accreditation exists where there are both a professional drive to set and maintain standards and either regulatory or market pressures that support accreditation as an alternative to regulation or nonstandardized reporting to each entity demanding information.

Although a full discussion of the relative merits of accreditation versus government regulation in ensuring accountability is beyond the scope of this chapter, the following points describe a few of the relative advantages of accreditation.

- Standards can be created, changed, and updated frequently on the basis of science and professional norms rather than on the basis of the political process required for amending laws or government regulations.
- The bar can be set above the minimum required for licensure or mandatory government review without unduly constraining entry into the field.
- The feedback provided to the entity or individual being evaluated usually is richer than pass/fail licensure decisions and can include substantial information the entity can use to improve quality and safety.

The following points describe a couple of the relative disadvantages of accreditation.

- If the accrediting body is perceived to be controlled by the industry being evaluated, there may be concern that the standards and evaluation process are not rigorous enough to serve the public's interest.
- If multiple accrediting bodies provide accreditation for the same type of healthcare entity, the competition—which in most circumstances drives continuous improvement in products and services—creates the potential for each body to set more easily achievable standards to gain market share.

The Process and Content of Accreditation

Accreditation is based on the premise that it is possible both to define attributes critical (either required or highly desirable) to the quality and safety of a healthcare product or service and to create a method to measure whether a threshold of performance has been achieved. Critical attributes can be defined for both administrative and clinical activities, and they can be based on expert opinion, consensus (of providers or multiple stakeholders), or research studies (qualitative or quantitative studies). Measurement can involve on-site observation, review of policies, review or abstraction of data from administrative or clinical records, surveys, and interviews with provider staff or patients (see Figure 18.1). Many accreditation programs still rely on only on-site observation and review of reports and policies, but other types of measurement are feasible.

Following the measurement phase—data collection by the accrediting body—the accreditor analyzes the data to transform them into information about the evaluated entity's performance. An accreditation decision usually includes an overall assessment of the entity (organization or service) as a whole. It also may include assessment of specific components, functions, or services that compose the larger entity.

To complete the process, the accrediting body shares information concerning the results of the evaluation to both the evaluated entity and the parties (e.g., consumers, patients, purchasers, insurers, government agencies)

FIGURE 18.1
Potential
Sources of
Data for Use in
Accreditation

Observation
Direct observation of structures or processes used by an entity

Interviews
Structured and unstructured interviews with patients and staff

Audits
Verification of the integrity and accuracy of data, including data collection and reporting processes

Review of written documentation (reports, policies, medical records)
Review, either on-site or remotely, and abstraction of data that have been recorded for either administrative or clinical purposes

Surveys
Collection and analysis of data from surveys of those using services (e.g., consumers, patients, physicians in HMOs) or supplying services (e.g., nurses, doctors, pharmacists in hospitals)

Derived information (claims, clinical reports)
Collection and analysis of data contained in either paper or electronic form and used in claims (e.g., office visit, laboratory, pharmacy, other services) or in reports on clinical processes (e.g., laboratory, pathology results)

requesting the accountability. The level and quantity of information the accrediting body shares with the evaluated entity and outside groups vary. The information can range from a simple list of organizations that passed (with no indication of organizations that did not apply or applied but failed to be accredited) to relatively detailed information on comparative performance, including performance on specific subsets of the requirements. The subject of the evaluation often receives more in-depth information. If this information is timely and sufficiently detailed, the subject can use it in activities to improve quality and safety. Most accreditation bodies expect that the accredited organization will use this feedback to improve.

Scope and Use of Accreditation in Healthcare: Successes and Failures

Hospitals

Accountability for hospital quality in the United States has relied primarily on regulation and accreditation, both of which are highly influenced by professionalism and professionals. Similarly to licensure for physicians, hospital licensure is codified in laws at the state level and usually overseen by state-appointed medical or hospital boards, the majority of whose members are physicians. However, the federal government, in its role as the largest purchaser of hospital care in the United States (through the Medicare program), has played the most prominent government role in defining hospital accountability. To participate in Medicare, the 1964 legislation that created the program required hospitals to undergo a federal regulatory review and certification by the organization now called the Centers for Medicare & Medicaid Services (CMS). As an alternative to federal review, the legislation allowed hospitals to participate in Medicare through *deemed status* based on accreditation by a private body, The Joint Commission. Thus, the accreditation of hospitals is tightly linked to the creation and evolution of The Joint Commission.[3] Today, over 80 percent of U.S. hospitals are accredited by The Joint Commission, and these hospitals contain over 96 percent of hospital beds in the United States.

Because Medicare pays for nearly 40 percent of all hospital bed days, the viability of most hospitals depends on their ability to participate in the Medicare program. In their distrust of direct government oversight and need to participate in Medicare, most U.S. hospitals seek Joint Commission accreditation (Greenberg 1998). In addition, 46 states and 1 territory license hospitals on the basis of attainment of Joint Commission accreditation.

Accreditation by The Joint Commission is based on a set of standards. These standards encompass the requirements set out by CMS that organizations must meet to participate in the Medicare program (called Conditions of Participation). In addition to meeting basic standards, The Joint Commission requires hospitals to conduct activities to improve the quality and safety of patient care, including activities based on the collection and use of nationally standardized (core) performance measurement sets called ORYX. These sets measure a large number of clinical conditions related to hospital admission (e.g., heart failure, acute myocardial infarction, pneumonia, childbirth, surgical infections). Each hospital selects a subset of ORYX measures to report to The Joint Commission on a quarterly basis. The Joint Commission uses these measurements to focus its onsite survey of the hospital and examine the hospital's use of the measurement results to improve the quality and safety of care.

The National Quality Forum evaluates and endorses all ORYX measures. This forum represents the various users of performance measurement results—consumers, purchasers, healthcare organizations, healthcare professionals, and government. In addition, the Hospital Quality Alliance approved many of these measures, which are now reported publicly on The Joint Commission and CMS websites.

For accreditation reviews beginning in January 2004, The Joint Commission made seven significant changes designed to make accreditation a more continuous process for maintaining and improving a healthcare organization's performance and to provide more useful information about healthcare organizations to the public.

1. It rewrote and reorganized standards to make them as clear as possible and eliminated those not strongly linked to patient safety and quality of care. It also reformatted the standards to itemize the elements of performance in each, clarifying what an organization must do to comply with each standard.

2. It introduced a requirement that organizations conduct a performance evaluation annually on its compliance with all the standards. Organizations must submit this self-assessment, a corrective action plan to address standard(s) not in compliance, and objective measures to be used in demonstrating successful correction to The Joint Commission for review, consultation, and approval. To encourage a rigorous self-assessment and full disclosure, The Joint Commission does not use these findings and plans, if approved, to revoke an organization's accreditation status.

3. It feeds information from multiple sources, including MedPar and ORYX data, into a priority focus tool—an algorithm that identifies critical areas on which the organization can focus internal assessment and improvement activities and on which The Joint Commission can focus during the on-site survey.

4. During the on-site survey, surveyors examine these priority focus areas by using a tracer methodology—that is, following patients' care throughout their hospitalization by observing care, interviewing patients and staff, and examining documents.

5. The surveyors use their findings to conduct system analyses to identify and consult on strengths and weaknesses in the hospital's clinical and organizational systems.

6. If an organization is out of compliance with only a few standards, it has 45 days to provide evidence of compliance to The Joint Commission. If The Joint Commission accepts the evidence, it accredits the organization. If the organization fails to provide sufficient evidence, The Joint Commission places it on provisional accreditation. If it has too many standards out of compliance during the on-site survey or does not emerge from provisional accreditation in a timely manner, The Joint Commission accredits the organization conditionally; if poor performance continues, The Joint Commission does not accredit the organization. Thus, *accredited* means that The Joint Commission found the organization to be in compliance with all the standards.

7. The report of an organization's performance placed on The Joint Commission's public website includes not only the organization's accreditation status but also absolute and comparative performance with respect to discrete national patient safety goals and to quality goals based on ORYX data (i.e., for acute myocardial infarction, heart failure, community-acquired pneumonia, pregnancy and related conditions, surgical infections, childhood asthma care, and, as they are developed, additional national standardized core measures for other diseases and conditions).

In addition, this quality report indicates whether the hospital has earned special certification for disease-specific services such as diabetes, asthma, or heart disease, or other quality awards, such as the Baldrige National Quality Award.

In 2006, all on-site accreditation surveys became unannounced. Previously, full surveys, usually occurring at three-year intervals, were announced a few months in advance.

In addition to hospitals, The Joint Commission accredits an array of other healthcare organizations including home care organizations, hospices, nursing homes, ambulatory surgery centers, ambulatory office practices, behavioral health programs, and laboratories.

Insurers

Before the emergence of HMOs, insurers were regulated primarily though state insurance laws. Through the 1980s, accountability for HMOs, which emerged in the late 1970s and early 1980s and combined insurance with varying degrees of oversight of clinical delivery functions, remained largely within an insurance regulatory framework. Accountability for care in HMOs that employed physicians or ran hospitals was subject to the same licensing and accreditation standards as those of other hospitals and physicians. Initially, there was little or no oversight of HMO functions related to utilization or quality management or contractually imposed controls on physicians or other providers.

Not motivated by these limited regulatory requirements, HMO accountability instead grew in response to market forces, specifically pressures from the purchasers of healthcare for more detailed information on the quality of services provided by HMOs. One manifestation of this pressure was the creation of a voluntary accreditation process by the National Committee for Quality Assurance (NCQA). Although other organizations including URAC (previously called the Utilization Review Accreditation Commission) and the Accrediting Association for Ambulatory Health Care (AAAHC) accredit HMOs, NCQA accredits most of them. More recently, health plans' participation in the Medicare program and more widespread and detailed regulation, especially of HMO plans, have raised regulatory pressures as well.

Although some large employers (about half of the *Fortune* 100) and the federal Office of Personnel Management require health plan accreditation, relatively few other employers do. Largely because voluntary accreditation by NCQA and others developed before states' movement to increase regulation of HMOs, about 35 states now recognize private accreditation as fulfilling all or part of state HMO licensure requirements. In addition, CMS has issued rules that allow HMOs and preferred provider organizations (PPOs) to substitute deemed status by accrediting bodies approved by CMS for most CMS requirements related to HMO and PPO participation in the Medicare Advantage program. However, because Medicare is a much smaller proportion of HMO or PPO enrollment, Medicare requirements for PPOs and HMOs—or deemed status for these requirements—have not affected health plan accountability as significantly. Thus, in contrast to nearly universal hospital accreditation, only half of all HMOs (although most of the largest plans) are accredited by a private accrediting group. Finally, for non-HMO forms of managed care, such as the PPO or consumer-directed health plan (most of which are basically high-deductible PPO plans) markets, little accountability for quality exists beyond the market and basic state insurance regulations. Although NCQA and other accreditors offer voluntary accreditation programs for PPOs, fewer than 10 percent of PPOs are accredited. However, as a result of the participation of PPO plans in the Medicare Advantage program and a growing interest of some employers to be able to compare PPO and HMO plans, the percentage of accredited PPOs is growing.

Like most other accrediting bodies, NCQA began as a committee of a trade organization related to health plans—the Group Health Association of America, the predecessor of the current Association of American Health Plans (AAHP). However, in addition to the interest from health plans themselves, private purchasers' demands for accountability strongly influenced NCQA's early development. As a result, NCQA became independent of AAHP in 1990 and has evolved independently; its current board of directors includes representatives from consumer, purchaser, provider, and other healthcare sectors. Only 1 of the 16 current board members is affiliated with an HMO or other organization now accredited by NCQA—an unusual board composition among accrediting organizations.

Another factor that marked the early development of NCQA was the development and implementation of a set of clinical performance measures originally called the Health Plan Employer Data and Information Set, recently changed to the Healthcare Effectiveness Data and Information Set (HEDIS). With input from clinicians and purchasers, a small group of HMO leaders began to create this data set. The goal was to create a reliable, valid, and standard set of clinical performance measures that would provide useful information on quality for purchasers and limit large purchasers' uncoordinated and disparate demands for clinical information from HMOs. HEDIS now includes more than 100 performance measures, most of which are specified for use at both plan and physician office practice levels.

Since 1999, NCQA accreditation has changed in important ways. The addition of measures related to management of major chronic illnesses has expanded the HEDIS measurement set substantially. In addition, HEDIS now includes a version of the Consumer Assessment of Healthcare Providers and Systems (CAHPS 2.0H) developed by a research team coordinated and funded by the Agency for Healthcare Research and Quality. More than

80 percent of HMOs, including plans that do not opt for NCQA accreditation, now report most or all of the HEDIS measures annually to NCQA (Dybkare 1994). Although some plans do not report on all measures (e.g., some plans do not have enough members or lack critical data), the population base of the plans that do report a given measure usually exceeds 50 million people. Beginning in 2008, NCQA is implementing a broad array of standards for health plans (termed Accreditation 08) in three new areas:

1. How plans educate and involve their members (enrollees)
2. How plans use and evaluate disease and care management
3. How plans measure and reward high-quality care in hospitals and physician office practices

In 1999, NCQA began to incorporate performance on selected HEDIS measures as an integral and substantial portion (35 percent in 2007) of the overall accreditation score, representing a major change in accreditation practice. As noted previously, nearly all accreditation and certification have relied exclusively on adherence to standards or on cognitive testing rather than on an analysis of quantitative performance measures. A major criticism of accreditation is that little empirical evidence links compliance with accreditation standards to outcomes of the service or care delivered. The inclusion of reliable measures of clinical processes and outcomes of care in the accreditation process increases the likelihood that accreditation status is a valid indication of the quality of care delivered.

NCQA now reports its accreditation decisions on a public website as *excellent, commendable, accredited, provisional,* or *denied* (Romano 1993). The website also includes plan-specific information about performance on accreditation standards and HEDIS measures grouped in five categories understandable to consumers (*access-service, qualified providers, staying healthy, getting better,* and *living with illness*). NCQA HEDIS and health plan accreditation data now are linked to major commercial websites such as Medscape, America OnLine (AOL), and Compuserve and have been used as the basis of an annual "Best Health Plans" issue of *U.S. News and World Report*. This level of reporting begins to provide the level of detail that purchasers and consumers need to select health plans on the basis of differential quality.

NCQA also created a web-based reporting and self-assessment system for many of its accreditation processes, minimizing the need for on-site review of materials and programs. Finally, like The Joint Commission, NCQA has expanded its scope of accreditation programs to include managed behavioral health, disease management, and physician group practices.

In summary, for HMOs, the market—driven primarily by private purchasers and voluntary accreditation—has played a larger role in the evolution of accountability than in the physician or hospital sectors. Regulation by state and federal governments is moving beyond insurance regulation but is still not widespread or consistent, and beyond HMOs, little accountability of insurers exists.

Nursing Homes

Nursing home accreditation has been limited, largely because of the dominance of state Medicaid programs (Medicare accounts for less than 10 percent of nursing home expenditures) and self (private) pay as the means of financing nursing home care. CMS (Medicare and Medicaid) and the states (Medicaid) have developed an extensive set of regulatory standards and a government survey and certification program to enforce nursing home regulations. Given the less-than-adequate quality of nursing home care and, in some instances, outright abuse of patients in nursing homes in the past, most public advocacy groups have been strongly opposed to allowing deemed status out of fear that the largely for-profit nursing home industry would try to lower current regulatory standards. Thus, no legislation authorizes CMS or states to allow deemed status in Medicare or Medicaid for private accrediting bodies to substitute for governmental survey and certification of nursing homes.

This regulation contrasts with that of hospitals, traditionally not-for-profit entities with strong professional involvement, and of HMOs, for which private purchasers played a major role in requiring or encouraging accreditation. The Joint Commission and others offer accreditation to nursing homes, but few apply because the deemed status and market benefits are not present. Nevertheless, government surveys have shown that accredited nursing homes have significantly fewer serious deficiencies than do unaccredited nursing homes.

Ambulatory Care

Accreditation of ambulatory care practice (e.g., in sites where ambulatory surgery is performed) is growing, but it remains far less developed than in the hospital or HMO sector. One exception is in renal dialysis, where the dominance of Medicare as a payer and the creation of deemed status for some parts of the program by CMS have created close to universal accreditation of programs. However, most insurers, including Medicare, have few, if any, requirements other than licensure for ambulatory care sites (e.g., physician groups, individual offices) to participate in their programs. Moreover, the traditional reliance on professionalism for assurance of high quality is arguably stronger in ambulatory care, which has been dominated by small physician-owned practices. (The median size of a physician office practice is still under four physicians.)

The emergence of large regional or national for-profit entities providing imaging (MRI, mammography), renal dialysis, cancer treatment, and other services, combined with the growing recognition of purchasers, insurers, and the public of the wide variation in the quality and cost of ambulatory care services, is prompting a number of programs and entities to offer accreditation of ambulatory care programs. Some examples include accreditation of office-based surgery (e.g., by AAAHC or The Joint Commission) and imaging centers (e.g., by the American College of Radiology or The Joint Commission), but none of these activities has achieved close to universal acceptance, even when deemed by CMS (e.g., office-based surgery accreditation), with the exception of the deemed accreditation of mammography centers by the American College of Radiology. A notable and ultimately unsuccessful attempt in ambulatory care accreditation was the American Medical Accreditation Program, created by the American Medical Association to offer accreditation to physician office practices. A lack of regulatory and market incentives from the public and private sectors and the concern of some specialty boards that a physician's office accreditation would be redundant to board certification of the individual physician appear to have been major factors in the program's demise.

The Future of Accreditation: Challenges and Changes

If accreditation is to remain an important part of ensuring accountability, accreditation will need to evolve in response to market forces and the evolution of the healthcare system. One of the most important challenges to accreditation is the proliferation of new services and products and the types of organizations that provide them.

For example, most of the growth in hospital revenues since the mid-1990s has been in ambulatory and ancillary services; some hospitals now receive the majority of their income from services other than inpatient care. This movement also has given rise to myriad outpatient facilities that provide some component of inpatient services, such as urgent care centers, ambulatory surgery centers, and office-based surgery sites. An accreditation process for hospitals that focuses largely on inpatient standards would not address this new reality.

In addition, services like disease management, mental health benefits management, and pharmacy benefits management, which were included in the services of a staff- or group-model HMO, are now provided by contract with separate entities—entities for which no system of accountability for quality and safety currently exists. Accreditation that focuses on hospitals or HMOs, even if it addresses delegated functions, does not capture these new activities and sites fully.

Accreditation will need to evolve quickly toward a more flexible, multi-entity, performance-based process to serve both the public interest and that of these new activities. Accreditation also will need to address issues related to coordination of services for patients and data sharing between the increasingly fragmented entities involved in healthcare.

Another factor that continues to gain momentum is public demand for information that allows comparison of individual clinicians, clinical groups, hospitals, and health plans regarding clinical quality and cost. The need for quality measurement data to use as the basis for payment in the growing number of pay-for-reporting or performance programs has further accelerated the demand for this information (Rosenthal et al. 2006). Reliance on structural and process standards to provide a range of accreditation decisions for a single entity provides only a limited amount of meaningful information to consumers or purchasers relevant to their decision making. In other words, although this information helps to differentiate between accredited and unaccredited organizations, it is less helpful in differentiating accredited organizations with respect to specific services or programs. This lack of differentiation is especially evident in the hospital sector, where virtually all hospitals are accredited. Furthermore, creating comparative information at the physician group or individual level would be even more costly and difficult than creating similar information with respect to HMOs or hospitals.

Given the costs of information gathering and the lower fiscal margins in virtually all sectors of healthcare, accreditors and others will need to find ways to reduce the number of redundant standards and measures and the cost of data collection. Without these developments, efforts to enhance accountability at the provider level are likely to result in redundant and dysfunctional evaluations—and unnecessary costs—and to increase the resistance of those being evaluated even further.

As noted, NCQA now includes performance measures as part of HMO accreditation and reports information on accreditation of HMOs and PPOs at multiple levels of performance. Likewise, as noted, The Joint Commission reports comparative data on its website that are more useful to the public and purchasers in selecting healthcare provider organizations, especially at the hospital or large group level. At present, however, because of issues with small sample size (especially within a given health plan), information on clinical performance measures, although already collected at the individual physician level for some measures, cannot be reported for most measures at the physician level reliably. In addition, the system in which a physician provides care can influence his or her patient outcomes (Krein et al. 2002). Pennsylvania's release of surgeon-specific mortality data demonstrated that some surgeons who operated in multiple hospitals had better-than-average (statewide) results in one hospital and worse-than-average (statewide) results in another hospital. Thus, collection of the depth and quantity of information necessary to prepare reports that are reliable and valid at the physician small group or individual physician level will pose a formidable challenge.

Nevertheless, with the increasing demand for value-based purchasing—purchasing healthcare services on the basis of quality and safety, not just costs—interest in measuring performance in physician offices has increased. CMS has announced a program in which physician offices that voluntarily report on standardized performance measures will receive bonus payments under Medicare. Accreditation cannot play a central role in accountability in the future unless it can provide the public (purchasers, insurers, consumers, and patients) with reliable and valid comparative information on quality and safety.

A number of other groups not tied directly to accreditation have created report cards of varying types. Most rely on consumer surveys of varying reliability or validity. Few use random samples or have large enough sample sizes to offer valid comparisons between entities. Some larger HMOs rate providers, and others furnish basic demographical information about physicians in their clinical networks. In another effort, the Pacific Business Group on Health created a more sophisticated set of measures to rate HMOs and providers; this set includes physician group practice information for larger physician groups in the California market.

Although some large purchasers are able to use current information on HMO quality as part of their purchasing decisions, most consumers feel overwhelmed by the number of sites and are distrustful of conflicting report cards or ratings. The result is that consumers still rely largely on word-of-mouth information from friends, relatives, coworkers, or their physicians in making healthcare choices.

The long-term hope for more effective accreditation and information about quality depends on enhancement of information technology use in healthcare. The wide availability of broadband, web-enabled data collection eventually may enable accreditation based on real-time measurement of a rich array of clinical structure, process, and outcome performance measures that also can be used for quality monitoring, rather than on retrospective measures or survey-assessed compliance with standards alone.

Accreditation Sets the Bar Too Low

Issue

Accreditation, especially where it is a prerequisite for participating in large insurance programs such as Medicare, must be constructed to set a basic level of acceptable quality that at least encompasses the minimal level required by law and regulation. If the threshold is set too far above this minimal level, many or most providers will not be able to achieve accreditation, thus reducing the information about them that enables consumer choice and adversely affecting access for many consumers. Most important, the fewer organizations enrolled in the accreditation process, the less influence accreditation has in improving the quality and safety of care. On the other hand, if the threshold is set too close to the regulatory minimum, providers with serious quality defects may gain access to the insurance program and patients will be less protected from harm. This dilemma is similar to that seen in licensing and has led some to see accreditation as a basic floor of requirements that everyone doing business in a given area should achieve. Thus, if regulatory requirements are considered the minimum level of performance that must be achieved to remain in business, accreditation could be described as a basic level of quality and safety that should be achieved.

Where accreditation is optional, those who do not attempt to achieve accreditation avoid the cost of accreditation and the risk of not passing. With no pressure to participate, a high threshold could discourage providers from seeking accreditation because the risk of failure is far worse than not being evaluated at all. Even more challenging is the situation in which multiple accrediting bodies compete. Purchasers or consumers may or may not distinguish one body's accreditation from that of another. A move by one accrediting body to raise standards may be seen by its competitor(s) as an opportunity to gain market share by retaining a lower standard. When neither strong pressure from state regulation nor incentives (e.g., differential payment or selection) from private purchasers exist to encourage accreditation and push standards to high levels, provider organizations tend to move to the easiest accreditation program or drop accreditation altogether.

Finally, the governance of many accrediting organizations is a concern. As noted earlier in this chapter, accreditation traditionally has been a bridge between professionalism and regulation. In many instances, professionals have created accrediting bodies to drive quality assessment and improvement and to reduce the need for direct government regulation. Many accrediting organizations emanate from professional groups themselves. Although involvement of those within the profession is important in setting credible standards, if the interests of other stakeholders, particularly consumers, do not balance this involvement, there may be pressure to refrain from setting standards that could disadvantage members of the professional organization that controls, or strongly influences, the accrediting organization. Accrediting bodies given deemed status by the federal government must be not for profit; regardless of the composition of their governing boards, they must act in the interest of the public.

Analysis and Response

Given these disparate forces, the decision on where to set the threshold of acceptable performance can be challenging. The problem of setting the bar too low often resolves itself over time because nearly all accreditation programs implement new standards and requirements that periodically raise the bar. NCQA's new Accreditation 08 program and The Joint Commission's revision of the hospital accreditation program in 2004—with an overall update to be implemented in 2009—are examples of how accreditation programs can introduce substantial numbers of new and more challenging standards over time. Even more important in terms of raising the bar over time are the inclusion of quality improvement standards that emphasize demonstration of improvement on clinical measures, the relative performance of an entity on clinical measures as part of its accreditation score, and the incremental inclusion of specific patient safety goals in the accreditation process.

The decision on where to set the "passing" level may be even more problematic to the degree that accrediting bodies are strongly influenced or controlled by the providers they accredit or, in contrast, by those that advocate higher quality but nevertheless are not willing to pay more to attain it. One approach to addressing this challenge is to seek broad input from those being accredited and those desiring accountability though formal groups such as multi- and single-stakeholder advisory councils. Structuring the accrediting body's board of directors or committees that have decision-making authority so that they are representative of all the relevant stakeholder groups is also helpful in addressing this challenge. In addition, the accrediting body's collaboration with other multi-stakeholder groups, such as the National Quality Forum, helps to create stakeholder buy-in.

An important factor in the usefulness of accreditation is the careful determination of a standard's importance and evidence base. Good standards must be based on a carefully structured determination of what evidence can be found and documented to support a conclusion that the standard in question is critical to good quality and safety. The standards also must be linked to collective definitions of quality. IOM's (2001) definition is used most widely: the degree to which healthcare services for individuals or populations increase the likelihood of desired outcomes and are consistent with current professional knowledge.

In the case of endpoint outcomes, any endpoint seen as important and desirable by those with an interest in the action should be a standard. However, a more formal, consensual process is valuable in determining the scope and definition of critical outcomes. Although outcomes often are considered the most desirable type of requirement or standard, numerous instances exist in which outcomes are not measurable, so infrequent (e.g., death from wrong-site surgery), or so remote in time (e.g., myocardial infarction from untreated hypertension) that using a process or structural standard as a proxy is more desirable. Any standard, and its corresponding metric based on a structure, process, or intermediate outcome, must be linked to some desired end outcome. Structural or process standards can relate to either administrative or clinical systems.

In the administrative realm, few, if any, experimental studies suggest links to health outcomes, and most links rely on face validity (including laws) and expert opinion (e.g., Baldrige National Quality Award criteria for managing and improving quality, or advisory group expert advice on the role of organizational leadership in improving safety). To avoid meaningless and burdensome administrative standards, careful dialog and review by experts *external to* the staff of the accrediting body are critical. In clinical services, evidence should come from experimental studies (e.g., studies on safe practices and infection-control procedures such as hand washing) and, when possible, from randomized controlled trials (e.g., the guideline that HbA1c levels in diabetics should be lower than 9.0).

To transform standards into information about an organization's performance, accreditation must include some metric or verification process to ensure that the organization has met the required standards and criteria. Few means of gathering data exist (see Figure 18.1). Most accreditation in the past has included only structural or process standards measured by reviews of documentation, interviews with patients or staff, or observation of certain processes. Because this type of review is subjective, the reviewers' levels of expertise, experience, and survey training are crucial to valid measurement.

Since 1999, in assessing health plan accreditation, NCQA has included scores of plans' relative performance on measures of clinical processes or intermediate outcomes (HEDIS) and on surveys of patient experience of care (CAHPS). Since 2001, The Joint Commission has included similar measures of intermediate and physiological outcomes in the ORYX measures that hospitals use, and in the future, it plans on incorporating results from a hospital CAHPS to survey patient experience. Relative performance scores on these measures are not currently included in Joint Commission accreditation scores. Clinical performance measures and patient experience-of-care surveys, especially when used for public accountability, are, in most cases, based on higher levels of scientific evidence than are on-site reviews of structures or processes. This scientific evidence links them directly to final outcomes (e.g., survival, quality of life). Thus, clinical performance measures and patient experience-of-care surveys provide a view of quality unavailable in structure and administrative process review alone. In addition, if these performance measures are collected from a sufficient sampling frame and reported in a timely manner, those being evaluated can use them as internal quality improvement measures. Thus, the potential exists for performance measures to serve as an effective and efficient means for both external reporting and internal quality improvement purposes.

If a measure is not useful for internal quality improvement because it measures a process or an outcome that is not under the control of the measured entity, the measure is probably not relevant as an accountability measure either; accountability is based on the ability to control—at least in part—the things for which one is held accountable.

External measurement of outcomes may be the ultimate goal in most instances, but in some areas, such as safety, structural or process measures of risk reduction are necessary even if the undesirable outcome never occurs.

In such cases, verification of structural or process elements critical to quality and safety is part of accreditation. In addition, because of coding and reporting problems, insufficient sample sizes, or a lack of robust electronic information systems, reliable or valid performance measures on many aspects of quality are currently impossible or prohibitively expensive to collect. Thus, metrics other than performance measures still play a central and critical role in providing accountability for quality.

Accreditation Fails to Provide Critical Information Needed for Either Consumer Choice or Quality Improvement

Issue

In the past, most accreditation has been reported as pass/fail or, in many instances, as a list of those who received accreditation, with no reporting of those who attempted and failed or those who did not even attempt accreditation. Although this pass/fail information can be considered as meeting the basic intent of accreditation (to ensure that a basic floor— beyond the minimum—has been met), most accreditation processes now include a rich set of information that can be used for comparison or choice. Moreover, the scoring or determination of achieving a set threshold is not an exact science. Reasonable individuals can disagree on which requirements are most critical or should contribute most to the scoring. Finally, the level of data publicly reported may reflect the relative influence of those who want to limit external reporting and those who want more public accountability.

Analysis and Response

In most traditional forms of accreditation, the only information provided to those outside the entity being accredited was whether the entity received accreditation. In some cases, this information did not include whether a group had been evaluated but was denied accreditation. In some cases, such as airline safety, public knowledge that a given airline, airplane, and pilot are certified may be enough, but where personal services are involved, a reasonable argument can be made that the public needs more detailed information. Although accreditation itself is an important differentiation from nonaccredited status, consumer and payer demand for more in-depth information about quality in healthcare is increasing, and the fact that an entity is accredited is no longer sufficient. Given the strength of evidence of substantial variation in the quantity and quality of services provided by accredited healthcare providers (IOM 2001), purchasers and patients would benefit from more information on which to base their choices.

By using the information gathered in accreditation in a more robust manner, organizations can use accreditation as more than a basic floor and can provide the public with information critical to making choices about quality. As noted, some accreditation programs have expanded their set of metrics beyond inspection and verification. In addition, NCQA and The Joint Commission no longer submit simple reports of "accredited or not." NCQA reports accreditation status in one of its annual publications (the *State of Health Care Report*) on the NCQA website. It also reports accreditation status in a publicly available data set (Quality Compass) both as ranked categories based on accreditation scores (excellent, commendable, accredited, provisional) and as specific ranked areas of accreditation (one to four stars in access-service, providers [credentials], staying healthy, getting better, and living with chronic illness). Using NCQA data, the *U.S. News and World Report* annual "Best Health Plans" issue and website also have featured numerical plan ranking along with star ratings.

The Joint Commission provides similar levels of accreditation status and, as described above, provides disease-specific performance information on selected ORYX measures on its public website. In 2007, The Joint Commission began publication of an annual report on quality and safety that analyzes performance and trends for ORYX measures and specific national patient safety goals both nationally and by state. At present, other accrediting bodies (e.g., URAC, AAAHC) disclose only whether the organization has achieved accredited or certified status.

The Cost of Accreditation Is Not Worth the Benefit

Issue

The concern that the cost of accreditation is not worth the benefit it provides is raised most frequently by those undergoing (and directly paying for) accreditation. However, purchasers and consumers who benefit from (as well as indirectly pay for) accreditation should see a net benefit. The costs of accreditation, both indirect (e.g., preparation, data collection, reports) and direct (e.g., the fee paid to be reviewed), can be considerable—especially of accreditation that relies exclusively or heavily on paper documentation of large quantities of data or on extensive on-site inspections. If purchasers or consumers do not use or require accreditation, providers may feel that accreditation is not a cost-effective use of their resources. If accreditation is required, concerns still exist about whether the standards reflect critical components of quality and safety and whether the evaluation methods are the most efficient means for determining compliance with those standards. Any quality improvement or regulatory process has associated costs, but given the high and rising costs of healthcare, investment in a form of accreditation that does not bring real value, either to providers though quality improvement or to those using the services through assurance of quality or choice, should be questioned.

Analysis and Response

In its traditional form, accreditation is a mechanism for enhancing improvement in the quality and safety of healthcare and for providing accountability of the entity to other stakeholders (e.g., patients, consumers, purchasers, insurers, regulators). Ultimately, those who pay for the healthcare services and ask for accountability for those services must determine whether the benefits of accreditation exceed its costs. A healthcare organization may choose to *undergo* accreditation by an outside entity as a benchmark for its overall internal quality improvement processes, but this benefit may not be sufficient—if purchasers and consumers do not use the results—for the organization to *maintain* its accreditation. Some public purchasers (CMS and a few Medicaid programs), some regulators (26 states), and some private purchasers (mostly *Fortune* 100 companies) require accreditation of health plans as a precursor to contracting with them, but the majority do not. Likewise, most states and CMS accept (deem) hospital accreditation in lieu of government survey and certification, but they do not require accreditation of hospitals; a (free) state survey for licensure and Medicare certification is always available. Surveys of consumers and private purchasers (specifically those selecting health plans) indicate a minimal understanding of the value or use of accreditation in decision making, which presents a mixed picture of how, in actual practice, the costs and benefits of accreditation are weighed.

However, given the ongoing concerns about healthcare insurers and about the quality and safety of care in hospitals, organizations need some form of accountability. The value of the most common alternatives to accreditation (i.e., reliance on professionalism and voluntary quality improvement, government regulation, or contractually defined performance measures) in ensuring accountability is far from proven.

Some feel that government regulation may be more desirable than, or a replacement for, voluntary (or deemed) accreditation. However, regulation is fraught with political problems and frequently lags behind changes in healthcare. The history of healthcare licensure, state mandates, and other regulatory processes shows ample evidence of the limitations of regulation as a means of providing accountability. Regulation is often an adversarial process in which political power, rather than evidence-based analysis, determines the outcome.

In contrast, accreditation can create an active dialog between those being held accountable and those desiring the accountability. In addition, because action by a legislature is not required, accrediting bodies can adjust more quickly to changes in the scope, modes, and technologies of delivered services. Finally, a healthcare provider that seeks voluntary accreditation has a desire to take ownership of and responsibility for its performance rather than only to meet an outside party's requirements. Ultimately, these providers, not government agencies and accrediting bodies, control the quality and safety of care for the public.

Conclusion

This chapter traces the development of accreditation as an approach to addressing accountability in healthcare. In the past, accreditation in its traditional form has, in some areas of healthcare, provided a successful approach to measuring and reporting accountability. Healthcare clearly needs enhanced accountability. This need demands a more robust set of metrics and accountability at multiple levels of the healthcare system. The challenge is whether accreditation can evolve to meet this expanded demand for accountability. An expanded scope of accreditation can help to meet that challenge, but major barriers first must be overcome for that expanded scope to meet its potential.

Study Questions

1. Compare and contrast the use of licensure and accreditation in terms of accountability and quality improvement.
2. What role can/should accreditation play in the future, given the prospect of a huge amount of information from electronic clinical and administrative data sources?
3. What roles do the market, regulation, and professionalism play in defining and promoting the use of accreditation as a means of accountability? How would a more prominent market for medical services affect the usefulness of accreditation? How would the implementation of a single-payer, government-financed system affect it (e.g., if Medicare coverage were extended to everyone living in the United States)?
4. If the ultimate goal is better health outcomes for individuals and populations, can measurement of health outcomes alone substitute for structure and process measures? Why or why not?

Notes

1. For example, hospital accreditation by The Joint Commission or certification by CMS is a prerequisite for hospitals to participate in the Medicare program. In this situation, accreditation by The Joint Commission is deemed (accepted as a substitute) for most elements of the CMS review and certification process.
2. Thirty-five states currently require HMOs to be accredited to sell insurance within the state or offer insurance to state employees. PPOs also face such requirements. In addition, 46 states and 1 territory use Joint

Commission accreditation to make hospital licensure decisions.

3. First called The Joint Commission on Accreditation of Hospitals (JCAH) and then The Joint Commission on Accreditation of Healthcare Organizations (JCAHO), The Joint Commission was founded in 1951 as an outgrowth of the American College of Surgeons (ACS) Hospital Standardization Program established in 1918 to improve the quality of care in U.S. hospitals, which at that time were largely unlicensed and unregulated. The JCAH Board of Commissioners was appointed by the ACS, American College of Physicians (ACP), American Hospital Association (AHA), and American Medical Association (AMA). The Canadian Medical Association also was a founding member but later withdrew and was replaced in 1969 by the American Dental Association (ADA). In the past decades, six voting public members; a voting nurse at large; and nonvoting representatives of home care, long-term care, and behavioral health have been added to the board, and 21 of the board's remaining 22 members still are appointed by ACP, ACS, ADA, AMA, and AHA.

References

Dybkare, R. 1994. "Quality Assurance, Accreditation, and Certification: Needs and Possibilities." *Clinical Chemistry* 40 (7, Pt. 2): 1416–20.

Emanuel, E. J., and L. L. Emanuel. 1996. "What Is Accountability in Health Care?" *Annals of Internal Medicine* 124 (2): 229–39.

Emanuel, L. L. 1996. "A Professional Response to Demands for Accountability: Practical Recommendations Regarding Ethical Aspects of Patient Care." Working Group on Accountability. *Annals of Internal Medicine* 124 (2): 240–49.

Greenberg, E. L. 1998. "How Accreditation Could Strengthen Local Public Health: An Examination of Models from Managed Care and Insurance Regulators." *Journal of Public Health Management and Practice* 4 (4): 33–37.

Institute of Medicine. 2001. *Crossing the Quality Chasm: A New Health System for the 21st Century*. Washington, DC: National Academies Press.

Krein, S. L., T. P. Hofer, E. A. Kerr, and R. A. Hayward. 2002. "Whom Should We Profile? Examing Diabetes Care Practice Variation Among Primary Care Providers, Groups and Health Facilities." *Health Services Research* 37 (5): 1159–80.

Romano, P. M. 1993. "Managed Care Accreditation: The Process and Early Findings." *Journal of Healthcare Quality* 15 (6): 12–16.

Rosenthal, M. B., B. E. Landon, S. L. Normand, R. G. Frank, and A. M. Epstein. 2006. "Pay for Performance in Commercial HMOs." *New England Journal of Medicine* 355 (18): 1895–902.

Other Useful Resources

Bell, D., and E. N. Brandt, Jr. 1999. "Accreditation by the National Committee on Quality Assurance (NCQA): A Description." *Journal of the Oklahoma State Medical Association* 92 (5): 234–37.

Braun, B. I., R. G. Koss, and J. M. Loeb. 1999. "Integrating Performance Measure Data into the Joint Commission Accreditation Process." *Evaluation & the Health Professions* 22 (3): 283–97.

Carlson, D. A. 1996. "Point of Care Testing: Regulation and Accreditation." *Clinical Laboratory Science* 9 (5): 298–302.

Flanagan, A. 1997. "Ensuring Health Care Quality: JCAHO's Perspective. Joint Commission on Accreditation of Healthcare Organizations." *Clinical Therapeutics* 19 (6): 1540–44.

Gonen, J. S., and S. L. Probyn. 1996. "The Evolution of Accreditation." *HMO* 37 (1): 52–57.

Halverson, P. K., R. M. Nicola, and E. L. Baker. 1998. "Performance Measurement and Accreditation of Public Health Organizations: A Call to Action." *Journal of Public Health Management and Practice* 4 (4): 5–7.

Irvine, D. 1997. "The Performance of Doctors: I: Professionalism and Self Regulation in a Changing World." *British Medical Journal* 314 (7093): 1540–42.

The Joint Commission. 2000. *Benchmarking in Health Care: Finding and Implementing Best Practices.* Oakbrook Terrace, IL: The Joint Commission.

Kassebaum, D. G., R. H. Eaglen, and E. R. Cutler. 1997. "The Meaning and Application of Medical Accreditation Standards." *Academic Medicine* 72 (9): 808–18.

Lansky, D., and S. Purdy. 1995. "Public Accountability for Health: New Standards for Health System Performance." *Managed Care Quarterly* 3 (3): 17–24.

Markson, L. E., and D. B. Nash. 1995. *Accountability and Quality in Health Care: The New Responsibility.* Oakbrook Terrace, IL: The Joint Commission.

O'Leary, D. S., and P. M. Schyve. 1994. "The Role of Accreditation in Quality Oversight and Improvement Under Healthcare Reform." *Quality Letter for Healthcare Leaders* 5 (10): 11–14.

O'Leary, M. R. 1996. *Clinical Performance Data: A Guide to Interpretation.* Oakbrook Terrace, IL: The Joint Commission.

O'Malley, C. 1997. "Quality Measurement for Health Systems: Accreditation and Report Cards." *American Journal of Health-System Pharmacy* 54 (13): 1528–35.

Scanlon, D. P., and T. J. Hendrix. 1998. "Health Plan Accreditation: NCQA, JCAHO, or Both?" *Managed Care Quarterly* 6 (4): 52–61.

Schyve, P. M. 1998. "Joint Commission Perspectives on Accreditation of Public Health Practice." *Journal of Public Health Management and Practice* 4 (4): 28–33.

Scrivens, E. 1998. "Widening the Scope of Accreditation—Issues and Challenges in Community and Primary Care." *International Journal for Quality in Health Care* 10 (3): 191–97.

Shaw, C. D. 2000. "External Quality Mechanisms for Health Care: Summary of the ExPeRT Project on Accreditation, EFQM and ISO Assessment in European Union Countries. External Peer Review Techniques. European Foundation for Quality Management. International Organization for Standardization." *International Journal for Quality in Health Care* 12 (3): 169–75.

Viswanathan, H. N. 2000. "Accrediting Organizations and Quality Improvement." *American Journal of Managed Care* 6 (10): 1117–30.

Walshe, K. 2000. *Accreditation in Primary Care: Towards Clinical Governance.* Abingdon, UK: Radcliffe.

HOW PURCHASERS SELECT AND PAY FOR QUALITY

Francois de Brantes

ealthcare cost trends continue to outpace inflation, and a study by RAND confirms that quality of care is highly deficient (McGlynn et al. 2003; Schuster, McGlynn, and Brook 1998; Wennberg 1999). Costs are increasing, and quality is stagnating. Faced with the decreasing value of resources committed to healthcare, purchasers have developed new strategies to select and pay for quality in the delivery of healthcare services.

In healthcare, the concept of value-based purchasing (VBP) was imported and applied on the basis of the premise that plans would compete for employer/employee premium dollars by demonstrating greater effectiveness in caring for covered members and greater efficiency in paying for care services. The latter was achieved by consolidating the purchasing power of payers and health plan sponsors and obtaining discounts from physicians, hospitals, and ancillary care providers. The former was achieved by standardizing measures of quality across plans and creating a common way of assessing plan quality. Efforts by the National Committee for Quality Assurance (NCQA) described in the previous chapter helped create the methodology for assessing plan performance on effectiveness of care in a standard way.

Even before VBP at the plan level lost its ability to improve quality and control costs for the majority of Americans covered by health insurance, purchasers had started to understand that providers did not change their behaviors for one plan alone. They changed their behaviors for all plans. As a result, there was little difference in the quality of care between managed care networks and nonmanaged networks (McGlynn et al. 2003; Schuster, McGlynn, and Brook 1998; Wennberg 1999), especially as purchasers demanded that plans increase the size of their networks. With the expansion of networks came the reduction in relative purchasing power. Purchaser focus has, as a result, shifted from individual plan performance to individual provider performance, evidenced by the creation of the Leapfrog Group (Birkmeyer et al. 2000).[1] With the release of the Institute of Medicine's (IOM 2001) *Crossing the Quality Chasm* report, purchasers also realized that serious gaps remained in the quality of care in the United States and that variations in quality at the individual provider level were significant. Reducing the variation and increasing the overall level of quality have become purchasing imperatives, especially with renewed and rampant cost increases.

Although Joint Commission accreditation of hospitals provides a baseline for measuring individual provider performance, it is insufficient to meet the needs of purchasers and consumers in relation to the new definition of VBP because accreditation hides significant variations in quality performance. However, The Joint Commission's individual measures of performance provide a robust answer as it continues to make them increasingly public.

Today, VBP has the ability to create competition at the provider level regarding effectiveness and efficiency of care. If quality is equal, purchasers want to reward the most efficient provider. If there are different degrees of quality, purchasers want to reward providers that demonstrate a higher level of quality. In addition, consumers show little or no interest in plan performance (they continue to select their plans on the basis of premium differences, not quality differences) but are increasingly interested in and motivated by provider performance (Hibbard and Jewett 1997; Marshall et al. 2000). Use of financial incentives, such as different coinsurance or co-pay levels, or use of tiering to differentiate providers is causing consumers to demand comparative provider performance data, which, until recently, were not available.

This chapter describes the efforts of General Electric (GE) and other large purchasers, in cooperation with health plans, leading provider organizations, and NCQA, to create a sustainable framework for VBP at the physician level. The effort is called Bridges to Excellence[2] because its objective is to create a bridge to cross the quality chasm. The primary components of that bridge are performance measures. Without them, there is no way to understand the gaps in quality nor any way to distinguish levels of performance from one provider to another with respect to the effectiveness of the care they deliver. Because cost of care is an imperfect way of measuring overall provider performance, purchasers' initial efforts should focus on defining measures of effectiveness and creating a business case for providers to compete on the basis of quality (Galvin 2001).

Background and Terminology

These concepts and initiatives already have had consequences in healthcare organizations and have the potential for more. Summaries of a few of these consequences follow.

- Managed care organizations (MCOs)—MCOs have touted their provider quality initiatives as a competitive advantage to increase their market share by winning new customers. However, many of these initiatives have failed to demonstrate robust returns on investment. In addition, they create dissonance at the provider level because of the disparity of initiatives among MCOs and the differences in the performance measures they use. Starting with the Leapfrog Group (Birkmeyer et al. 2000), purchasers continue to urge plans and providers to focus on standardizing measures of effectiveness of care and creating a level playing field for the comparison of physicians and hospitals. This standardization is especially important to purchaser-employers that offer multiple plans in a single geographic location. How can they explain to employees that each plan has identified a different set of top-quality providers? As a result, plans have agreed to come together under the Ambulatory and Hospital Quality Alliances and to harmonize the ways in which they measure quality. However, they will continue to compete on maximization of efficiency of care scores through innovative contracting mechanisms and benefit designs.

- Provider organizations (i.e., integrated delivery networks or large group practices)—Having a standardized means of assessing internal performance and a business case for improving effectiveness of care will help organized provider groups compete for patients. They have more resources to deploy in information technology and other support programs to help their physicians meet quality goals. In addition, the redesign of payment systems that encourage physicians to adopt better processes will put the decision making about use of new technologies back into their hands. If they are judged and rewarded on the basis of the effectiveness and efficiency of the care they provide, physicians and hospitals will have a vested interest in using technologies that are proven effective and efficient. However, individual physician practices continue to struggle with the transformation of their care processes because the fee-for-service volume is difficult to slow down enough to afford the time and financial resources to engage in practice reengineering.

- Accreditation organizations (NCQA, The Joint Commission)—To meet purchaser and consumer needs, accreditation organizations have adapted their performance measurement systems to make them more transparent and more detailed. The Joint Commission has started to disclose full hospital report cards instead of overall accreditation scores, which can mask significant variations in quality within an institution. Similarly, NCQA continues to move toward individual physician measurement as opposed to plan-wide accreditation.

- Disease management and care management/coordination vendors—Over time, vendors that currently provide a purchaser-based service to manage individual cases or populations with a specific condition should shift their sales and marketing strategy to the provider. If providers are measured on and rewarded for effectiveness of care, they will need to reengineer internal care processes and use the services of these vendors. Purchasers, on the other hand, no longer should need to buy the services of these vendors because they will be paying for them at the point of care.

- Technology vendors—In a real VBP model, the bundling of payments around episodes of care creates a mechanism for providers to reap the benefits of adopting technologies that are proven effective and efficient in managing patients and delivering better outcomes. Technology vendors should focus their products and services on these factors. At the same time, technology vendors no longer will have to rely on the approval of various managed care organizations to deploy their products because physicians will be able to adopt them directly.

Case Study: Bridges to Excellence: Building a Real Business Case for Better Quality Care

IOM's 2001 report, *Crossing the Quality Chasm*, documented the quality shortfalls in the U.S. healthcare system and provided a road map for change. Subsequent publications have substantiated the quality issues, including a paper that indicated 20 percent of physicians and 25 percent of the public have had personal experiences of serious harm resulting from avoidable errors (Blendon et al. 2002). IOM pointed out that the reimbursement system does not encourage, and frequently discourages, quality improvement. Healthcare purchasers, concerned about the rising costs of healthcare, believed that improving quality would mitigate unnecessary cost increases. Through the Leapfrog Group, a voluntary organization of 130 healthcare purchasers, they established reward for quality as a fundamental principle of purchasing healthcare services. Leading providers and provider organizations also recognized the instability of the status quo.

Although several studies have demonstrated that quality can reduce overall costs, there is no consensus on this theory. Part of the problem in establishing a business case is that results vary by type of quality improvement (reduction in overuse, misuse, or underuse), reimbursement system (fee for service or prepaid), and reward recipient (payers or providers). A fundamental premise in the Bridges to Excellence initiative is that both payers and providers must experience a positive return on investment for the project to be sustainable.

In sectors outside healthcare, there is an underlying belief that higher quality lowers cost, and there is a growing consensus in healthcare that better quality should be rewarded (see Table 19.1 for details on various pay-for-quality initiatives). GE, through its adoption of a quality improvement methodology called Six Sigma (Harry and Schroeder 1999), has demonstrated billions of dollars of savings over the past few years. Working with a group of organizations and individuals representing different stakeholders of the healthcare system (provider, payer, plan, measurement experts), GE applied the same Six Sigma methodology (called Design for Six Sigma [DFSS]) to develop Bridges to Excellence that it uses to design all new products, from jet engines to long-term care insurance products. The program defined a clear mission: to create an adaptable healthcare model that rewards quality performance, in particular, but not exclusively, for chronic care, simultaneously for providers or provider organizations and purchasers. The rewards were based on objective measures of processes of care that (1) prevent defects—misuse, overuse, and underuse—and (2) are valued, actionable, and auditable by providers, consumer-patients, and purchasers.

TABLE 19.1
Pay-for-Quality Initiatives

Inpatient	Outpatient
Anthem cardiac surgery recognition program: Anthem's program is one of the largest in the United States. It rewards hospitals that meet certain performance measures for cardiac surgery and gives them a benchmark against which to compare their performance.	**CMS—Physician group practice demonstration:** In this demonstration project, CMS bundles payments for Parts A and B and ties them to selected HEDIS measures (e.g., A1c, LVEF, and ECG for CHF). The goal is to create an incentive for physicians to manage their patients better and to reward physicians by decreasing hospitalizations.
Blue Shield of CA hospital tiering program: Blue Shield of CA, like many plans across the country, tiers its hospitals on the basis of how well they perform with respect to both cost and quality. It uses a combination of Leapfrog measures and other statewide hospital performance data in assessing quality.	**The Integrated Healthcare Association (IHA):** This organization includes the largest plans in California. They have agreed to measure physician performance in a common way, although each plan independently determines the rewards. IHA uses HEDIS indicators, measures of use of information technology to decrease errors, and patient experience of care surveys.
Hannaford Brothers hospital co-pay program: Employers as diverse as Hannaford Brothers and Boeing are using benefit design changes to vary the co-pays between hospitals according to certain quality measures, driving more patients to higher-quality facilities.	**Plans—Aetna, CIGNA, Highmark, Anthem, BCBS IL, BC CA, Ind. Health:** Many plans across the country reward physicians for meeting certain performance measures (primarily HEDIS indicators), though for the most part this performance is not made public.
Empire Blue Cross and Blue Shield's Leapfrog program: Empire was the first plan to launch a reward program for hospitals that meet the Leapfrog measures. Rewards are bonuses that represent a certain percentage of existing fees (up to 4 percent).	**Anthem of New England's PCP incentive program:** Anthem of New England developed a comprehensive incentive program that assesses a physician's performance through a series of process and outcome measures and ties future fee schedule increases to the performance score.

This framework is the building block of VBP. You need mutual measures of quality and rewards linked to them to encourage providers to participate. Bridges to Excellence focuses on a design that gives bonuses to those who meet standard performance measures. An extension would be to redesign the overall payments to providers, baking in the bonuses.

Design for Six Sigma

The DFSS process, summarized in Figure 19.1, lays out a series of steps, grouped in tollgates (TGs), and statistical tools that guide the development of a new product or service. Unique concepts in Six Sigma are CTQs—program attributes that are "critical to quality" and define what the customer needs—and CTPs—design attributes of the product or service that are "critical to process" and ensure that CTQs are met. The application of these concepts increases the likelihood of success of new products or services.

Defining the CTQs

This step in the DFSS process is the most important because it requires all the stakeholders to agree on a core set of important principles (customer and stakeholder needs) that will define the program's design. Given the nature of the Bridges to Excellence program—a performance-based incentive program with publicly reported performance measures—both physicians and consumer-patients are considered customers; all other parties, including

FIGURE 19.1
DFSS Process

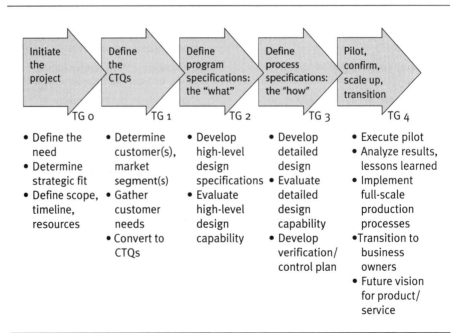

SOURCE: The General Electric Company. Used with permission.

purchasers, are stakeholders. This distinction is critical because customers' needs drive most of the product's design.

GE identified, sorted, and ranked customer needs (CTQs) through a combination of interviews, focus groups, and literature searches. In previous work (De Brantes and Galvin 2001), GE defined key attributes that consumer-patients require of healthcare-related information and of their interaction with consumers. Through focus groups, it collected information on physician needs, which work done by Bailit and Dyer (2002) on incentive programs validated. It reached consensus that rewards and incentives have to be (1) meaningful enough to more than compensate for the added cost associated with data collection and measurement of processes, (2) perceived to be fair and equitable, (3) attainable, (4) periodically reviewed, and (5) incremental, with small step increments as opposed to a "cliff." Incentives should be based on measures that are standard and well accepted by experts, and they should measure only what is actionable by the physician or provider being assessed. Finally, if performance measures are linked to outcomes, patient incentives should be deployed to align patient behavior with the performance measures. These provider CTQs are summarized in Table 19.2.

Incentives and Rewards	Performance Measures
• Meaningful provider incentives	• Performance measures that are well defined and within the provider's control
• Clear expectations for performance	
• Timely rewards	
• Regular evaluation of the incentive program and modification as needed	• Thresholds that are a stretch but attainable over time
• Incentive focus on a limited number of measures	• Accurate and comprehensive data
• Collaboration and consultation with providers to obtain and retain buy-in	• Timely data that provides feedback to the provider and staff on what to improve
• Incentive approach that is easy to understand and administer	• Absolute benchmarks of performance
• Predictable cost and benefit of program	• Use of an independent entity for performance measurement
• Incentives that occur regularly for action over which providers have control	• Patient incentives to address noncompliance
• Collaboration of insurers and purchasers to overcome small market share	• Minimization of burden on staff and duplication of effort
• Enough meaning to more than compensate for the added cost associated with data collection and measurement of process	
• Fair and equitable rewards and incentives	
• Inclusion of small step increments as opposed to a cliff	
• Nonpunitive process	

TABLE 19.2
Provider CTQs

Other key attributes of successful physician-based incentive programs include: simplicity and standardization of processes; no added burden on staff or office; low intensity of data requirements; increased income while providing high-quality care; ability to (1) educate and motivate patients to seek out high-quality providers and (2) educate staff and enable them to be better teachers; and avoidance of putting the physician at odds with the patient.

As the design of the program evolved from high-level to detailed design, providers were interviewed and consulted regularly to make sure that the incentives and rewards would meet their needs and stimulate their desire to achieve the performance measures.

Defining the Program Specifications—Measures, Specific Incentives, and Consumer-Focused Elements

1. Performance Measures

The performance measures had to meet specific requirements. They had to help achieve the six aims for better care identified in IOM's report: safe, timely, effective, efficient, equitable, and patient centered. They also had to be clearly measurable, actionable, and under the control of the provider being measured.

After defining these critical attributes, the cross-functional team identified a series of processes that could influence these attributes to varying degrees. The Six Sigma tool used in this phase of the design is called a Quality Functional Deployment, the results of which are summarized in Figure 19.2.

The team took several weeks to agree on how to rank each of the key processes of care with respect to how they affected the critical attributes. The consensus on how each process would affect a customer need—high, medium, or low impact—and the importance of that need relative to others yielded a ranking of 16 processes. The highest was "information and resources for both clinicians and patients in managing specific, high-intensity conditions—typically, but not always, after an acute episode or hospitalization." The rest of the processes were grouped in three tiers; the top two tiers included 11 different processes that fit into three distinct categories shown in Figure 19.3: clinical information systems with evidence-based decision support, patient education and support, and care management. These three categories of processes are consistent with the areas of focus identified by IOM (2001) in its *Crossing the Quality Chasm* report, have been highlighted in a number of recent studies, and are the focus of similar initiatives.

Conversion of these three categories of care processes into meaningful measures led to a canvassing of existing performance measures to

FIGURE 19.2
Quality Functional Deployment

Customer Expectation	Importance	Data capture and management for patient tracking	Data capture and management of patient compliance with standards of care	Data capture and management of provider compliance with standards of care	Evidence-based clinical treatment decision support focused on error prevention	Evidence-based clinical treatment decision support focused on guidelines for care	Value-based decision support focused on an integrated radiology program	Value-based decision support focused on an integrated PBM program	Information and resources enabling the patient to make fully informed decisions for treatment of condition	Information and resources enabling the patient to make fully informed decisions for managing health	Proactive management of patient care—Disease management programs	Proactive management of patient care—Coordination of multi-specialty teams	Proactive management of patient care—Effective systems of communication across providers	Proactive management of patient care—Effective systems of communication between patients and providers	Proactive management of patient care—Risk factor screenings	Proactive management of patient care—Support systems for patient lifestyle changes	Information and resources for both clinicians and patients in managing specific, high-intensity conditions—typically, but not always, after an acute episode or hospitalization	Total
Safe—care does not harm the patient	5	L	H	M	H	M	L	H	M	L	M	H	H	M	L	L	H	370
Effective—care is evidence based and designed to help the patient get better as soon as appropriate	5	M	H	H	M	M	M	H	H	M	H	H	M	M	H	M	M	480
Patient centered—focused on the patient's values, physiology, respecting the patient's needs for information and support	5	L	M	L	L	H	M	M	H	H	H	H	H	H	H	H	H	470
Timely—care is given when needed, with minimum delays, efficient flow, as appropriate	4	L	M	M	L	M	M	M	L	L	M	H	H	H	M	H	H	256
Efficient—care given represents the best use of resources to get the best value for money spent	5	M	H	H	M	H	H	H	M	M	H	H	H	M	M	H	H	440
Equitable—appropriate standards of care are applied to all irrespective of gender, color, creed, socioeconomic background, culture, etc.	4	H	H	H	H	H	H	H	M	M	H	M	M	L	H	L	H	368
Measurable—processes used are measurable	4	H	M	M	M	H	H	H	L	L	M	L	L	M	H	M	M	328
Portable—processes defined are adaptable from one care system/setting to another	3	H	H	M	L	H	L	M	H	H	M	L	M	H	H	H	H	288
Actionable—processes defined are implemented by providers or provider organizations	5	H	H	H	H	M	H	H	H	H	H	M	H	H	H	H	H	690
Impactful—processes defined favorably affect the largest number of patients possible	2	H	H	L	M	H	M	H	M	M	M	M	H	H	H	M	L	176
Customer-centric—convenient to the patient and delivered with a high level of customer service	3	L	M	L	L	L	L	M	H	H	M	H	H	H	M	H	H	258
Total		209	309	257	189	273	211	333	253	205	249	253	301	259	293	195	335	

SOURCE: The General Electric Company. Used with permission.

FIGURE 19.3

Process
Groupings

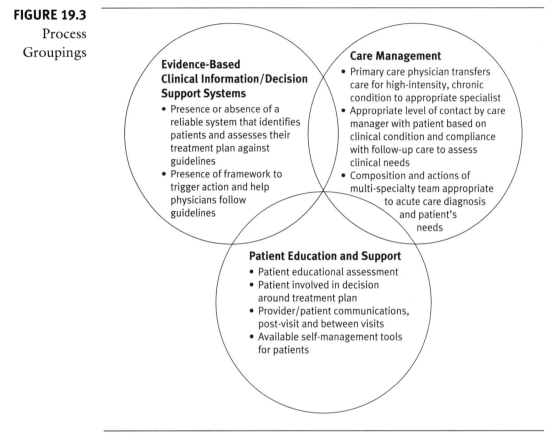

**Evidence-Based
Clinical Information/Decision
Support Systems**
- Presence or absence of a
  reliable system that identifies
  patients and assesses their
  treatment plan against
  guidelines
- Presence of framework to
  trigger action and help
  physicians follow
  guidelines

Care Management
- Primary care physician transfers
  care for high-intensity, chronic
  condition to appropriate specialist
- Appropriate level of contact by care
  manager with patient based on
  clinical condition and compliance
  with follow-up care to assess
  clinical needs
- Composition and actions of
  multi-specialty team appropriate
  to acute care diagnosis
  and patient's
  needs

Patient Education and Support
- Patient educational assessment
- Patient involved in decision
  around treatment plan
- Provider/patient communications,
  post-visit and between visits
- Available self-management tools
  for patients

SOURCE: The General Electric Company. Used with permission.

determine whether any set would map back to the three groups of processes.
One program emerged as a good candidate: the American Diabetes
Association-NCQA Diabetes Physician Recognition Program (DPRP). This
program is a self-report (with audit) by individual physicians of their practices' performance on a set of measures of the care of diabetes patients.
The DPRP has shown that performing physicians systematically improve
their performance on resubmission. Although the criteria used to score certifying physicians are primarily outcomes based, achieving these outcomes
requires practice reengineering.

Because only 6 percent of consumers under age 65 have diabetes,
measuring provider performance on this dimension only cannot achieve the
broad impact specified in the original mission statement. As such, the Bridges
to Excellence program decided to divide its effort. It (1) adopted the DPRP
and turned it into an incentive program (Diabetes Care Link) and (2) refined
the three groups of core measures into measurable performance indicators
(Physician Office Link) by using existing surveys developed in similar efforts
in other parts of the country as a guide. The results of these efforts are summarized in Figure 19.4.

FIGURE 19.4
Summary of Physician Office Link Measures

Clinical Information Systems/ Evidence-Based Medicine		Patient Education and Support		Care Management	
Basic Registries and Follow-Up	**Pts**	**Education Resources**	**Pts**	**Care of Chronic Conditions**	**Pts**
1. Type of registry used for chronic conditions	10	1. Assessment of patient language preferences and risk factors	30	1. Identification of the practice's top three chronic conditions	10
2. Percentage of patients in registry	10	2. Identification of preferred languages in patient population	35	2. Structured process for disease management for patients with the top three conditions	45
3. Use of registry to identify patient populations	40	3. Provision of educational resources in preferred languages for risk factors and chronic conditions	35	3. Use of resources to assist with medication compliance, appointments, and barriers to care	45
4. Use of paper or electronic system to track and follow up on referrals and test results	40				
	100		100		100
Electronic Registries, Prescriptions, and Test Ordering	**Pts**	**Referrals for Risk Factors and Chronic Conditions**	**Pts**	**Preventable Admissions**	**Pts**
1. Types of patient information in registry	10	1. Percentage of patients who have specific risk factors	50	1. Using data to identify patients who are at risk for emergency admissions	20
2. Capabilities of an electronic system for prescriptions and tests	20	2. Provision of referrals for education and support to patients with risk factors and chronic conditions	50	2. Identification of the reasons for and prevalence of emergency admissions	20
3. Use of electronic system for ordering prescriptions and checking for safety and efficiency	40			3. Structured system to prevent emergency admissions	60
4. Use of electronic system to order and retrieve tests	10				
5. Use of electronic system to track missing test results, distinguish abnormal results, and prompt follow-up on test results	20				
	100		100		100
Electronic Medical Records	**Pts**	**Quality Measurement and Improvement**	**Pts**	**Care of High-Risk Medical Conditions**	**Pts**
1. Types of patient information in an EMR	10	1. Identification of opportunities for improving outcomes or processes	20	1. Resources for managing patients with high-risk conditions	5
2. Percentage of patients who have information in the EMR	20	2. Setting goals for performance for identified opportunities of improvement	20	2. Number and percentage of patients who receive high-risk care management	5
3. EMR's capability to report across practice on multiple fields	30	3. Measurement of performance and identification of goals not met	20	3. Contents of the high-risk care management program	30
4. EMR's capability to use decision support to prompt physician interventions	30	4. Implementation of improvement activities	40	4. Qualifications of the high-risk care manager	10
5. EMR's capability to capture services ordered, delivered, or paid	5			5. Types of information in database of patients with high-risk conditions	15
6. Use of EMR to track referrals and test results	5			6. Frequency of communication between physician and care manager	5
				7. Frequency of communication between care manager and patient	30
	100		100		100

SOURCE: The General Electric Company. Used with permission.

2. Incentives and Rewards

In the focus groups, physicians defined three broad categories and types of incentives, as well as their importance—direct financial incentives (most important), indirect financial incentives, and nonfinancial incentives (least important).

The existing data on cost savings resulting from improvements in treating diabetics or managing information flow in a physician office are not definitive. However, purchasers, with their bias toward action, believe that there is sufficient evidence to move forward. Actuarial models indicate that potential short- and long-term savings of about 7 percent of total costs can be achieved by improving outcomes for diabetes patients. In addition, potential short-term savings of 4 percent of total cost of care (or overall premiums) can be achieved by a more thorough reengineering of physician practices (i.e., adoption of the processes in the Physician Office Link).

Purchasers will require a return on additional monies paid to physicians, so they reasonably can keep 50 percent of the expected savings and set the other 50 percent aside as the incentive pool available to those who meet the performance measures.

This analysis and parsing of the savings pool resulted in a $100 bonus per diabetes patient per year for physicians meeting the DPRP performance measures and $55 per patient per year for physicians meeting the Physician Office Link performance measures.

The DPRP performance bonus is not the preferred bonus method among physicians because it is a "cliff"; they either receive it or do not receive it (see incentive CTQs in Table 19.2). In contrast, the Physician Office Link bonus is structured to be gradual and to provide the physician with money to invest in better systems of care. Figure 19.4 contains nine modules of measures, each independent of the other. The bonuses are structured to encourage physicians to meet an increasing number of modules over three years. In the first year, they can qualify for the full bonus ($55) by meeting any one of the modules in each column, for a total of three modules. In the second year, they must meet two out of three in each column, for a total of six modules. In the third year, they must meet all nine modules. If physicians do not improve their performance from one year to another, they still qualify for a bonus, albeit lower than the previous year's bonus. This system of providing a graduated increase in performance while providing an opportunity to qualify for the maximum bonus resonates more with physicians than do the cliff-type bonuses.

Although nonfinancial rewards—in particular public recognition programs via some form of rating system—are not of uniform importance to providers (some providers have expressed strong antipathy for public data dissemination), purchasers and consumers have demonstrated a need for and are demanding comparative provider performance data. To meet the needs of consumer-patients in this domain, a research project was launched to gather critical input from consumers, enabling the design of an enhanced provider directory that could incorporate all the data elements necessary for consumers to make informed decisions. An initial series of focus groups was conducted during which consumers delineated the data elements they wanted and then categorized those data into intuitive groupings. Subsequent focus groups used a "pencil and paper" exercise to test the groups of measures and associated labels. The result was the prototype shown in Figure 19.5. This prototype needs further validation and testing to determine its effectiveness in helping consumers select physicians and hospitals.

FIGURE 19.5
Physician
Report Card
Prototype

Doctor Information	Address	Staffing	Credentials	Hospital Affiliation
Dr. Robert Smith Family Practice ID NO. 0004668833 03 My Philosophy of Care 518.472.4584 518.472.4620 fax dr.smith@aol.com	997 Glen Cove Avenue Glen Head, NY 11545 Monday–Thursday 10–5 Friday, Saturday 11–4	• 2 nurses • 3 technicians • 1 on-call doctor	NY Medical College, MD, 1989 St. Lukes–Roosevelt, 1992 AM Board of Internal Medicine, 1994	Mt. Sinai Medical Center Westchester Medical Center Columbia Presbyterian Medical Center

Performance Report:

Effectiveness of Care

	Diabetes care	Cardiac care
Overall		

Doctor: 5
Average score: 6

Patient Experience of Care

Overall	

Doctor: 4
Average score: 5

Doctor-Patient Interactions

Communication
Interpersonal treatments
Knowledge of patient
Health promotions
Integration
Patient trust
Relationship duration

Access and Office Systems

Organizational access
Visit-based continuity
Clinical team

Key

Your provider | Average provider

Clinical Information Systems and Evidence-Based Medicine		Patient Education and Support		Care Management	
Basic registries and follow-up	✓ 100%	Educational resources		Care of chronic conditions	✓ 70%
Electronic registries, prescription and test ordering		Referrals for risk factors and chronic conditions		Preventable admissions	
Electronic medical records		Quality measurement and improvement		Care of high-risk medical conditions	

Key

✓ Provider has fulfilled the requirements for the measure

SOURCE: The General Electric Company. Used with permission.

3. Consumer-Based Elements

Consumer-patients are engaged in the program by providing them information on physicians that they did not have previously, as illustrated earlier. In addition, consumer-patients with diabetes want to increase their understanding of their condition and are encouraged to improve or stabilize it. Work by Bodenheimer, Wagner, and Grumbach (2002a, 2002b) has demonstrated that a chronic care management model's potential cannot be realized without robust patient involvement. Physicians who reviewed Bridges to Excellence strongly echoed that opinion. If part of their performance measure was based on patient outcomes, they were adamant that patients should have similar incentives to improve outcomes.

A novel program called Diabetes Care Rewards resulted from this perspective. It includes tools with which diabetes patients can monitor their self-care activities and provides them with points for lowering their HbA1c and following care guidelines. They can accumulate these points to qualify for rewards offered by the participating employer-purchasers. In some cases, these rewards are vouchers for lower co-payments on physician office visits or prescriptions. In other cases, they are coupons that they can redeem on sites that offer products not covered by health benefits (e.g., sugar-free candy).

In focus groups, consumer-patients indicated that having a monetary or quasi-monetary reward was very important to them and would keep them focused on achieving better outcomes. These rewards did not have to be big, just achievable (echoing what physicians said was important for their incentives).

Designing the Program's Implementation

The following three CTQs drove the majority of the operational design of Bridges to Excellence:

1. Make the rewards as meaningful as possible by consolidating the bonuses in a single payment
2. Make the program administratively simple for purchasers, plans, and providers
3. Do not cause the plans to open up their provider contracts or do anything that would disrupt current network arrangements

These CTQs forced Bridges to Excellence to eliminate many options (e.g., having each plan administer and pay the bonuses) that would have been easy for purchasers to implement but would have countered what the customers and other stakeholders wanted. One of the core principles in designing a new program using the Six Sigma methodology is not to retrofit a solution into an existing infrastructure because the existing infrastructure may not meet customers' needs.

As a result, Bridges to Excellence hired an independent third party, Medstat (a subsidiary of the Thomson Company), as the "general contractor." Medstat's role was to aggregate data files from plans and create a master patient/physician/purchaser grid that defined the number of patients per physician for whom a bonus could be paid. This grid enabled participating purchasers to gauge quickly what their maximum exposure would be if all physicians met the performance measures.

On a quarterly basis, Medstat sent invoices to each purchaser that reflected the bonuses it had to pay to physicians who met the performance measures and then paid each physician a lump-sum bonus, across all participating purchasers.

This structure was administratively simple because it was not dependent on a specific health plan or network arrangement and did not require a plan to modify its existing contractual arrangements with network physicians. In fact, the health plan's role was limited to sending the data file to Medstat (although it could help physicians in its network meet the performance measures and market enrollment in the self-care tools to patients with diabetes). The structure did require employers to sign a few agreements so that the data could flow between their plans and Medstat, and employers were bound by the terms of the program to pay the bonuses and engage their employees in better self-care.

Program Evolution

The successful pilots of Bridges to Excellence have led to a wide adoption of what is now widely known as *pay for performance* throughout the U.S. healthcare system. In 2006, Congress passed a budget reconciliation act that enshrined pay for performance for hospitals and laid the foundation for pay for performance for physicians. In response to this growth in program demand, Bridges to Excellence converted its implementation model from one that relies on a third-party intermediary (Medstat, which is not a health plan administrator) to a plan-managed model. In this model, health plans are responsible for paying physician rewards directly, on behalf of either their fully insured members or their self-insured customers. Physicians still benefit from focusing on a parsimonious set of measures, and employers throughout the country can deploy the programs of Bridges to Excellence more readily.

Conclusion and Key Lessons

Designing a new product or service in a system as fragmented as healthcare, and with stakeholders that can have, at times, highly divergent needs, is not easy. However, the framework provided by the DFSS process enables all stakeholders to make trade-offs between their needs and other stakeholder needs, and it appeals to all—purchasers, providers, plans, and patients.

Key principles of a successful design ensure that:

- the incentives meet provider CTQs (in particular, they need to be attainable and meaningful);
- the measures meet provider and purchaser CTQs, create a return on investment for purchasers, are achievable yet not easy, and are standard as opposed to custom; and
- the operational structure meets purchaser and plan CTQs, is simple and easy for purchasers to implement, and keeps the administrative burden on plans to a minimum.

Study Questions

1. Why are purchasers increasingly interested in a new model for VBP?
2. Once purchasers and plans have created enough rewards to attract physicians to meet high performance measures, and enough of them do, what is the next phase in creating a robust VBP model?
3. What would a VBP model look like compared to the existing plan-based delivery system?

Notes

1. For more information, see www.leapfroggroup.org.
2. For more information, see www.bridgestoexcellence.org.

References

Bailit, M., and M. B. Dyer. 2002. *Provider Incentive Models for Improving Quality of Care.* Washington, DC: National Health Care Purchasing Institute.

Birkmeyer, J. D., C. M. Birkmeyer, D. E. Wennberg, and M. Young. 2000. *Leapfrog Patient Safety Standards: The Potential Benefits of Universal Adoption.* Washington, DC: Leapfrog Group.

Blendon, R. J., C. M. DesRoches, M. Brodie, J. M. Benson, A. B. Rosen, E. Schneider, D. E. Altman, K. Zapert, M. J. Herrmann, and A. E. Steffenson. 2002. "Views of Practicing Physicians and the Public on Medical Errors." *New England Journal of Medicine* 347 (24): 1933–40.

Bodenheimer, T., E. H. Wagner, and K. Grumbach. 2002a. "Improving Primary Care for Patients with Chronic Illness." *Journal of the American Medical Association* 288 (14): 1775–79.

————. 2002b. "Improving Primary Care for Patients with Chronic Illness: The Chronic Care Model, Part 2." *Journal of the American Medical Association* 288 (15): 1909–14.

De Brantes, F., and R. S. Galvin. 2001. "Creating, Connecting and Supporting Active Consumers." *International Journal of Medical Marketing* 2 (1): 73–80.

Galvin, R. S. 2001. "The Business Case for Quality." *Health Affairs* 20 (6): 57–58.

Harry, M., and R. Schroeder. 1999. *Six Sigma: The Breakthrough Management Strategy Revolutionizing the World's Top Corporations.* New York: Doubleday.

Hibbard, J. H., and J. J. Jewett. 1997. "Will Quality Report Cards Help Consumers?" *Health Affairs* 16 (3): 218–28.

Institute of Medicine. 2001. *Crossing the Quality Chasm: A New Health System for the 21st Century.* Washington, DC: National Academies Press.

Marshall, M., P. Shekelle, S. Leatherman, and R. Brook. 2000. "The Public Release of Performance Data: What Do We Expect to Gain? A Review of the Evidence." *Journal of the American Medical Association* 283 (14): 1866–74.

McGlynn, E. A., S. M. Asch, J. Adams, J. Keesey, J. Hicks, A. DeCristofaro, and E. A. Kerr. 2003. "The Quality of Health Care Delivered to Adults in the United States." *New England Journal of Medicine* 348 (26): 2635–45.

Schuster, M. A., E. A. McGlynn, and R. Brook. 1998. "How Good Is the Quality of Healthcare in the United States?" *Milbank Quarterly* 76 (4): 517–63.

Wennberg, J. A. 1999. "Understanding Geographic Variations in Health Care Delivery." *New England Journal of Medicine* 340: 52–53.

INDEX

ABOUT THE AUTHORS

About the Editors

Elizabeth R. Ransom, MD, received her BS in microbiology and immunology from McGill University in Montreal, and her MD from Wayne State University School of Medicine in Detroit. She completed her residency in otolaryngology—head and neck surgery in 1994 at Henry Ford Hospital and became a senior staff physician there. In 1996 she was appointed as residency program director of Otolaryngology. She served on the graduate and undergraduate medical education committees and was a member of the admissions committee for Wayne State University School of Medicine.

Dr. Ransom's administrative and leadership activities at Henry Ford Health System included division director, Ear, Nose, and Throat, Northeast Region (1994–2006); chair, Credentials Committee of the Henry Ford Medical Group (HFMG) (2000–2006); member of the Board of Governors of the HFMG (1999–2006); and vice chair of the Board of Governors (2004–2006). She also served as program chair of the Michigan Otolaryngological Society (2004–2006) and vice chair of the Michigan Chief Medical Officer Consortium (2003–2006).

After moving to Texas, Dr. Ransom took a position in 2007 as physician engagement consultant with Texas Health Resources (THR). THR is one of the largest faith-based nonprofit health organizations in the country, with 13 hospitals and 3,700 physicians in the Dallas-Fort Worth metroplex. She is responsible for strategic feasibility assessment and development of a systemwide graduate medical education program, and contributes to the growth of strategic alignment among physicians, hospitals, and corporate entities.

Maulik S. Joshi, DrPH, is president of the Health Research & Educational Trust (HRET) and senior vice president for research at the American Hospital Association. Before joining HRET, Dr. Joshi served as president and chief executive officer of the Network for Regional Healthcare Improvement and was a senior adviser for the office of the director at the Agency for Healthcare Research and Quality. He also served as president and chief executive officer of the Delmarva Foundation. During his tenure with the Delmarva Foundation, the organization was the recipient of the 2005 U.S. Senate Productivity award. This award, based on the national Malcolm Baldrige criteria for performance excellence, is the highest of its kind in the state of Maryland. In addition, Dr. Joshi was vice president of the Institute for

Healthcare Improvement, cofounder and executive vice president of DoctorQuality, senior director of quality for the University of Pennsylvania Health System, and executive vice president of The HMO Group.

Dr. Joshi received his DrPH and MHSA from the University of Michigan and earned his BS in mathematics from Lafayette College. He is currently editor in chief for the *Journal for Healthcare Quality*. His most recent publication is *Healthcare Transformation: A Guide for the Hospital Board Member*, published in 2009 by CRC Press and AHA Press. Dr. Joshi also serves on numerous governance and advisory boards.

David B. Nash, MD, MBA, is dean of the Jefferson School of Population Health and the Dr. Raymond C. and Doris N. Grandon professor of health policy at Thomas Jefferson University in Philadelphia. Dr. Nash, a board-certified internist, founded the original Office of Health Policy in 1990. From 1996 to 2003, he served as the first associate dean for health policy at Jefferson Medical College. In 2004 he was named co-director of the master's program in public health at Jefferson and was named a finalist in the 15th Annual Discover Awards for Innovation in Public Health by *Discover* magazine.

Scott B. Ransom, DO, FACHE, is the fifth president of the University of North Texas (UNT) Health Science Center at Fort Worth. As president, Dr. Ransom leads a growing academic health science center that includes four schools: the Texas College of Osteopathic Medicine, the Graduate School of Biomedical Sciences, the School of Public Health, and the School of Health Professions. He also leads the largest multi-specialty clinical practice in Tarrant County, which includes over 240 clinicians. More than 375 full-time and 550 part-time faculty members work with over 1,200 students who are training to be osteopathic physicians, researchers, public health officers, physician assistants, and other health professionals. As vice chancellor for health affairs, Dr. Ransom leads all health-related programs for the 36,000-student, three-campus UNT system.

Dr. Ransom earned a medical degree from the University of Health Sciences in Kansas City, an MBA from the University of Michigan in Ann Arbor, and an MPH from Harvard University.

He completed a residency in obstetrics and gynecology at Oakwood Hospital in Dearborn, Michigan, and completed the program in clinical effectiveness at Harvard University. Dr. Ransom is also a graduate of the U.S. Marine Corps Officer Candidate School.

Dr. Ransom is a fellow in many professional organizations, including the American College of Obstetrics and Gynecology, the American College of Surgeons, the American College of Physician Executives, and the American College of Healthcare Executives.

Before joining the UNT Health Science Center, Dr. Ransom served as the executive director of the program for healthcare improvement and leadership development, and professor with tenure in obstetrics, gynecology, health management, and policy at the University of Michigan in Ann Arbor. His research efforts have garnered significant grant funding from the National Institutes of Health, the National Science Foundation, the Department of Veterans Affairs, and others.

Before joining the University of Michigan, Dr. Ransom was vice president of medical affairs, and then senior vice president and chief quality officer, at the Detroit Medical Center, a $1.8 billion, seven-hospital healthcare system.

Dr. Ransom has published more than 130 articles, chapters, and abstracts and eight books on topics related to clinical improvement, women's health, quality, and leadership.

He is a past president of the American College of Physician Executives and past chair of the Certifying Commission in Medical Management. He has served on several national boards, including the Healthcare Leadership Institute for General Electric Corporation, Center for Innovation of the National Board of Medical Examiners, Institute for Research on Women and Gender, and Botanical Research Institute. He serves on several community boards, including the Fort Worth Chamber of Commerce, Longhorn Council's Boy Scout Foundation, and Fort Worth Library Foundation.

About the Contributors

Kimberly D. Acquaviva, PhD, MSW, is assistant professor in the Department of Nursing Education and director of the National Collaborative on Aging at George Washington University.

A. Al-Assaf, MD, CQA, is regents' professor, and professor and associate dean, for international health at the College of Public Health, University of Oklahoma Health Sciences Center in Oklahoma City.

David J. Ballard, MD, PhD, is senior vice president and chief quality officer of Baylor Health Care System (BHCS), and executive director and BHCS endowed chair at the Institute for Health Care Research and Improvement in Dallas, Texas.

Donald Berwick, MD, is chief executive officer of the Institute for Healthcare Improvement and professor of health management and policy at Harvard University.

John Bulger, DO, is director of inpatient services for general internal medicine and associate chief academic officer for Geisinger Health System in Danville, Pennsylvania.

John J. Byrnes, MD, is senior vice president, system quality at Spectrum Health System and clinical associate professor at Michigan State University College of Human Medicine in Grand Rapids, Michigan.

Ellen M. Dawson, PhD, ANP, is chair, Department of Nursing Education, at George Washington University.

Francois de Brantes is chief executive officer of the nonprofit Bridges to Excellence and based in Fairfield County, Connecticut.

Susan Edgman-Levitan, PA, is executive director of the John D. Stoeckle Center for Primary Care Innovation at Massachusetts General Hospital in Boston and a fellow of the Institute for Healthcare Improvement in Boston.

Adam Evans, MD, MBA, is a second-year anesthesiology resident at New York Presbyterian Hospital-Weill Cornell Medical College.

Thomas J. Fairchild, PhD, is the vice president of strategy and measurement at the University of North Texas Health Science Center in Fort Worth, where he oversees institutional performance management and quality improvement.

Frances A. Griffin, RRT, is director at the Institute for Healthcare Improvement located in Cambridge, Massachusetts.

Linda S. Hanold, MHSA, is director of the department of quality at The Joint Commission in Oakbrook Terrace, Illinois.

Carol Haraden, PhD, is vice president, Institute for Healthcare Improvement.

Robert S. Hopkins III, MPH, PhD, is a medical risk management consultant with LifeWings Partners, LLC, in Memphis, Tennessee.

Richard Jacoby, MD, is a clinical associate professor in the department of health policy at Jefferson Medical College.

Jean E. Johnson, PhD, RN, FAAN, is senior associate dean of health sciences and professor at George Washington University.

Richard G. Koss is director of the department of health services research at The Joint Commission in Oakbrook Terrace, Illinois.

Robert C. Lloyd, PhD, is executive director, performance improvement, at the Institute for Healthcare Improvement in Boston.

Jerod M. Loeb, PhD, is executive vice president for the division of quality measurement and research at The Joint Commission in Oakbrook Terrace, Illinois.

David Nicewander is with the Institute for Health Care Research and Improvement at Baylor Health Care System in Dallas, Texas.

L. Gregory Pawlson, MD, MPH, is executive vice president of the National Committee for Quality Assurance in Washington, DC.

Michael D. Pugh is president and chief executive officer of Verisma Systems, Inc., and has over 30 years of CEO experience in hospitals, healthcare systems, managed care, and healthcare consulting. He is a senior faculty member of the Institute for Healthcare Improvement and a lecturer for the graduate health administration program at the University of Colorado.

James L. Reinertsen, MD, is senior fellow at the Institute for Healthcare Improvement in Boston and president of the Reinertsen Group in Alta, Wyoming.

Stephen Schmaltz, PhD, is an associate director and senior statistician at The Joint Commission in Oakbrook Terrace, Illinois.

Paul Schyve, MD, is senior vice president at The Joint Commission in Oakbrook Terrace, Illinois.

Richard E. Ward, MD, MBA, is vice president of clinical programs and medical informatics at Blue Cross Blue Shield of Michigan in Southfield.

Kevin Warren, MHA, CPHQ, is senior vice president of operations at TMF Health Quality Institute in Austin, Texas.

Valerie Weber, MD, is director of general internal medicine and vice chair, division of medicine, Geisinger Medical Center.

Leon Wyszewianski, PhD, is associate professor in the department of health management and policy at the University of Michigan School of Public Health in Ann Arbor.